PULMONARY FUNCTION TESTING
INDICATIONS AND INTERPRETATIONS

PULMONARY FUNCTION TESTING
INDICATIONS AND INTERPRETATIONS

A Project of the California Thoracic Society

Edited by

Archie F. Wilson, M.D., Ph.D.

Professor of Medicine and Physiology
Chief, Pulmonary and Critical Care Medicine
University of California School of Medicine
Irvine, California

Grune & Stratton
(Harcourt Brace Jovanovich, Publishers)
Orlando   San Diego   New York   London
Toronto   Montreal   Sydney   Tokyo

GRUNE & STRATTON, INC.
Orlando, FL 32887

Distributed in the United Kingdom by
GRUNE & STRATTON, LTD.
24/28 Oval Road, London NW 1

Library of Congress Catalog Number 84-73389
International Standard Book Number 0-8089-1692-0

PRINTED IN THE UNITED STATES OF AMERICA
85 86 87 88   10 9 8 7 6 5 4 3 2 1

Contents

Preface

Pulmonary Function Testing: Indications and Interpretations is meant to serve as a sequel to *Pulmonary Function Testing: Guidelines and Controversies*. Like its predecessor, this handbook is a product of the California Thoracic Society and was compiled prior to, during, and immediately after a postgraduate course that was given by leaders in this field. The chapters were written by individual members of the Pulmonary Physiology Committee after prolonged discussion with the faculty of the postgraduate course and other committee members.

It was our purpose to provide a handbook that would be useful to the pulmonary clinician who uses the laboratory to study disordered respiratory physiology for clinical purposes. We have included not only discussions of all tests likely to be obtained in both community and medical center pulmonary function laboratories but also applications of the testing to a number of nontraditional sites including the work place, intensive care units, and exercise and sleep laboratories. Evaluation of respiration testing for preoperative assessment, occupational disability, and pediatric patients is included. We have also discussed the use of the computer in pulmonary function interpretation.

We hope this handbook will provide a clear guide to diagnosis of pulmonary disorders by function testing. We also hope that we have adequately pointed the way to understanding both the limitations and some of the new areas in which pulmonary function testing is likely to expand.

Acknowledgments

Special thanks to Elma Plappert for her many years of guidance and support as Executive Secretary of the California Thoracic Society; Roberta Langenfeld for her secretarial support; and Karla Peterson for her editorial assistance.

Contributors

Pulmonary Physiology Committee

Larry N. Ayers, M.D.   Private Practice, El Cajon, California

Jack L. Clausen, M.D.   Assistant Professor of Medicine, Division of Pulmonary and Critical Care Medicine, University of California Medical Center, San Diego, California

Arthur Dawson, M.D.   Senior Consultant, Division of Chest and Critical Care Medicine, Scripps Clinic and Research Foundation, La Jolla, California

Robert J. Fallat, M.D.   Associate Professor, University of California School of Medicine; Director, Pulmonary Medicine, Pacific Presbyterian Medical Center, San Francisco, California

James E. Hansen, M.D.   Co-director of Clinical Respiratory Physiology Laboratory, Harbor/University of California Medical Center, Los Angeles, California

John G. Mohler, M.D.   Associate Professor of Medicine, University of Southern California School of Medicine; Director, Pulmonary Physiology Laboratory, Los Angeles County/University of Southern California Medical Center, Los Angeles, California

Arnold C. G. Platzker, M.D.   Director, Neonatal-Respiratory Disease Division, Childrens Hospital of Los Angeles; Associate Professor of Clinical Pediatrics, University of Southern California School of Medicine, Los Angeles, California

Antonius L. Van Kessel, B.Sc.R.C.P.T. Technical Director, Pulmonary Physiology and Respiratory Therapy Departments; Research Associate, Division of Respiratory Medicine, Stanford University Medical Center, Stanford, California

Archie F. Wilson, M.D., Ph.D. Professor of Medicine and Physiology; Chief, Pulmonary Disease; Department of Medicine, University of California School of Medicine, Irvine, California

Other Contributors

William Michael Alberts, M.D. Fellow, Pulmonary Medicine, University of California School of Medicine, San Diego, California. Currently Assistant Professor, Division of Pulmonary and Critical Care Medicine, James A. Haley Veterans Hospital, Tampa, Florida.

Clarence R. Collier, M.D. Professor of Medicine, Physiology, and Biophysics, University of Southern California School of Medicine, Los Angeles, California

Ronald D. Fairshter, M.D. Associate Professor of Medicine, University of California School of Medicine, Irvine, California

Christian Guilleminault, M.D. Staff Neurologist; Associate Professor of Psychiatry and Behavioral Sciences, Stanford University School of Medicine, Stanford, California

Thomas G. Keens, M.D. Associate Director, Pulmonary Function Laboratory, Childrens Hospital of Los Angeles; Assistant Professor of Pediatrics, University of Southern California School of Medicine, Los Angeles California

Kaye H. Kilburn, M.D. Ralph Edgington Professor of Medicine; Director, Environmental Sciences Laboratory, University of Southern California School of Medicine, Los Angeles, California

John F. Murray, M.D. Chief, Chest Service, San Francisco General Hospital; Professor of Medicine, University of California School of Medicine, San Francisco, California

Joe W. Ramsdell, M.D.   Associate Adjunct Professor of Medicine, Division of Pulmonary and Critical Care Medicine, University of California School of Medicine, San Diego, California

Andrew L. Ries, M.D.   Assistant Professor of Medicine, Division of Pulmonary and Critical Care Medicine, University of California Medical Center, San Diego, California

Michael G. Snow, R.C.P.T.   Technical Director, Pulmonary Funtion Laboratory, Pacific Presbyterian Medical Center, San Francisco, California

Myron Stein, M.D.   Clinical Professor of Medicine, University of California, Los Angeles; Co-director, Pulmonary Department, David M. Brotman Memorial Hospital, Culver City, California

Susan A. Ward, D.Phil.   Assistant Professor, Department of Anesthesiology, University of California School of Medicine, Los Angeles, California

Raphael Warshaw, B.A.   Research Associate, Environmental Sciences Laboratory, University of Southern California School of Medicine, Los Angeles, California

Brian J. Whipp, Ph.D.   Professor of Physiology and Medicine, Division of Respiratory Physiology and Medicine, Harbor/University of California School of Medicine, Los Angeles, California

Gary A. Wolff, M.S.E.E.   Senior Programmer Analyst, Los Angeles County/University of Southern California Medical Center, Los Angeles, California

Terms and Abbreviations

The variety of abbreviations used in clinical pulmonary function reports (e.g., MEF 50%, FEF 50%, V̇max 50%, and V̇ 50%) often leads to considerable confusion, especially for physicians without specific training in pulmonary medicine. Although not perfect, the terminology and abbreviations suggested by an American College of Chest Physicians/American Thoracic Society (ACCP/ATS) joint committee are the best available and should be used whenever possible. Those most relevant to subsequent chapters are given below. Abbreviations marked with an asterisk were not cited by the ACCP/ATS joint committee, but are used in this book.

A	Alveolar
a	Arterial
an	Anatomic
ATPD	Ambient temperature and pressure, dry
ATPS	Ambient temperature and pressure, saturated with water vapor at these conditions
B	Barometric
BTPS	Body conditions: Body temperature, ambient pressure, and saturated with water vapor at these conditions
C	A general symbol for compliance, volume change per unit of applied pressure
c	Capillary
C/V_L	Specific compliance
CD*	Cumulative inhalation dose. The total dose of an agent inhaled during bronchial challenge testing; it is the sum of the products of concentration multiplied by the number of breaths at that concentration
C_{dyn}	Dynamic compliance, compliance measured at point of zero gas flow at the mouth during active breathing. The respiratory frequency should be designated; e.g., $C_{dyn}40$
C_{st}	Static compliance, compliance determined from measurements made during conditions of prolonged interruption of air flow
D	Dead space or wasted ventilation (qualifying symbol, e.g., V_D)

D/V_A	Diffusion per unit of alveolar volume
D_k	Diffusion coefficient or permeability constant as described by Krogh; it equals $D \cdot (P_B - P_{H_2O})/V_A$
D_m	Diffusing capacity of the alveolar capillary membrane (STPD)
D_x (or $D_{L_{CO}}$)	Diffusing capacity of the lung expressed as volume (STPD) of gas (x) uptake per unit alveolar-capillary pressure difference for the gas used. Unless otherwise stated, carbon monoxide is assumed to be the test gas, i.e., D is D_{co}. A modifier can be used to designate the technique, e.g., D_{SB} is single breath carbon monoxide diffusing capacity and D_{SS} is steady state CO diffusing capacity. (Editor's note: This recommendation has not widely been accepted. $D_{L_{CO}}$, $D_{L_{CO}}SB$, and $D_{L_{CO}}SS$ are still the most commonly used abbreviations.)
E	Expired
ERV	Expiratory reserve volume; the maximal volume of air exhaled from the end-expiratory level
est	Estimated
f	Respiratory frequency per minute
F	Fractional concentration of a gas
FEF_{max}	The maximal forced expiratory flow achieved during an FVC
$FEF_{25-75\%}$	Mean forced expiratory flow during the middle half of the FVC (formerly called the maximum mid-expiratory flow rate)
$FEF_{75\%}$	Instantaneous forced expiratory flow after 75% of the FVC has been exhaled
$FEF_{200-1200}$	Mean forced expiratory flow between 200 ml and 1200 ml of the FVC (formerly called the maximum expiratory flow rate)
FEF_x	Forced expiratory flow, related to some portion of the FVC curve. Modifiers refer to the amount of the FVC already *exhaled* when the measurement is made
FET_x	The forced expiratory time for a specified portion of the FVC; e.g., $FET_{95\%}$ is the time required to deliver the first 95% of the FVC and $FET_{25-75\%}$ is the time required to deliver the $FEF_{25-75\%}$
$FEV_t/FVC\%$	Forced expiratory volume (timed) to forced vital capacity ratio, expressed as a percentage
FIF_x	Forced inspiratory flow. As in the case of the FEF, the appropriate modifiers must be used to designate the volume at which flow is being measured. Unless otherwise specified, the volume qualifiers indicate the volume inspired from RV at the point of the measurement
FRC	Functional residual capacity; the sum of RV and ERV (the volume of air remaining in the lungs at the end-expiratory position). The method of measurement should be indicated as with RV

G_{aw}	Airway conductance, the reciprocal of R_{aw}
G_{aw}/V_L	Specific conductance, expressed per liter of lung volume at which G is measured (also referred to as SG_{aw})
I	Inspired
IRV	Inspiratory reserve volume; the maximal volume of air inhaled from the end-inspiratory level
IC	Inspiratory capacity; the sum of IRV and V_T
L	Lung
max	Maximal
MIP*	Maximal inspiratory pressure
MEP*	Maximal expiratory pressure
MVV_x	Maximal voluntary ventilation. The volume of air expired in a specified period during repetitive maximal respiratory effort. The respiratory frequency is indicated by a numerical qualifier; e.g., MVV_{60} is MVV performed at 60 breaths per minute. If no qualifier is given, an unrestricted frequency is assumed
p	Physiological
P	Pressure, blood or gas
PA*	Pulmonary artery
PD*	Provocative dose; the dose of an agent used in bronchial challenge testing which results in a defined change in a specific physiologic parameter. The parameter tested and the percent change in this parameter is expressed in cumulative dose units over the time following exposure that the positive response occurred. For example, $PD_{35}SG_{aw}$ = x units/y minutes, where x is the cumulative inhalation dose and y the time at which a 35% fall in SG_{aw} was noted
PEF	The highest forced expiratory flow measured with a peak flow meter
P_{st}	Static transpulmonary pressure at a specified lung volume; e.g., $P_{st}TLC$ is static recoil pressure measured at TLC (maximal recoil pressure)
Q_c	Capillary blood volume (usually expressed as V_c in the literature, a symbol inconsistent with those recommended for blood volumes). When determined from the following equation, Q_c represents the effective pulmonary capillary blood volume, i.e., capillary blood volume in intimate association with alveolar gas: $$1/D = 1/D_m + 1/(\Theta \cdot Q_c)$$
R	A general symbol for resistance, pressure per unit flow
R_{aw}	Airway resistance
rb	Rebreathing
RQ*	Respiratory quotient

R_{us} — Resistance of the airways on the alveolar side (upstream) of the point in the airways where intraluminal pressure equals Ppl, measured under conditions of maximum expiratory flow

RV — Residual volume; that volume of air remaining in the lungs after maximal exhalation. The method of measurement should be indicated in the text or, when necessary, by appropriate qualifying symbols

SBN* — Single breath nitrogen test; a test in which plots of expired N_2 concentration versus expired volume after inspiration of 100% O_2 are recorded. The closing volume and slope of Phase III are two parameters measured by this test

STPD — Standard conditions: temperature 0° C, pressure 760 mm Hg, and dry (0 water vapor)

t — Time

T — Tidal

TGV* — Thoracic gas volume; the volume of gas within the thoracic cage as measured by body plethysmography

TLC — Total lung capacity; the sum of all volume compartments or the volume of air in the lungs after maximal inspiration. The method of measurement should be indicated, as with RV

V — Gas volume. The particular gas as well as its pressure, water vapor conditions, and other special conditions must be specified in text or indicated by appropriate qualifying symbols

v — Venous

$\bar{v}$ — Mixed venous

$\dot{V}_A$ — Alveolar ventilation per minute (BTPS)

$\dot{V}_{co_2}$ — Carbon dioxide production per minute (STPD)

$\dot{V}_D$ — Ventilation per minute of the physiologic dead space (wasted ventilation), BTPS, defined by the following equation:
$$\dot{V}_D = \dot{V}_E(PaCO_2 - P_ECO_2/(PaCO_2 - P_ICO_2)$$

V_D — The physiologic dead-space volume defined as $\dot{V}_D/f$

$V_D an$ — Volume of the anatomic dead space (BTPS)

$\dot{V}_E$ — Expired volume per minute (BTPS)

$\dot{V}_I$ — Inspired volume per minute (BTPS)

Viso$\dot{V}$* — Volume of isoflow; the volume when the expiratory flow rates become identical when flow–volume loops performed after breathing room air and helium–oxygen mixtures are compared

$\dot{V}_{O_2}$ — Oxygen consumption per minute (STPD)

$\dot{V}_{max}X$ — Forced expiratory flow, related to the total lung capacity or the actual volume of the lung at which the measurement is made. *Modifiers refer to the amount of lung volume remaining when the measurement is made.* For example: $\dot{V}_{max}$ 75% is instantaneous forced expiratory flow when the lung is at 75% of its

TLC. $\dot{V}_{max}3.0$ is instantaneous forced expiratory flow when the lung volume is 3.0 liters. [Editor's note: It is still common to find reports in which modifiers refer to the amount of VC remaining.]

V_T Tidal volume; TV is also commonly used

XA or Xa   A small capital letter or lowercase letter on the same line following a primary symbol is a qualifier to further define the primary symbol. When small capital letters are not available on typewriters or to printers, large capital letters may be used as subscripts, e.g., $X_A = XA$

Blood-Gas Measurements

Abbreviations for these values are readily composed by combining the general symbols recommended earlier. The following are examples:

$PaCO_2$ Arterial carbon dioxide tension

$C(a-v)O_2$ Arteriovenous oxygen content difference

CcO_2 Oxygen content of pulmonary end-capillary blood

F_ECO^* Fractional concentration of CO in expired gas

$P(A-a)O_2$ Alveolar-arterial oxygen pressure difference; the previously used symbol, $A-aDO_2$ is not recommended

SaO_2 Arterial oxygen saturation of hemoglobin

Q_{sp} Physiologic shunt flow (total venous admixture) defined by the following equation when gas and blood data are collected during ambient air breathing:

$$Qsp = \frac{CcO_2 - CaO_2}{CcO_2 - CvO_2} \cdot Q$$

$P_{ET}O_2$ PO_2 of end tidal expired gas

$TCPO_2$ Transcutaneous PO_2

CHAPTER 1

The Limitations of Pulmonary Function Testing

JOHN F. MURRAY

Pulmonary function tests are widely used in the evaluation and management of patients with known or suspected disorders of respiration. The clinical application of these studies rests on knowledge of pulmonary physiology, which has a sound experimental foundation, although we need more information about the relationship between the structure and function of the lungs in health and disease. Despite having a scientific basis, the results of pulmonary function tests must be interpreted empirically, and the temptation to use certain abnormalities to deduce the presence of specific underlying pathologic changes has proved irresistible, albeit often misleading. In a recent editorial, Butler[1] reviewed the inherent limitations that may involve each step of the testing continuum: the apparatus, the patient, the technician, and the interpreter. The purpose of this discussion is (1) to consider why we perform pulmonary function tests and what we are trying to measure; (2) to remind the reader about certain measurement inaccuracies that are frequently overlooked; and (3) to emphasize the enormous problems that plague interpretation, particularly those concerning the concept of *normality* and how to isolate a *specific abnormality.*

WHAT ARE WE MEASURING?

The main reasons for performing pulmonary function studies are listed in Table 1-1. Each of these indications deals with some aspect of the consequences of how particular disorders affect respiratory function. Thus, to examine in

PULMONARY FUNCTION TESTING
INDICATIONS AND INTERPRETATIONS

Table 1-1   Uses of Pulmonary Function Tests

Detection and quantification of respiratory disease.
Evolution of disease and/or response to therapy.
Preoperative evaluation (to identify a high-risk patient or to define extent of
   resectability).
Assessment of disability and/or impairment.

greater detail how presently available tests actually assess respiratory function, we need to define respiration and the mechanisms by which it is carried out.

Respiration can be defined as those processes concerned with gas exchange between an organism and its environment. In humans, respiration has been subdivided into four components: (1) *ventilation*—the active movement of gas from the environment into the lungs and its distribution to the sites of gas exchange; (2) *blood flow*—the active movement of mixed venous blood into the lungs and its distribution to the sites of gas exchange; (3) *diffusion*—the passive movement of molecules of O_2 and CO_2 between inspired gas and incoming blood at the sites of gas exchange; and (4) *control of breathing*—the regulation of ventilation, usually to satisfy metabolic requirements and/or to meet certain voluntary needs.

When viewed in this context, it becomes obvious that no available test of pulmonary function satisfactorily measures respiration much less the totality of any one of its subdivisions. To examine ventilation, we subdivide it further into several components in the hope that by studying the offspring we will gain information about the parent. By this means, we use tests such as the measurement of static lung volumes or of maximal expiratory flow rates to provide insight into the adequacy of the movement of gas in and out of the lungs. Many laboratories can measure the diffusing capacity of the resting lungs for carbon monoxide (DL_{CO}) but this does not tell us what we would like to know about the diffusion of O_2 and CO_2 across the alveolar-capillary membrane during exercise or other stressful conditions. Pulmonary physiologists tend to neglect the pulmonary circulation, and our ability to assess the control of breathing is limited to measuring total central nervous system output and overall chemoreception. The results of one of the most commonly used tests of pulmonary function—measurement of arterial PO_2 and PCO_2—are hopelessly nonspecific because the values are affected by abnormalities in each of the four subdivisions of respiration and to some extent by changes in cardiac output as well.

Nevertheless, from a practical point of view the present approach works fairly well. Of the patients referred for study in hospital-based pulmonary function laboratories, the most common abnormality is a disorder of ventilation: either of airflow obstruction, which is detected by tests of forced expiratory volume in 1 second (FEV_1); or of pulmonary restriction, which is signified by a decrease in vital capacity (VC). And when it comes to managing patients with respiratory failure, the PO_2 and PCO_2 values are often of more immediate concern than the underlying pathologic abnormalities to the attending physician.

Thus, users of the results of pulmonary function tests must realize that they are viewing an extremely complex process—respiration—through tiny windows that provide limited glimpses of what is going on but never of exactly what they would like to see. And, as will be pointed out, our already restricted vision becomes clouded by measurement errors. This further blurs the ultimate distinction that physicians are trying to make between normal and abnormal.

INACCURACIES OF MEASUREMENT

All laboratories, even the best, are subject to technical inaccuracies. These may involve common and simple measurements (e.g., spirometry) that, according to published standards, should have a high degree of accuracy and reproducibility[2]. For example, the results of five frequently used tests of pulmonary function performed in five different, highly respected, university-based pulmonary function laboratories *on the same healthy subjects* are shown in Table 1-2. If we assume that the true value is the mean of the five values for a given test, then the asterisks indicate the individual values that differ from the true value by more than 5%. An accuracy of $\pm$ 5% is applicable to measurements of forced VC (FVC) and FEV_1,[2] but may be too strict for such tests as total lung capacity (TLC) (although, surprisingly, this criterion was met in each of the values in Table 1-2), residual volume (RV), and diffusing capacity (observe that all the values of diffusing capacity were "erroneous" because they all fell into either a high or low group, neither within 5% of the mean). Better reproducibility of FVC and FEV_1 but equally poor DL_{CO} results were recently reported in a study that explored the possibility of using trained subjects to identify interlaboratory variances and to effect proficiency control.[3]

Table 1-2   Results of Studies of Pulmonary Function Tests of the
Same Subject in Five Different Laboratories

Test	A	B	C	D	E	Mean
FVC	5.64	5.06*	5.83*	5.35	5.65	5.51 liter
FEV_1	4.44	3.73*	4.65	4.19	4.15	4.23 liter
TLC	7.12	7.46	7.47	7.61	7.18	7.37 liter
RV	1.34	2.20*	1.48*	2.30*	1.78	1.82 liter
DL_{CO}	28*	29*	35*	34*	29*	31.1 liter/min/mm Hg

FVC = forced vital capacity, FEV_1 = forced expiratory volume in 1 second, TLC = total lung capacity, RV = residual volume, and DL_{CO} = single breath diffusing capacity for carbon monoxide; *Differs from the mean by > $\pm$ 5%.

Some of the variations in recorded VC values in the same subject may be accounted for by differences in the techniques of the measurement. It is known, for example, that the results of slow (relaxed) and fast (forced) VC maneuvers may differ by as much as 1 liter, especially in patients with obstruction of airflow.[4] Furthermore, there seems to be a diurnal variation in VC and FEV_1 that can be masked or augmented by environmental pollutants, cigarette smoking, drugs, and exercise. Serial pulmonary function tests are seldom standardized for these important variables.

Another part of the difficulty is attributable to the fact that our notions about the magnitude of analytic error come from meticulous studies in a few high-powered, usually research-oriented laboratories. This experience does not appear to reflect that of pulmonary function laboratories in general. For example, we would like to believe that we can measure the PCO_2 of a given blood specimen to within ± 2 mm Hg.[5] But the results of analyses of PCO_2 of the same unknown solution by 814 laboratories in California reveal a range of ± 4 mm Hg from the mean for 95% of the values (Fig. 1-1). A bicarbonate-phosphate solution was used in these studies, which probably caused the results to be more widely dispersed than if tonometered blood had been used; however, 3% of the values differed from the mean by 7 > mm Hg and, in the same series, values of 20 and 60 mm Hg were reported. The results of similar studies using an unknown for PO_2 were even worse (Fig. 1-2).

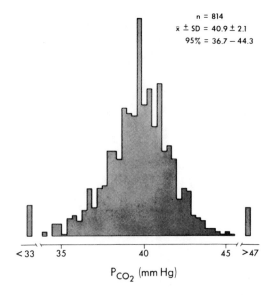

$n = 814$
$\bar{x} ± SD = 40.9 ± 2.1$
$95\% = 36.7 - 44.3$

Figure 1-1. Frequency distribution curve of the report from 814 laboratories of the results of PCO_2 analyses of some unknown specimen.

$< 33 \quad 35 \quad\quad\quad 40 \quad\quad\quad 45 \quad >47$

P_{CO_2} (mm Hg)

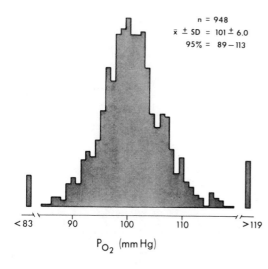

Figure 1-2. Frequency distribution curve of the reports from 948 laboratories of the results of PCO_2 analyses of the same unknown specimen.

NORMAL VERSUS ABNORMAL

Even if we assume perfect accuracy in a given test, there is still the problem of determining whether the resulting value is normal or abnormal. The method in widest use for making this distinction involves comparing the measured value with a predicted value. But this creates a whole new set of problems because we simply do not have sufficient knowledge of the determinants of lung function to provide reliable predictions.

It is not surprising that the major determinant of lung function is a person's size and, to a lesser extent, his or her strength. Accordingly, lung volumes and expiratory flow rates are *size corrected* by dividing the observed values by predicted ones for a person of the same gender, age, and height. A wide range of normality still occurs: $\pm$ 20%–25% of the predicted value for most lung volumes. Part of this large variation results from marked differences in body build and strength among healthy subjects of the same height, attributes that are likely to vary even more among sick patients. Furthermore, it is now known (Fig. 1-3) that substantial differences exist in lung volumes among various ethnic groups.[6] This has created a problem for the large number of users of computer-based pulmonary function testing systems that incorporate prediction equations derived from North American whites because these are not valid for blacks, Asians, and other races.

The data on the effect of age on pulmonary function are far from complete. There clearly seems to be a decline in VC and in FEV_1 during senescence, but whether this is linear or curvilinear and at what age the effect begins, estimates

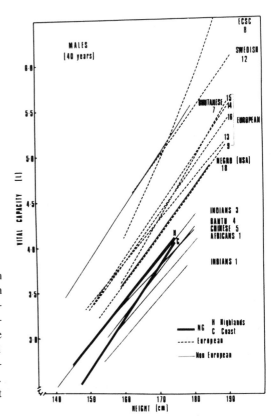

Figure 1-3. VC as a function of height in 40-year-old men from New Guinea (NG) compared with those from other ethnic groups. Note that at the same height, VC varies by more than 1 liter. The numbers refer to references in the original article. (Reproduced from Woolcock et al.[6]. With permission.)

vary from 20 to 40 years of age, are not known with certainty. Although there is more agreement on male–female differences in pulmonary function, even this is not completely settled.[7]

To avoid the pitfalls of size correction, other approaches have been tried. An observed value is *size compensated* when it is divided by another volume measured at the same time (e.g., RV/TLC, FEV_1/FVC, or specific conductance). Size compensation has disadvantages when size has different effects on numerator and denominator as observed in restrictive ventilatory disorders.

The effects of interperson variations in strength, and hence in effort, are taken into account by attempting to standardize for them (e.g., exhorting a "maximal" effort, by measuring it, or by ensuring reproducibility of successive maneuvers). A unique opportunity is afforded in forced expiratory maneuvers because the maximal velocity of airflow at a given lung volume becomes *effort independent* after only modest, not maximal, effort is generated. Unfortunately, the potential benefits of this phenomenon are largely offset by the inadequacy of size correction and size compensation in these tests; after compensation by dividing maximal expiratory flows at a given volume by observed VC or TLC, there is still nearly a fourfold range of corrected flow rates among normal subjects of the same age and gender.[8]

Let us assume that a pulmonary function test has been accurately performed and that the result is clearly abnormal. Can this finding be used to identify the pathologic cause of such an abnormality if one exists? This is seldom possible because as Mead[9] succinctly states, one "cannot get there (i.e., to specific pathology) from here (i.e., from common tests of pulmonary mechanical function)." The same is true of tests of other types of function.

The lack of physiologic discrimination of abnormalities of arterial PO_2 and PCO_2, apart from indicating a disturbance in one or more of the multiple processes that contribute to gas exchange, has already been mentioned. Obviously, no conclusions concerning anatomic alteration are possible from the results of blood-gas analysis. Greater pathologic identification might be expected from studies of the components of ventilation because tests of lung volumes should reflect parenchymal disturbances and tests of expiratory airflow should indicate airway caliber. Unfortunately, this is not always true because of the marked interdependencies that exist between the airways on the one hand and the parenchyma on the other. Inflation and deflation of the parenchyma are wholly dependent on gas flowing through airways, whereas the size of the airways is greatly influenced by the elastic recoil properties of the parenchyma. The quintessential clinical example of this pathophysiologic interaction is pulmonary emphysema, a disease chiefly of the lung parenchyma, in which the airways are nearly normal anatomically. The physiologic hallmark of emphysema, however, is limitation of expiratory airflow.

SUMMARY

Quality control is essential to pulmonary function testing and requires frequent checks and calibrations of all instruments. The pulmonary technologist must be trained to ensure that each patient will perform reliably. A satisfactory performance requires cooperation and understanding, both of which require time. The effects of drugs, breathing maneuvers, and smoking should be controlled whenever possible. The adequacy of performance can usually be inferred by inspecting successive maximal expiratory maneuvers for contour and reproducibility. The prediction equations used should take account of ethnic origin, but even so, the limitations of size correction and size compensation should be recognized.

When accurately performed and properly reported, pulmonary function tests provide valuable clinical information. For example, spirometry is important in the selection of drugs for the treatment of patients with obstruction of airflow and in the identification of patients at high risk of developing postoperative complications. Bronchial provocation tests can identify patients with hyperactive airways, and tests during exercise are helpful in assessing disability and/or impairment. Blood-gas measurements are essential in the diagnosis and treatment of respiratory failure.

Serial studies in the same patient avoid some of the problems in interpretation caused by the wide range of intersubject variability, and are a useful way to study the course of disease and its response to treatment. More specialized tests, such as measurement of diffusing capacity and TLC, serve to detect patients with infiltrative disorders or pulmonary vascular diseases. It should also be recognized that commonly observed combinations of abnormalities or patterns of disturbances are more discriminatory than any single finding. Thus, expiratory obstruction of airflow plus decreased diffusing capacity is likely to, but does not necessarily, indicate the presence of emphysema; in contrast, either abnormality alone only indicates certain generic categories of disburbances.

The physician who uses the results of any pulmonary function test, however, should realize that these values present problems in interpretation that are far greater than those presented by the results of many other commonly used laboratory tests. More precise analytic methods and ways of handling the data will help, but the time when these tests will define specific pathology seems far in the future.

Supported in part by a SCOR grant from the National Heart, Lung and Blood Institute (HL 19155)

REFERENCES

1. Butler J: The pulmonary function test. Cautious overinterpretation. *Chest* 79:498–500, 1981.
2. American Thoracic Society: ATS Statement—Snowbird workshop on standardization of spirometry. *Am Rev Respir Dis* 119:831–838, 1979.
3. Snow M, Stein C, Fallat R: Interlaboratory variability of pulmonary function tests. *Am Rev Diagnostics* 2:43–45, 1983.
4. Tweeddale PM, Merchant S, Leslie MJ, et al.: Quality control in pulmonary function testing. A help or hindrance? *Bull Europ Physiopath Resp* 18:485–490, 1982.
5. Severinghaus JW, Bradley AF: Electrodes for blood PO_2 and PCO_2 determination. *J Appl Physiol* 13:515–520, 1958.
6. Woolcock AJ, Colman, MH, Blackburn CRB: Factors affecting normal values for ventilatory lung function. *Am Rev Respir Dis* 106:692–709, 1972.
7. Buist AS: Evaluation of lung function: Concepts of normality. in Simmons DH (ed): *Current Pulmonology IV.* Boston, Houghton Mifflin, 1982.
8. Green M, Mead J, Turner JM: Variability of maximum expiratory flow-volume curves. *J Appl Physiol* 37:67–74, 1974.
9. Mead J: Problems in interpreting common tests of pulmonary function, in: Macklem PT, Permutt S (eds): *The lung in the transition between health and disease.* New York, Marcel Dekker, Inc, pp 43–51, 1978.

CHAPTER 2

Spirometry

ARTHUR DAWSON

HISTORIC DEVELOPMENT

In 1846, Hutchinson[1] described a water spirometer similar in its main features to the instrument used today, and used it to analyze his data on measurement of the vital capacity (VC) in more than 2000 people. He developed a regression equation to predict the VC from the height of the subject and showed that spirometry could identify pulmonary tuberculosis before it was detectable by the clinical methods of the time.

The test that is now called the maximum voluntary ventilation was described in 1933 by Hermannsen. After Baldwin and associates established normal predicted values in 1948, it was commonly used to quantify pulmonary insufficiency.

Spirometry became much more useful for the diagnosis of bronchial obstructive disease when Tiffeneau and Pinelli introduced a timed measurement of the forced expiratory vital capacity in 1947, a method improved and popularized in America by Gaensler. A number of spirometric indices were proposed to describe the relationship between expired volume and time but, apart from the FEV_1, the measurement that has gained the widest acceptance is the "maximal midexpiratory flow" (now known as the $FEF_{25-75\%}$) introduced by Leuallen and Fowler in 1955.

In the last 25 years, spirometry has become so generally used that it is almost part of the complete physical examination. Computer-assisted methods have made possible a great enhancement of the speed and sophistication of the calculations. In 1979, the recommendations of the Snowbird Workshop were published by the American Thoracic Society, establishing standards for the performance of spirometric systems and the details of how the test should be done[2].

PULMONARY FUNCTION TESTING
INDICATIONS AND INTERPRETATIONS

REVIEW OF METHODS

A spirometer is a device that measures the volume of air inspired or expired and records the time over which the volume change occurs. The classic water-sealed bell and dry bellows spirometers measure the change of volume with a drum kymograph or a moving stylus on a sheet of paper. A second class of devices provides an output proportional to air flow and the volume change is determined by integration of an electronic flow signal. Examples are the Fleisch pneumotachograph, the hot-wire anemometer, and the turbine flowmeter. A volumetric spirometer mechanically coupled to a recording device has a certain built-in reliability because its performance can be checked relatively easily. This instrument remains the standard against which flowmeters, devices with electrical outputs, and computerized spirometry systems can be evaluated. All types can produce reliable data and the choice of a system depends mainly on considerations of cost and the type of work to be done. For busy hospital laboratories and for testing of large groups, the speed of a computerized system unquestionably justifies the high initial cost. The price of microprocessor-assisted spirometers is still too great for the majority of physicians in office practice, so small, dry spirometers selling in the $1500 to $2000 range are most commonly used. However, digital spirometers are rapidly decreasing in price and improving in performance, and it is probably only a matter of a few years before the water spirometer is found only in a few specialized laboratories.

The performance of spirometric equipment has received much attention in the last decade, but the most important factors in obtaining reliable data are the training of the technician and the cooperation of the patient; the latter depends largely on the former. Many hospital laboratories are still supervised by physicians who have little training or interest in lung function testing and provide only perfunctory direction to the respiratory therapists or ECG technicians who occasionally run a spirogram. Data obtained under such conditions may be worthless at best and at times seriously misleading. Consider what might happen if a group of workers in a potentially hazardous occupation were given a careless spirometer test as part of their pre-employment physical examination. If there were later a question as to whether one of these workers had developed an industrial disease, the spurious data would assume great medicolegal importance and might lead to a serious injustice to the worker or employer, depending on the direction of the error. The standards recommended by the Snowbird Workshop should apply to all spirometry testing whether it is done in the hospital, in the private medical office, or at the workplace. There is no justification for slipshod spirometry and it is essential that everybody performing the test be sufficiently trained to obtain the full cooperation of the subject and to recognize technical artifacts in the results.

Spirometry without a graphic tracing is of relatively little value as a diagnostic test. Only by seeing the record can one evaluate the adequacy of the patient's effort, and the tracing can often demonstrate subtle features of disease that are not evident when only numeric data are reported. The graph should be available not only to the physician interpreting the test but should also be part of the final report. A spirometry report consisting only of numbers is not much more useful than a radiologist's interpretation of a chest film without the original roentgenogram.

CALCULATIONS

Figure 2-1 represents the same forced expirogram in both volume-versus-time and flow-volume formats, and demonstrates the spirometric indices that can be derived from them. The volume-time curve is rotated 90° from its usual orientation so that the two curves share a common volume axis. The volume expired over a specific time cannot be calculated directly from the flow-volume tracing but the FEV_1, for example, can be represented by a tic on the curve. It should be emphasized that the two curves contain the same information. The U.S. Social Security Administration requires that tracings be presented in the volume-time format, presumably because it is difficult for an independent consultant to be sure from inspection of the flow-volume curve whether the forced expiration was sustained for an adequate time. Therefore, it is best that an instrument be able to present the data in both ways. In this volume we show

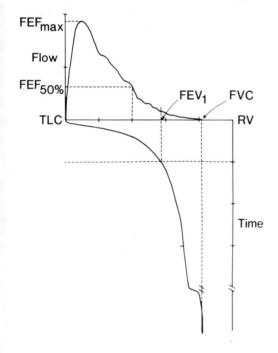

Figure 2-1. The same forced expiration shown above the horizontal axis as a flow-volume curve and below in the volume-time format.

mostly flow-volume curves which make certain clinically interesting features more obvious.

PATHOPHYSIOLOGICAL RATIONALE

DETERMINANTS OF THE VITAL CAPACITY

In the normal adult the VC is essentially a measure of stature. It shows a positive correlation with height and a negative correlation with age. Consideration of weight adds little accuracy to a linear regression equation because of the opposing effects of a large frame and of obesity. The vital capacity is the difference between the total lung capacity (TLC) and the residual volume and therefore it is determined by the factors governing these volumes which represent the limits of voluntary inspiration and voluntary expiration. The TLC is the volume at which the tension generated by the diaphragm and the other inspiratory muscles is balanced by the elastic recoil of the lungs and the chest wall. In disease, the TLC may be restricted by abnormalities of the bony thorax, the inspiratory muscles or the pleura as well as by loss of functioning alveoli. In practice, chest pain, fatigue and poor effort may prevent the patient from attaining as full an inspiration as possible with a maximum effort and the measured vital capacity will be correspondingly reduced.

In young adults the residual volume is, like the TLC, determined mainly by the compliance of the thoracic cage and by the limits of shortening of the muscles of expiration. In addition, in the dependent regions of the lungs small airways closure prevents further emptying of some alveoli even as air continues to be expelled from regions whose airways remain open.[3] In older persons the lung elastic recoil diminishes and the small airways close at a higher lung volume. Alveolar emptying is delayed in other regions whose airways are narrowed but still open. As a result the terminal part of forced expiration is so much slower that flow continues for as long as expiratory effort can be maintained.[4] Therefore the "true" residual volume is more a hypothetical than a real volume in older adults and in most individuals with obstructive lung disease. Expiratory effort should be continued for at least 6 and preferably for 10 seconds to obtain valid measurements of the expiratory vital capacity. Some very cooperative bronchitic patients can sustain a forced expiration for as long as 25 seconds but there is a risk of fainting with such prolonged expiratory effort.

In obstructive lung disease (OLD) the residual volume characteristically increases while the TLC remains unchanged or increases only slightly. Therefore the vital capacity is diminished. In many pathological states causing a reduction of the vital capacity there is both a low TLC and an increased residual volume. For example, the vital capacity diminishes in many types of heart disease, especially congestive heart failure, probably owing to a combination of increased intrathoracic blood volume, increased heart size, reduced alveolar distensibility and small airways closure.

DETERMINANTS OF FORCED EXPIRATORY FLOW

During a forced expiration the driving pressure to expel air from the lungs is the alveolar pressure which is equal to the sum of the pleural pressure and the static recoil pressure.

$$Palv = Ppl + Pst$$

The intraluminal pressure in the airways falls progressively "downstream" from the alveoli and at some "equal pressure point" is equal to the pleural pressure, which is approximately the same as the extraluminal pressure of the intrathoracic airways.[5] The greater the resistance of the peripheral airways the more distally the equal pressure points will be located. If the equal pressure points are within the thorax then the "downstream" airways will tend to collapse during a forced expiration. Greater expiratory effort will increase both the pleural and the alveolar pressures, but since the increment is transmitted equally to the intraluminal and extraluminal pressures, the equal pressure points do not change their location. Therefore, if the resistance of the small airways of the "upstream segment" is sufficient to cause the intraluminal pressure to fall below the pleural pressure, the effective driving pressure for expiration is the static recoil pressure. The static recoil pressure is normally sufficient at high lung volumes to prevent compression of the intrathoracic airways. At low volumes "dynamic compression" appears so that, after perhaps 75 to 80 percent of the vital capacity has been expelled, forced expiratory flow is independent of effort and depends on the recoil pressure. The recoil pressure diminishes with decreasing lung volume and so flow falls progressively as forced expiration continues (Figure 2-2).

In OLD the resistance of the small airways is increased and the static recoil pressure may be reduced. Both of these factors cause dynamic compression to appear at a higher lung volume. Therefore, expiratory flow will be not only diminished but also less influenced by effort. Patients with markedly reduced lung elastic recoil may show "negative effort dependence" and flow will actually diminish with a more forcible expiration.

DETERMINANTS OF INSPIRATORY FLOW

During inspiratory effort the patency of the intrathoracic airways is maintained by the subatmospheric extraluminal pressure. The driving pressure for inspiratory flow is the difference between the atmospheric pressure at the mouth and the negative alveolar pressure. With increasing effort the airways resistance is the same or even decreased as the driving pressure is augmented. Therefore

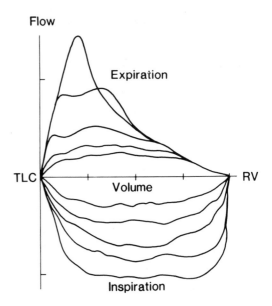

Figure 2-2. Effect of variable effort on the flow-volume loop of a normal subject. Inspiratory flow is below and expiratory flow above the horizontal axis. Flow in the terminal part of expiration is independent of effort.

inspiratory flow is dependent on effort and relatively uninfluenced by the recoil pressure and by the properties of the intrathoracic airways (Figure 2-2). Inspiratory flow is relatively fixed only if there is an obstruction of the trachea or extrathoracic airways when, presumably, most of the effect of increased effort is dissipated because of energy loss through turbulence at the obstruction. Measurement of maximal inspiratory flow, therefore, may be helpful in recognizing obstruction of the extrathoracic airways and in demonstrating the high ratio of inspiratory to expiratory flow in obstructive lung disease, but it is of much less clinical interest than the "forced expirogram".

INDICATIONS FOR SPIROMETRY TESTING

To establish baseline ventilatory function.   This subject is discussed in the "Controversies" section at the end of this chapter.

To detect disease.   Obstructive lung disease is one of the most common disabling conditions in this country. It is probably largely preventable. Spirometry is close to being an ideal screening test for the detection of obstructive lung disease. Almost by definition there are few, if any, false positive and false negative results, and abnormalities can be detected years in advance of the appearance of symptoms at a stage when cessation of smoking offers the maximum hope of avoiding severe disability. Spirometry is also valuable in the diagnosis of a variety of other conditions affecting the lungs, such as interstitial lung disease and other restrictive lung disorders, but it must usually be supplemented by more specialized tests of lung function.

To follow the course of disease. Spirometry is essential for following the progress of many chronic lung diseases and its value is much enhanced if a test is done prior to the onset of symptoms or early in the course of the illness. The normal values for spirometry are so variable that detection of a change on serial testing of an individual may be a much more sensitive indicator of abnormality than comparing his or her data with reference values.

To monitor treatment. In asthma, with its rapid variations in airways obstruction, spirometry is indispensable in assessing the response to therapeutic interventions. It is equally valuable to follow the short-term and long-term responses to treatment in chronic obstructive lung disease. Additional tests may be required to evaluate therapy in interstitial lung disease but spirometry is most practicable for following patients in the intervals between more comprehensive tests because of its availability and relatively low cost (see also Chapter 4 this volume).

Evaluation of impairment. Chronic obstructive lung disease ranks second among the reasons for disability payments in this country. The Social Security Administration requires spirometry to quantify the impairment in persons claiming disability due to chronic bronchitis or emphysema and most other governmental and nongovernmental sources of disability payments have similar requirements. Spirometry is likewise necessary to support a disability claim for other forms of diffuse lung disease, such as pneumoconiosis and pulmonary fibrosis (see also Chapter 20 this volume).

Preoperative evaluation. Because this subject is much debated, a complete discussion is deferred until the end of this chapter (see also Chapter 19 in this volume).

Identifying the high-risk smoker. A number of attempts have been made to recognize specific risk factors that will identify the smokers most likely to develop disabling obstructive lung disease later in life.[6] At present, no method seems more reliable than serial spirometry. Those who show a more rapid decline of the forced vital capacity or the FEV_1 than the average smoker (about 50 ml/yr) may be candidates for special efforts to get them to quit the tobacco habit.[7,8]

Occupational surveys. Modern technology has generated a host of new and potentially toxic airborne chemicals and particulate materials. It is economically, if not physically, impossible to prevent industrial workers from inhaling low levels of these substances, and various government agencies are charged with the responsibility of establishing maximum permissible concentrations for the working environment. These are necessarily based on a combination of guesswork and short-term animal toxicity studies. It is not feasible to consider all of the possible complicating influences, such as interactions of airborne pollutants with each other and with nonoccupational risk factors such as cigarette smoking, nor is it possible to estimate accurately the full range of individual susceptibillity. Therefore, in any potentially hazardous industrial environment, it is necessary that individual workers be periodically monitored for developing respiratory problems. Spirometry is an essential part of such testing (see also Chapter 20 in this volume).

INTERPRETATIONS

PATTERNS OF ABNORMALITY

The two basic items of information in the spirometric test are a measurement of volume, the vital capacity, and a measurement of respiratory air flow. Spirometric abnormalities may be broadly divided into those manifested by decreased VC (i.e., loss of *ventilable lung volume*) and by diminished flow (i.e., *obstructive disease*). When the VC is reduced without a comparable decrease in flow, one can suspect *restrictive disease,* but this term should be reserved for conditions in which the lung volume is reduced (see also Chapter 15 in this volume). For reasons considered previously, obstructive disease may reduce the VC so that when a low VC is associated with diminished flow, the diagnosis of a "true" restrictive abnormality may require a measurement of lung volume by another method. Conversely, when VC is markedly diminished, there tends to be a more or less proportionate reduction of flow so that even if the FEV_1 is much below the predicted value, the ratio of FEV_1 to FVC may be normal or even higher than usual. At times when a severe loss of ventilable lung volume is combined with obstructive disease, it may be impossible to identify the obstructive component confidently without more extensive lung function testing.

The Slow and the Forced VC

The spirometric test should include a measurement of the slow or nonforced expiratory VC in addition to the forced vital capacity (FVC). Normally the two are identical and when they differ substantially, for example, by more than 0.2, it is evidence of what has been called *air trapping*. The difference between slow and the forced VC is mainly due to the phenomenon of *dynamic compression* resulting from increased resistance of intrathoracic airways and loss of lung elastic recoil. When it is marked, it suggests pulmonary emphysema but it can also be seen in uncomplicated bronchospasm.

Ventilable Volume Loss

When the spirogram is interpreted without other lung function data, the term *ventilable volume loss* can be used operationally to describe a heterogeneous group of disorders whose main common feature is reduction of the VC. Spirograms showing volume loss can be separated into those in which a normal or supernormal maximum expiratory flow is preserved and those in which the flow is reduced in proportion with the VC. In the first type there is a high likelihood of true restrictive disease because the airways tend to be kept dilated by an increased elastic recoil pressure, as in early interstitial lung disease. Another feature that helps to identify restrictive disease is the steep descending limb of the flow-volume curve (Fig. 2-3A). The second pattern is typically seen after a lung resection when the remaining lung is normal (Fig. 2-3B). Figure 2-3C shows a patient with combined obstructive and restrictive disease. It is often impossible to distinguish these three patterns of loss of ventilable volume without clinical information and additional lung function measurements.

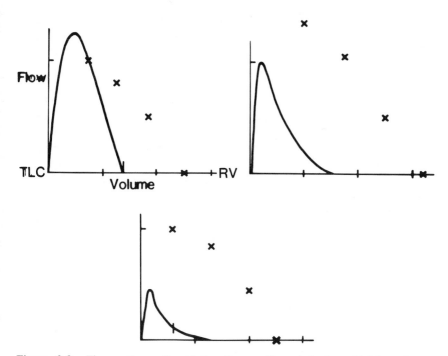

Figure 2-3. Three patterns of restrictive disease. Above left—interstitial lung disease with normal flow. The FVC was 1.48 l (58% of predicted), the FEV_1 was 1.42 l (67% predicted), and the $FEF_{25-75\%}$ was 3.96 l/sec (129%). Above right—restrictive disease in a patient who had a left lower lobectomy and right pneumonectomy. The FVC was 1.54 l (47%), the FEV_1 was 1.33 l (33%), and the $FEF_{25-75\%}$ was 1.59 l/sec (47%). Below—combined restrictive and obstructive disease in a heavy smoker who had a thoracoplasty for tuberculosis. The FVC was 0.97 l (38%), the FEV_1 was 0.66 l (33%), and the $FEF_{25-75\%}$ was 0.42 l/sec (15%).

Obstructive Lung Disease

Figures 2-4, 2-5, and 2-6 show representative curves of mild, moderate, and severe obstructive lung disease. In these examples, the FVCs all happen to be in the normal range but there is usually some decrease in the VC in severe obstruction. Many patients with severe obstructive disease show the "dog leg" flow-volume curve illustrated in Figure 2-6 with relatively high flow maintained for the first 15–25% of the expired volume and then an abrupt fall to very reduced flows through the rest of the breath. The inflection represents the onset of marked dynamic compression of the intrathoracic airways and it is less pronounced in a nonforced expiration.

Small Airways Obstruction

In the last 15 years, there has been much interest in recognizing disease of the small airways less than 2 mm in diameter. Early studies suggested that the small airways contributed only about 10% of the total airways resistance[9] but more recent work has shown that 33% is probably a better estimate.[10] It follows that there could be a moderate increase in the resistance of the small airways with little detectable effect upon expiratory flow.

Several methods have been developed to identify early disease of the small airways but for the most part they are too complex for routine diagnostic testing.[11] It may be possible, however, to identify the small airways' involvement from the spirogram if the expiratory flow at low lung volume is carefully analyzed.[12]

Because the small airways lack cartilaginous support they depend for their patency on the lung elastic recoil. Since the recoil pressure diminishes with decreasing lung volume, the resistance of the small airways increases relative to that of the central airways in the terminal part of the forced expiration. Therefore, small airways disease can be suspected if the FEV_1 and the FEF_{max} are

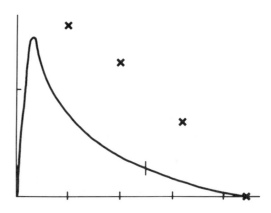

Figure 2-4. Mild obstructive lung disease. The FVC was 4.14 l (94% of predicted), the FEV_1 was 2.60 l (75%), and the $FEF_{25-75\%}$ was 1.63 l/sec (38%).

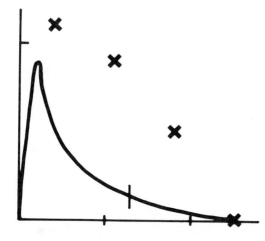

Figure 2-5. Moderate obstructive disease. The FVC was 2.77 l (95%), the FEV_1 was 1.27 (55%), and the $FEF_{25-75\%}$ was 0.60 l/sec (13%).

normal whereas measurements obtained at low lung volume are abnormally reduced. The $FEF_{25-75\%}$ has been recommended as a good way to identify small airways disease[13] but measurements obtained entirely from the terminal part of the expiration such as the $FEF_{75\%}$ or the $FEF_{75-85\%}$[14] should be more sensitive. The last two measurements are very much influenced by the patient's effort to expire completely and the normal values are extremely variable, which somewhat limits their clinical usefulness. Once one has become accustomed to looking at the flow-volume curve it is easy to identify the "slow tail" characteristic of early obstruction of the small airways (Fig. 2-7). It must be admitted that at present the prognostic significance of this pattern is unknown but it may serve to

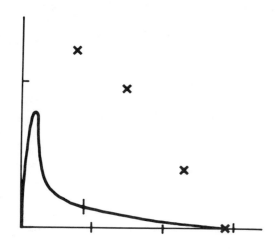

Figure 2-6. Severe obstructive disease. The FVC was 2.84 l (95%), the FEV_1 was 0.85 l (38%), and the $FEF_{25-75\%}$ was 0.29 l/sec (9%).

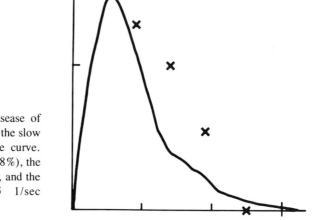

Figure 2-7. Early disease of the small airways. Note the slow tail on the flow-volume curve. The FVC was 3.95 l (118%), the FEV_1 was 2.49 l (97%), and the $FEF_{25-75\%}$ was 1.15 1/sec (33%).

alert the physician that patients will require more frequent follow-up spirometry and special efforts to persuade them to stop smoking.

Upper Airways Obstruction

Obstruction of the upper respiratory tract, the larynx, or the trachea produces the opposite effect from small airways disease. It is most readily identified in the initial most rapid part of the forced expiration when flow is dominated by the resistance of the major airways. Figure 2-8 shows an example of the typical pattern in a patient with a large substernal goiter. The *flat-topped* curve shown is seen when the obstruction is more or less fixed. The pattern is more variable if the obstruction involves major airways whose size varies with the intrathoracic pressure.[15] As noted above, upper airways obstruction also affects the inspiratory limb of the flow-volume curve. Though the features of upper airways obstruction have received a lot of attention in recent medical literature, in my experience the condition has been clinically obvious by the time the spirogram shows diagnostic abnormalities. The degree of obstruction necessary to affect the flow-volume curve was studied by Miller and Hyatt who measured inspiratory and expiratory flow in normal subjects breathing through a fixed external resistance. They showed that the orifice size had to be reduced to 8 mm or less before the flow-volume curve began to assume the characteristic flat-topped appearance.[16] It follows that spirometry should not be considered a reliable method to rule out obstruction of the upper airways when the condition is suspected on clinical grounds.

Negative Effort Dependence

Though forced expiration is an artificial respiratory maneuver, it has proven diagnostically useful because of its reproducibility and its relative independence

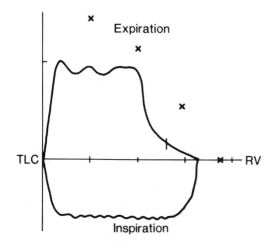

Figure 2-8. Upper airways obstruction. The FVC was 3.25 l (86%), the FEV_1 was 2.67 l (92%), and the $FEF_{25-75\%}$ was 3.25 l/sec (87%).

of patient effort. However, in patients with marked dynamic compression the results can be misleading. The solid curve in Figure 2-9 is from a patient with emphysema whose FEV_1 at a routine office visit had fallen from its usual level of 0.90 l. to 0.61 l. though he reported that he felt in his usual state of health. The dashed curve shows what happened when he performed a nonforced expiration; his FEV_1 rose to 0.91 l. In such a patient the forced expiratory flow is dominated by the compression of the intrathoracic airways and the results may even correlate negatively with the clinical findings because the patient may expire more forcefully when he or she is feeling better. Obviously, such changes could obscure the response to a therapeutic intervention and lead to an incorrect clinical decision, especially if the physicians managing the patient and interpreting the test are not the same. The problem has been recognized by a number of investigators and there have been attempts to analyze partial and nonforced expirations, but at present the technical details and normal values are not sufficiently established for these methods to be widely accepted. It is important when one is

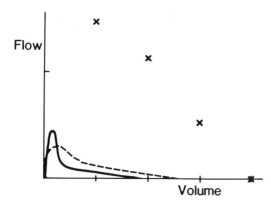

Figure 2-9. Negative effort dependence. The solid curve represents a forced and the dashed a nonforced expiration.

basing clinical decisions on the results of spirometry to be alert for such misleading data. An important clue is a marked difference between the slow and the forced vital capacity. If there is a question a nonforced expiration should be recorded.

The Gas Compression Effect

A phenomenon related to negative effort dependence that has been a source of confusion is the effect of changes in the alveolar pressure on lung volume. During a forced expiration, part of the decrease in the absolute lung volume is due to compression of the intrathoracic gas. The discrepancy between the volume expired at the mouth and the change in the thoracic gas volume, which can be measured with a body plethysmograph, tends to be greater with greater expiratory effort, especially when the airways resistance is abnormally increased.[17] It is important to remember that the volume measured on the spirometric flow-volume curve is the volume expired at the mouth and that it may differ substantially from the change in absolute lung volume. Errors in interpretation may result if one tries to predict the change in isovolume flows by comparing spirometer-generated flow-volume curves obtained before and after some intervention that affects the airways resistance or when expiratory effort has varied significantly.

Neuromuscular Disease

Spirometry may be helpful in detecting respiratory muscle involvement with neuromuscular disease at a time when clinical symptoms and signs are absent. The most useful spirometric indicators of abnormality in amyotrophic lateral sclerosis are the FVC and the maximum voluntary ventilation (MVV) but both inspiratory and expiratory flow are frequently reduced.[18] The flow-volume curve may suggest only submaximal effort but a variety of abnormal patterns have been described, especially in patients with bulbar involvement when incoordination of the glottal muscles can cause sudden interruptions of expiratory flow. Abnormalities of the pharyngeal tissues have been suggested as an explanation of a *saw-toothed* pattern on both inspiratory and expiratory limbs of the flow-volume loop recently described as characteristic of patients with obstructive sleep apnea.[19] Though spirometry may be useful in following the course of respiratory muscle involvement in neuromuscular disease, it is not the most sensitive means of detecting it at an early stage. Black and Hyatt have shown that the maximal static respiratory pressures can be reduced even when spirometry is normal.[20]

The Maximum Voluntary Ventilation

The MVV is less frequently performed than it was a few years ago. It is a fatiguing test and it is quite dependent on patient training and motivation. Because of these difficulties several formulas have been proposed to predict the MVV from the forced expiratory volume timed (FEV_t). This practice seems both illogical and misleading but it had some justification when the MVV was used more widely than it is now to assess respiratory impairment and as a criterion for offering or refusing thoracotomy. The MVV remains helpful in interpreting the ventilatory response to exercise during pulmonary stress testing, and in this instance an indicator such as the FEV_1 multiplied by 35 may be a useful check on whether the recorded MVV represented an adequate patient effort.[21]

The main advantage of the MVV is that it tests the ability to sustain a high level of ventilation. When it is normal clinically significant restrictive and obstructive disease are practically excluded, that is, there are few false negative results, but false positives are frequent.

When the MVV is performed it is important to keep a graphic record of the test including the change in lung volume during the MVV maneuver. Figures 2-10A and 2-10B show the classic obstructive and restrictive ventilatory patterns. The patient with restrictive disease hyperventilated without a change in the end-expiratory lung volume, increasing ventilation by augmenting respiratory rate rather than tidal volume (Fig. 2-10B). This pattern minimizes the work of breathing, most of which is performed in overcoming the elastic recoil pressure. The patient with airways obstruction selects a high volume at which the increased recoil pressure maintains the patency of the intrathoracic airways (Fig. 2-10A).

NORMAL VALUES AND QUANTIFICATION OF IMPAIRMENT

Traditionally, the normal range of most lung function measurements, including the spirometric indices, has been considered to be within plus or minus

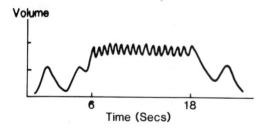

Volume

6   18
Time (Secs)

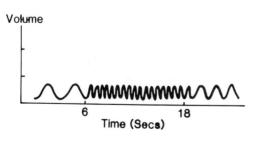

Volume

6   18
Time (Secs)

Figure 2-10. Two abnormal patterns of the MVV maneuver. Above—Obstructive disease. The tidal volume decreases and the end-expiratory volume increases during the maneuver. Below—Restrictive disease. The respiratory rate increases but the tidal volume and end expiratory volume are unchanged.

20% of the predicted value based on the gender, age, and height of the subject. This was a useful and easily remembered rule of thumb but it is no longer justified now that good data have been published giving confidence limits for the predicted values of a number of the standard lung function measurements.[22]

In clinical spirometry we are interested mainly in the lower limit of normal. If we define results falling below those of 95% of a comparable group of normal subjects as abnormal, we should perform a one-tailed test of whether the patient's measured value falls within the 95% confidence limits of a *referent population* of the same sex, age and body stature. The lower limit of normal, therefore, is defined as 1.64 standard deviations below the mean value for the referent population. It must be remembered, however, that this is an arbitrary definition and that in population studies it will stigmatize 1 in 20 individuals as diseased. A physician interpreting spirometry must have a clear understanding of what he or she means by abnormal when advising the patient, the employer, the insurance company, or the government agency at whose request the test is performed. Some of the problems in establishing normal values for spirometry are discussed in more detail in *Pulmonary Function Testing Guidelines and Controversies* in which we have also evaluated a number of the published equations used to calculate predicted values.[22] Crapo and associates have recently recommended some equations for reference values which include 95% confidence limits.[23] Their data have the advantage of being based on spirometry performed following the techniques and calculations recommended by the Snowbird Workshop.[2]

Once it is established that a spirometric measurement is abnormal, one has the problem of deciding whether the abnormality is mild, moderate, or severe. Some writers have suggested arbitrary limits depending on how many standard deviations below the mean the observed value falls. In my opinion, this is even less satisfactory than the traditional practice of quantifying impairment as a certain percentage below the predicted value. If a patient's VC were 4 standard deviations below the mean predicted value we could say with great confidence that he or she was not normal, but by itself this information would tell us nothing about whether the patient had any symptoms or whether his or her risk of premature disability or death was increased. At least the traditional grading was based on clinical impressions that roughly correlated the patient's symptoms with the degree of reduction of the observed measurement.

We need prospective studies in which the severity of various lung conditions is graded by criteria independent of spirometry, such as effort tolerance or subjective dyspnea. One could then look at a particular spirometric measurement in the patients with, for example, moderate impairment to determine the average percent reduction below the predicted value and its confidence limits. Unfortunately, few studies of this type have been done and we are left with the traditional approach which, it must be admitted, has served us reasonably well over the years.

The figures in Table 2-1 were taken from Morris[24] but they have been

Table 2-1 Spirometric Values as a Percentage of the Predicted and Severity of Functional Impairment

	Group 1	Group 2
Normal	> 5th percentile of normal reference population	
Mild	> 65	> 60
Moderate	50–64	45–59
Severe	35–49	30–44
Very severe	< 35	< 30

modified to avoid the arbitrary classification of anything above 80% of the predicted as normal. Slightly different figures were proposed by the intermountain Thoracic Society (Table 1).[25]

The numbers referring to the severity of abnormality are expressed as a percent of the predicted value. The tests in group I are the VC, FVC, FEV_1, and MVV. Group II includes the $FEF_{25-75\%}$. Other volume-dependent tests such as the $FEF_{25\%}$ and the $FEF_{50\%}$ probably belong in the same group.

A committee of the American Thoracic Society recently proposed that an individual should be considered severely impaired if his or her VC is 50% or less of the predicted value or if the FEV_1 or the FEV_1/FVC ratio is 40% or less of the predicted value based on the equations of Crapo et al.[26] If we defined the separation between mild and moderate as halfway between the lower limit of normal and the upper limit of severe impairment, we would have a method of grading the severity of disease, at least for these three commonly used measurements.

A person whose FEV_1 is less than 1.0 liter qualifies for a handicapped parking sticker in California. I have found this piece of intelligence remarkably effective in helping to persuade inveterate smokers that it is time to quit.

ARTIFACTS AND PITFALLS

IMPORTANCE OF PATIENT EFFORT AND COOPERATION

In order to be reliable the spirometric test must represent a true maximum effort. For most reasonably intelligent and cooperative patients a total of three trials has been shown to produce the maximum *training effect* and further trials result in little or no improvement.[27] An important check on the adequacy of the trials is that the best two should agree within 5% or 100 ml, whichever is greater.[2] Though three trials suffice for most patients, many more will be required for some subjects who require a great deal of careful coaching before they can produce an adequate performance. Much depends on the personality and skill of the technician. If he or she is abrupt or intimidating, patients will quickly become balky and the data will be useless. Technicians must be experienced enough to recognize unsatisfactory curves and to coach patients on how to alter their technique to achieve better results. Though the physician interpreting the test must also be alert to possible artifacts, only the technician can make a reliable assessment of the patient's performance and should record a comment on it to be included in the final report.

Special problems may be encountered in trying to get true maximal effort from patients being tested to evaluate lung function impairment when there is a question of disability, Workmen's Compensation, or personal injury. It is important for the referring physician to explain to the patient before the test that any attempt to give an inadequate performance will probably be obvious to the interpreter and will do his or her case more harm than good. This argument may carry some weight with the conscious malingerer but in the victim of a well-established "compensation neurosis" it may be impossible to get an adequate test. In such cases it may be necessary to ignore the spirometry and to rely on the tests that are relatively unaffected by patient effort (such as a normal functional residual capacity, diffusing capacity, and resting blood gases). On several occasions I have seen patients I was certain were malingerers who could produce a restrictive-appearing flow-volume curve with remarkable consistency. I have rarely seen a convincing simulation of the curve of severe obstructive disease.

Some of the following features of the tracing may be clues that the performance was not optimal.

1.   Submaximal effort may be suspected if the FEF_{max} is a much lower fraction of the predicted value than the FEV_1 or if the expired flow-volume curve shows an ill-defined peak resembling the nonforced curves in Figure 2-2.

2.   Incomplete expiration may be suspected if the flow abruptly falls to zero at the end of expiration but this pattern is sometimes seen in healthy adolescents and young adults (Fig. 2-11).

3.   A slow onset of forced expiration may result in an inaccurate determination of zero time causing major errors in the calculation of the FEV_1. An adequate method of back-extrapolation will correct this error but a curve should be rejected if the extrapolated volume is more than 10% of the FVC or 100 ml, whichever is greater.[2] Errors due to a slow onset may be especially difficult to detect in computer-assisted spirometry systems or when the flow-volume curve is recorded without a volume-time curve (Fig. 2-12). A good computer program should provide for rejection of trials requiring excessive back-extrapolation correction, but many commercially available systems do not include this feature.

4.   Technically satisfactory curves should be free of coughs, false starts, and interruptions of expiration by artificial teeth, tongue in the mouthpiece, and closure of the glottis. An experienced technician can usually pick up such problems by inspection of the tracing. Some patients are simply unable to provide an entirely satisfactory forced expiration and then it is a matter of judgment for the technician to select the best trials. At times even a very poor curve can give

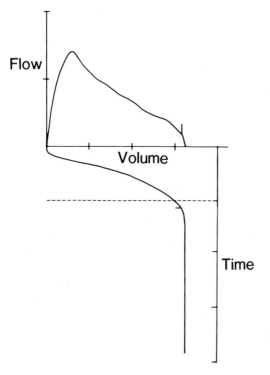

Figure 2-11. Abrupt termination of expiratory flow. One should suspect a poorly sustained expiration when one sees this pattern, but this depiction happens to be a good curve from a healthy young laboratory technician.

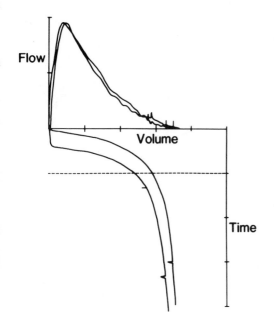

Figure 2-12. Two forced expirations from the same subject superimposed, one showing a slow onset. The flow-volume curves appear almost identical. The dashed line represents one second after the onset of flow while the tic marks one second after time zero determined by the back-extrapolation algorithm. The point where the dashed line intersects the volume-time curve indicates the large error in the FEV_1 without the back-extrapolation correction. Such errors are obvious on a hand-calculated curve but may not be evident when the calculations are done by a computer.

clinically useful information. For example, the descending limb of the flow-volume curve may show a typical obstructive pattern even though expiration was sustained for only a second or two.

Volume-Dependent Measurements of Expiratory Flow

Certain measurements of forced expiratory flow can be markedly influenced by how long expiration was sustained. For example, if the last few seconds of the forced expiration are cut off in a patient with a marked "slow tail" the $FEF_{25-75\%}$, which is the average flow over the middle 50% of the VC, will be measured over a higher range of lung volumes and the calculated value will be falsely elevated. There will be even greater errors in the $FEF_{75\%}$ and the $FEF_{75-85\%}$. This artifact can cause problems especially when the $FEF_{25-75\%}$ is compared before and after treatment with a bronchodilator or when serial tests are evaluated. Changes in the $FEF_{25-75\%}$ should always be interpreted with caution when the FVC differs between two tests. It has been suggested that the $FEF_{25-75\%}$ should be volume-adjusted so that measurements obtained before and after a bronchodilator can be compared over the same absolute range of lung volumes.[28,29] However, this requires an independent measurement of lung volume by body plethysmography and so the correction is not applicable to routine spirometry. The error due to volume changes can be reduced if the flows on two curves are compared by subtracting the same volume from the TLC. However, this correction is only valid if the TLC remains constant, which may not be the case if there is a marked change in flow.

Interpreting a Change in the FEV% —A Pons Asinorum

In assessing the response to an intervention, such as treatment with a bronchodilator, it is important to compare absolute values of the FEV_1 rather than the FEV_1/FVC. If the FVC increases after the treatment there may be no change or even a decrease in the FEV%, though the FEV_1 has improved significantly. I may seem to insult the intelligence of my readers by pointing out something so obvious but I have seen experienced chest physicians stumble over this pons asinorum.

Normal Spirogram in Obstructive Disease

Most of the time the spirogram is very sensitive to even minor degrees of bronchial obstruction. However, in occasional patients, usually young individuals with mild bronchospasm, there is more closure than narrowing of the airways. Because flow is relatively normal in the patent airways and it is zero in those which are occluded, the flow-volume curve does not show the concavity of the descending limb characteristic of bronchial obstruction. There is only a fall in the FVC and a rise in the residual volume. Comparing before and after broncho-dilator tests may or may not identify a significant response. The true state of affairs may only be revealed after the patient has received effective treatment. This is one reason why it is very useful to have baseline spirometry when a patient is first evaluated.

CONTROVERSIES

SHOULD SPIROMETRY BE INCLUDED IN THE PERIODIC HEALTH EXAMINATION?

Spirometry is a much underutilized test. I believe that every patient should have spirometry at the time the initial clinical data base is accumulated. If the first test is abnormal or in the presence of certain risk factors (respiratory symptoms, tobacco habit, family history of obstructive lung disease, or hazardous occupation) the test should be repeated periodically, perhaps every 1 to 5 years, depending on the estimated risk of progressive respiratory disease. Obviously, for this to be possible a spirometer must be available to every primary care internist and family practitioner. This may seem an irresponsible suggestion in this era of cost containment but a spirometer is as valuable a diagnostic tool as the electrocardiograph (ECG) and few physicians would attempt to practice primary medicine in this country without access to an ECG machine. Many physicians still consider spirometry a technically complex and expensive test which is only necessary when there is obvious respiratory impairment. Unfortu-nately, their opinion is lent some support by the arcane terminology that encum-bers the spirometric report and by the unreasonably high charges made for the test by some laboratories. The first objection can be overcome by continuing education of practicing physicians and perhaps by the more "friendly" appear-ance of a properly formatted flow-volume curve. The second should be mitigated as rapid computer-assisted spirometry increasingly competes with the slow hand-calculated methods. Until spirometry is more widely used chest specialists will continue to see heavy smokers with advanced obstructive lung disease who have faithfully gone through a periodic physical examination for years without sus-pecting that they had a preventable respiratory illness.

WHICH PATIENTS SHOULD HAVE PREOPERATIVE SPIROMETRY?

Spirometry is the most reliable means to identify high-risk patients for postoperative bronchopulmonary complications, especially pneumonia and atel-ectasis. There is general agreement that spirometry should be done in situations in which such complications are frequent, such as operations on the chest and upper abdomen and in the elderly, the obese, heavy smokers, and in those with respiratory symptoms.[30] Others have pointed out that these groups are obviously at risk and that spirometry can identify other patients with obstructive disease who are not symptomatic. Therefore, simple spirometry has been recommended as a routine part of the preoperative evaluation in most patients.[31]

Every internist must be familiar with the patient who was noted by the nurse three days after a cholecystectomy to be "congested" and "slightly dusky". At that point the chest film often shows bilateral basal atelectasis. The preoperative chest radiograph and ECG had, of course, been normal but no spirogram was requested although the patient had smoked two packs of cigarettes a day for 30 years.

Obviously, the appropriate indications for a chest radiograph and a spirogram are not the same but I find it useful in talking to my surgical colleagues to suggest that whenever they request a preoperative chest film they should probably do spirometry as well. A spirogram is much more sensitive than a chest radiograph in detecting the type of disease likely to lead to postoperative complications.

REFERENCES

1. Hutchinson J: On the capacity of the lungs and on the respiratory functions with a view of establishing a precise and easy method of detecting disease by the spirometer. *Trans Med-Chir Soc London* 29:137–252, 1846.
2. Gardner RM, Baker CD, Broennle AM Jr, et al.: ATS statement. Snowbird workshop on standardization of spirometry. *Am Rev Respir Dis* 119:831–838, 1979.
3. Engel LA, Grassino A, Anthonisen NR: Demonstration of airway closure in man. *J Appl Physiol* 38:1117–1125, 1975.
4. Leith DE, Mead J: Mechanisms determining residual volume of the lungs. *J Appl Physiol* 23:221–227, 1967.
5. Mead J, Turner JM, Macklem PT, et al.: Significance of the relationship between lung recoil and maximum expiratory flow. *J Appl Physiol* 22:95–108, 1967.
6. Madison R, Mittman C, Afifi AA, et al.: Risk factors for obstructive lung disease. *Am Rev Respir Dis* 124:149–153, 1981.
7. Fletcher CM, Peto R: The natural history of chronic airflow obstruction. *Br Med J* 1:1645–1648, 1977.
8. Bates DV: The fate of the chronic bronchitic: A report of the ten-year follow-up in the Canadian Department of Veterans' Affairs coordinated study of chronic bronchitis. *Am Rev Respir Dis* 108:1043–1065, 1973.
9. Macklem PT, Mead J: Resistance of central and peripheral airways measured by a retrograde catheter. *J Appl Physiol* 22:395–401, 1967.
10. Hoppin FG Jr, Green M, et al.: Relationship of central and peripheral airway resistance to lung volume in dogs. *J Appl Physiol* 44:728–737, 1978.
11. McFadden ER Jr, Kiker R, Holmes B, et al.: Small airway disease. An assessment of the tests of peripheral airway function. *Am J Med* 57:171–182, 1974.
12. Gelb AF, Zamel N: Simplified diagnosis of small-airway obstruction. *N Engl J Med* 288:395–398, 1973.

13. McFadden ER Jr, Linden DA: A reduction in maximum mid-expiratory flow rate. A spirographic manifestation of small airway disease. *Am J Med* 52:725-737, 1972.

14. Morris JF, Koski A, Breese J: Normal values and evaluation of forced end-expiratory flow. *Am Rev Respir Dis* 111:755-762, 1975.

15. Kryger M, Bode F, Antic R, et al.: Diagnosis of obstruction of the upper and central airways. *Am J Med* 61:85-93, 1976.

16. Miller RD, Hyatt RE: Obstructing lesions of the larynx and trachea: clinical and physiological characteristics. *Mayo Clin Proc* 44:145-161, 1969.

17. Ingram RH Jr, Schilder DP: Effect of gas compression on pulmonary pressure, flow, and volume relationship. *J Appl Physiol* 21:1821-826, 1966.

18. Fallat RJ, Jewitt B, Bass M, et al.: Spirometry in amyotrophic lateral sclerosis. *Arch Neurol* 36:74-80, 1979.

19. Sanders MH, Martin RJ, Pennock BE, et al.: The detection of sleep apnea in the awake patient. The 'saw-tooth' sign. *JAMA* 245:2414-2418, 1981.

20. Black LF, Hyatt RE: Maximal static respiratory pressures in generalized neuromuscular disease. *Am Rev Respir Dis* 103:641-650, 1971.

21. Spiro SG, Hahn HL, Edwards RHT, et al: An analysis of the physiological strain of submaximal exercise in patients with chronic obstructive bronchitis. Thorax 30:415-425, 1975.

22. Boushey HA, Dawson A: *Pulmonary Function Testing: Guidelines and Controversies*, (Chap. 7), San Diego, Academic Press, 1982.

23. Kass I, Bell WB, Epler GE, et al.: Evaluation of impairment/disability secondary to respiratory disease. *Am Rev Respir Dis* 126:945-951, 1982.

24. Morris JF: Spirometry in the evaluation of pulmonary function. *West J Med* 125:110-118, 1976.

25. Kanner RE, Morris AH (ed): *Clinical Pulmonary Function Testing*. Salt Lake City, Intermountain Thoracic Society, 1975.

26. Crapo RO, Morris AH, Gardner RM: Reference spirometric values using techniques and equipment that meet ATS recommendations. *Am Rev Respir Dis* 123:659-664, 1981.

27. Knudson RJ, Slatin RC, Lebowitz MD, et al.: The maximal expiratory flow-volume curve: normal standards, variability and effects of age. *Am Rev Respir Dis* 113:587-600, 1976.

28. Olsen CR, Hale FC: A method for interpreting acute response to bronchodilators from the spirogram. *Am Rev Respir Dis* 98:301-303, 1968.

29. Sherter CB, Connolly JJ, Schilder DP: The significance of volume-adjusting the maximal midexpiratory flow in assessing the response to a bronchodilator drug. Chest 73:568-571, 1978.

30. Tisi GM: Preoperative evaluation of pulmonary function. Validity, indications, and benefits. *Am Rev Respir Dis* 119:293-310, 1979.

31. Belman MJ, Mittman C: Preoperative pulmonary function evaluation and postoperative respiratory care (correspondence). *Am Rev Respir Dis* 120:706-707, 1979.

Density-Dependence of Maximal Expiratory Flow

RONALD D. FAIRSHTER

HISTORIC DEVELOPMENT

Physiologists and clinicians have been interested for years in the effects of a low-density gas mixture, 80% helium–20% oxygen (HeO_2), upon maximal expiratory flow ($\dot{V}_E$Max).[1-12] In 1941, Dean et al. demonstrated that under conditions of turbulent flow, resistance in a dog lung preparation was reduced by breathing HeO_2.[1] In 1960, Grape and colleagues found that pulmonary resistance was reduced in emphysematous patients breathing HeO_2.[2] Schilder and associates found, in 1963, that $\dot{V}_E$Max varied inversely with gas density in normal subjects.[3]

In 1972, Despas and associates demonstrated that $\dot{V}_E$Max increased less in some subjects with airflow obstruction after breathing HeO_2 than in normal subjects.[4] These investigators suggested that inhalation of HeO_2 could be utilized to demonstrate the predominant site of flow limitation within the lung.[4] Hutcheon and colleagues [5] and Dosman and co-workers[6] expanded upon that concept by suggesting that comparison of pulmonary function tests breathing air and breathing HeO_2 could be used to recognize very early, subclinical obstructive lung disease. Subsequently, Ingram and colleagues studied changes in the density-dependence of $\dot{V}_E$Max (response to breathing HeO_2) before and after bronchodilator.[7] Since that time, a number of clinical and physiologic studies have evaluated the density dependence of $\dot{V}_E$Max.[8-11] Although the results of these studies have been consistent with previous concepts, Mink and associates[12] have recently questioned the interpretation of density-dependence data.

Analyses of density-dependence data are based upon theoretical concepts that are compatible with a large body of data regarding the sites and mechanisms of flow limitation in normal and diseased lungs.[4-11] However, conclusive validation of these theoretical concepts is lacking. This chapter discusses HeO_2 flow-volume studies in terms of generally accepted concepts.[4-11] As already indicated, these concepts have been challenged.[12] Clinical applications of HeO_2 flow-volume data will be limited until the controversies (discussed further in this chapter) are resolved.

METHODS

Density-dependence measurements are usually made from maximal expiratory flow volume (MEFV) curves: MEFV maneuvers obtained while breathing air and HeO_2 are superimposed and compared. Two parameters are usually derived from the superimposed curves: volume of isoflow ($Viso\dot{V}$) and the percent increase in $\dot{V}_E Max$ at 50% of vital capacity (VC) during HeO_2 breathing ($\Delta \dot{V}_E Max_{50}$) (Eq. 1).

The equipment needed for measurement of air and the HeO_2 MEFV curves includes (a) an HeO_2 source with appropriate valves and connections; (b) a physiologic recorder (oscilloscope, rapidly responding X-Y recorder, computer); and (c) a spirometer, pneumotachygraph, or volume displacement plethysmograph to measure flow and volume. The spirometer has the advantage of simplicity. The pneumotachygraph requires separate calibration for HeO_2 and may have linearity problems over a wide range of flow rates. The volume displacement plethysmograph has the advantage of negating artifacts due to gas compression during MEFV maneuvers.[13] However, this apparatus is relatively complex and is not used in most clinical laboratories. Furthermore, mouth flow from the plethysmograph is usually measured with a pneumotachygraph (HeO_2 calibration and linearity problems). In addition, Benatar et al. have compared $\Delta \dot{V}_E Max_{50}$ values obtained simultaneously with a volume displacement plethysomograph and a spirometer.[8] The differences in results were small, leading the authors to suggest that spirometric determinations of density dependence are usually sufficient. Although the volume displacement plethysmograph remains the gold standard, it appears that density dependence of $\dot{V}_E Max$ can usually be reliably determined using spirometric techniques.

PROCEDURE

At least three satisfactory MEFV curves should be obtained breathing air and breathing HeO_2. The volume history of the lung should be identical for each MEFV maneuver. Patients should breathe enough HeO_2 to replace 95% or more of the alveolar nitrogen with helium. In normal or minimally obstructed patients, this is usually accomplished by three VC inhalations of HeO_2.[5] In subjects with more advanced airflow obstruction, five to ten minutes of tidal breathing of HeO_2 may be required.

CALCULATIONS

Air and HeO_2 MEFV curves exhibiting best flow rates at 50% and 25% of VC are identified and superimposed.[9] The curves may be superimposed at TLC or RV.[6] In either case, both VCs should be within 2.5–5% of the largest VC recorded. The $\Delta\dot{V}_E Max_{50}$ value is calculated as

$$\Delta\dot{V}_E Max_{50} = \frac{\dot{V}_E Max_{50}\,(HeO_2) - \dot{V}_E Max_{50}\,(Air) \times 100}{\dot{V}_E Max_{50}\,(air)} \qquad \text{Eq. 1}$$

Volume of isoflow is identified as the point at which HeO_2 flow rates first become and remain equal to, or less than, air flow rates. The volume between that point and residual volume is measured and expressed as a percent of VC (Figure 3-1).

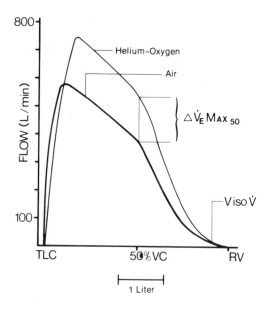

Figure 3-1. Maximal expiratory flow volume curves breathing air and helium in a normal person. The increment in flow at 50% of VC, calculated according to Equation 1 (see text), is $\Delta\dot{V}_E Max_{50}$. Volume of isoflow is also indicated.

PATHOPHYSIOLOGIC RATIONALE

In a system of converging tubes, flow is density dependent when the flow regime is turbulent (Reynolds numbers > 2000), or when pressure losses due to convective acceleration are high.[4-6] When the flow regime is fully developed laminar, pressure losses are due to viscosity and flow is independent of density.[4-6] In the lung, the mechanical and geometric characteristics of the peripheral and central airways differ; hence, the flow profile also changes between the peripheral and central airways. Ordinarily, flow is predominantly laminar in the peripheral airways and turbulent in the central airways.

In the normal human lung, flow is density dependent at high lung volumes.[3] At low lung volumes (< 25% of VC), density dependence is reduced or absent.[3,5] In some persons with obstruction to airflow, density dependence is reduced well above 25% of VC.[4,5] These observations are usually interpreted within the context of the prevailing theories of expiratory flow limitation in the lung:[14-16] at some flow-limiting segment of the airway (choke point), the local flow velocity equals the local speed of propagation of pressure pulse waves (wave speed). Because the velocity of flow cannot exceed the local wave speed, excess pressure is dissipated downstream (toward the mouth) from the choke point. The actual $\dot{V}_E$Max attained for any gas is thought to be a function of the cross-sectional area and compliance of the airway at the choke point (CP), lung elastic recoil (Pel), and lateral pressure losses within airways upstream (toward the alveoli) from the choke point.[14-16] The density dependence of $\dot{V}_E$Max (at any given lung volume) is generally thought to reflect the predominant flow regime upstream from the flow-limiting segment (choke point); that is, the amount of density dependence is probably determined by the relative proportions of density-dependent and density-independent pressure losses during maximal expiratory flow.[17]

In normal individuals, CP are located in the large airways during much of the forced vital capacity (FVC). Due to the small total cross-sectional area of the large airways, flow is turbulent in this segment of the bronchial tree. Furthermore, large convective pressure losses also occur in the central airways. Accordingly, flow is density dependent in normal persons for most (approximately 75%) of the expired FVC. At lower lung volumes (below approximately 25% of FVC), CP move to the periphery of the lung. Due to the large total cross-sectional area of the peripheral always, laminar flow regimes predominate, viscous pressure losses are important, and density dependence of flow is reduced or absent.

In some individuals with airflow obstruction, there is an accelerated drop in lateral airway pressure due to reduced Pel, increased peripheral airways resistance, or both; CP are displaced peripherally at higher than normal lung volumes and density dependence of $\dot{V}_E$Max is reduced. Accordingly, high Viso$\dot{V}$ or low $\Delta\dot{V}_E$Max$_{50}$ values (both of which indicate reduced density dependence) suggest an accelerated pressure drop within the airways and peripheral displacement of CP. In the case of $Viso\dot{V}$, the accelerated drop in lateral airway pressure is thought to be due to loss of Pel or increased peripheral airways resistance (R_P).[6] Hence, abnormally high $Viso\dot{V}$ values are consistent with both emphysema and peripheral airways obstruction. On the other hand, available evidence suggests that Pel is not an important determinant of $\Delta\dot{V}_E Max_{50}$.[6] Therefore, Dosman and associates have suggested that low $\Delta\dot{V}_E Max_{50}$ results are relatively specific for peripheral airways obstruction.[6]

Ingram and McFadden and associates have investigated changes in density dependence of $\dot{V}_E Max$ before and after bronchodilator administration.[7] Because these investigators found the same patterns of response at all lung volumes below 50% of VC, their principles are discussed in terms of $\dot{V}_E Max_{50}$. Ingram et al. suggested that the resistance upstream from the flow-limiting segment is actually composed of a large and a peripheral airways resistance in series ($R = R_L + R_P$). If a bronchodilator reduces R_P proportionately more than R_L, $\dot{V}_E Max$ will increase and R_P/R_L will decrease (R_P/R_L post $<$ R_P/R_L pre). Accordingly, compared to the prebronchodilator situation, a larger percentage of the pressure drop during postbronchodilator $\dot{V}_E Max$ would occur in large airways (turbulence, convective acceleration) and $\Delta\dot{V}_E Max_{50}$ would increase. If a bronchodilator reduces R_L proportionately more than R_P, $\dot{V}_E Max$ will increase and R_P/R_L will increase (R_P/R_L post $>$ R_P/R_L pre). Therefore, a larger percentage of the pressure losses during postbronchodilator $\dot{V}_E Max$ would occur in peripheral airways (high viscous resistance) and $\Delta\dot{V}_E Max_{50}$ would decrease. If a bronchodilator reduces R_P and R_L proportionately equally, then $\dot{V}_E Max$ will increase without changing R_P/R_L. Therefore, $\Delta\dot{V}_E Max_{50}$ will be unchanged from the prebronchodilator value.[7]

Interpretation of bronchodilator-induced changes in $\Delta\dot{V}_E Max_{50}$ are summarized in Table 3-1.

Table 3-1   Interpretation of Changes in $\dot{V}_E Max$ and $\Delta\dot{V}_E Max_{50}$ after Bronchodilators

$\dot{V}_E Max$*	$\Delta\dot{V}_E Max_{50}$*	Interpretation
Increased	Increased	Predominant peripheral airways bronchodilatation.
Increased	Decreased	Predominant central airways bronchodilatation.
Increased	Unchanged	Proportionately equal peripheral and central airways bronchodilatation.

*Compared to prebronchodilator values.

INDICATIONS

Possible indications for density-dependence measurements include early detection of peripheral airways disease (small airways obstruction); detection of the predominant site of flow limitation and/or bronchodilatation; and research. Several studies have suggested that measurement of $Viso\dot{V}$ and $\Delta\dot{V}_EMax_{50}$ are more sensitive than other physiologic methods of detecting early obstructive lung disease.[5,6,18] Volume of isoflow is generally considered the most sensitive test for peripheral airways obstruction.[5,6,18] The phenomena that lead to reduced density dependence also lower expiratory flow rates; however, $Viso\dot{V}$ and $\Delta\dot{V}_EMax_{50}$ often become abnormal at an earlier stage than $\dot{V}_EMax$. Unfortunately, there is no concrete evidence that early detection has any prognostic implications regarding the development of fixed irreversible airflow obstruction.[19] Therefore, the clinical value of an abnormal HeO_2 MEFV curve is uncertain. Density-dependence measurements are usually not recommended as screening tests in smoking populations.

HeO_2 MEFV curves may detect the predominant site of airflow limitation in patients with all stages of airflow obstruction. Such studies have been utilized in subjects with asthma and chronic airflow obstruction (CAO) to investigate the relationship between severity of disease, predominant site of airflow obstruction, and predominant site of bronchodilatation.[10,11,20] Although such data are useful in understanding the natural history of the diseases, differences in sites of flow limitation or sites of bronchodilatation do not, at this time, imply differences in therapy.

HeO_2 flow volume maneuvers are widely used for research purposes. It is possible that research may establish clinical indications for HeO_2 MEFV tests.

EXAMPLES

Case 1

An asymptomatic 30-year-old man has a history of smoking $1\frac{1}{2}$ packs of cigarettes daily since the age of 19 years. The patient is referred for pulmonary function tests as shown in Table 3-2.

Interpretation and discussion.   The only abnormal result is $Viso\dot{V}$; $Viso\dot{V}$ is higher than predicted.[6] The $\Delta\dot{V}_EMax_{50}$ is within the lower range of the predicted values.[6] Volume of isoflow is the most common pulmonary function abnormality in asymptomatic smokers.[5,6] Although $\Delta\dot{V}_EMax_{50}$ was within the predicted range for this individual, the value of 26% may represent a decrease from the patient's baseline (presmoking) value. Serial pulmonary function tests,

Table 3-2 Case 1

	Observed	Predicted
FEV$_1$ (liter)	3.6	3.9
FEV$_1$/FVC %	76.0	80.0
FEF$_{25-75\%}$(liter/sec)	3.4	4.3
FVC (liter)	4.8	4.7
R$_{aw}$ (cm/liter/sec)	2.2	< 3.1
FRC (liter)	2.7	2.6
RV (liter)	1.6	1.4
TLC (liter)	6.4	6.1
DL$_{CO}$SB (ml/min/mm Hg)	26.0	27.0
CV/VC%	8.0	< 10.6
$\Delta\dot{V}_E$Max$_{50}$ (%)	26.0	> 20.0
VisoV	33.0	< 27.4

when available, facilitate the evaluation of individual test results. The high Viso$\dot{V}$ result is consistent with subclinical emphysema or peripheral airway obstruction; however, the latter diagnosis is more likely because TLC and DL$_{CO}$SB are normal.[21]

CASE 2

A 66-year-old woman with a 50-year history of cigarette smoking and severe dyspnea with minimal exertion is referred for pulmonary function tests as shown in Table 3-3.

Table 3-3 Case 2

	Observed		Predicted
	PreBronchodilator	PostBronchodilator	
FEV$_1$ (liter)	0.76	1.10	1.9
FEV$_1$/FVC%	29.0	34.0	73.0
FVC (liter)	2.6	3.2	2.6
R$_{aw}$ (cm/liter/sec)	7.8	5.6	< 2.8
FRC (liter)	4.8	4.2	2.5
RV (liter)	3.7	2.9	1.8
TLC (liter)	6.3	6.1	4.4
DL$_{CO}$SB (ml/min/mm Hg)	8.0	—	21.0
$\dot{V}_E$Max$_{50}$ (liter/sec)	0.3	0.5	2.4
$\Delta\dot{V}_E$Max$_{50}$ (%)	0.	35.0%	> 20.0

Interpretation and discussion.   Prior to bronchodilator administration, the absence of density dependence suggests a predominantly peripheral site of airflow limitation. Low $\Delta\dot{V}_E Max_{50}$ values do not exclude central airways obstruction; in fact, it is likely that central airways obstruction is present in this severely obstructed patient. However, the absence of density dependence suggests that peripheral airways obstruction is predominant and is limiting flow.

Following inhalation of the bronchodilator, both flow rates and $\Delta\dot{V}_E Max_{50}$ increase. These results suggest that bronchodilatation has occurred predominantly in peripheral airways. Previous data from patients with chronic airflow obstruction suggests an inverse relationship between initial $\Delta\dot{V}_E Max_{50}$ and the change in $\Delta\dot{V}_E Max_{50}$ caused by bronchodilators (high prebronchodilator values of $\Delta\dot{V}_E Max_{50}$ decrease after bronchodilator; low prebronchodilator $\Delta\dot{V}_E Max_{50}$ values increase after bronchodilator).[11,20]

CASE 3

A 22-year-old woman with a 14-year history of asthma is referred for pulmonary function tests as shown in Table 3-4.

Interpretation and discussion.   Prior to bronchodilator administration, the high $\Delta\dot{V}_E Max_{50}$ suggests a predominantly central site of airflow limitation. The pressure losses are apparently primarily turbulent and convective. Following the bronchodilator, the increase in $\dot{V}_E Max$ and reduction in $\Delta\dot{V}_E Max_{50}$ are compatible with predominant large airway bronchodilatation. The relationship between initial $\Delta\dot{V}_E Max_{50}$ and change in $\Delta\dot{V}_E Max_{50}$ after bronchodilators is inverse in asthma[10] as well as in chronic airflow obstruction.[11,19]

Table 3-4   Case 3

| | Observed | | |
	PreBronchodilator	PostBronchodilator	Predicted
FEV_1 (liter)	2.6	3.2	3.0
$FEV_1/FVC\%$	70.0	80.0	83.0
FVC (liter)	3.7	4.0	3.6
R_{aw} (cm/liter/sec)	4.7	2.1	< 2.2
FRC (liter)	3.4	2.9	2.5
RV (liter)	2.2	1.7	1.7
TLC (liter)	5.9	5.7	5.3
$DL_{CO}SB$ (ml/min/mm Hg)	29.0	—	28.0
$\dot{V}_E Max_{50}$ (liter/sec)	2.3	3.2	3.8
$\Delta\dot{V}_E Max_{50}$ (%)	56.0	41.0	> 20.0

CASE 4

A 27-year-old asthmatic male is referred for pulmonary function tests as shown in Table 3-5.

Interpretation and discussion. Prior to inhalation of the bronchodilator, $\Delta\dot{V}_E Max_{50}$ is within the range of values predicted for normal individuals. This result (as well as the Viso$\dot{V}$ of 19%) indicates that airflow limitation was predominantly central. Following the bronchodilator, $\dot{V}_E Max$ increases but $\Delta\dot{V}_E Max_{50}$ changes very little, suggesting proportionately equal large and peripheral airways bronchodilatation.

ARTIFACTS

(1) Size of vital capacities breathing air and HeO_2. As previously noted, air and HeO_2 MEFV maneuvers chosen for comparison should both be within 5% (preferably 2.5%) of the largest VC recorded.

(2) Superimposition at RV or TLC. In the literature, air and HeO_2 MEFV curves have been superimposed both at RV and at TLC. Selection of very similarly sized air and HeO_2 VCs minimizes the problem of where to superimpose the curves. Mean values of Viso$\dot{V}$ were the same for a group of subjects compared by matching air and HeO_2 maneuvers at RV and at TLC (R. Fairshter, unpublished observations).

(3) Distribution effects. Incomplete replacement of alveolar nitrogen (N_2) with HeO_2 will reduce the apparent density dependence of $\dot{V}_E Max$. Subjects with

Table 3-5 Case 4

| | Observed | | Predicted |
	PreBronchodilator	PostBronchodilator	
FEV_1	1.8	2.5	3.3
$FEV_1/FVC\%$	47.0	58.0	80.0
FVC (liter)	3.8	4.3	4.1
R_{aw} (cm/liter/sec)	5.2	3.2	< 2.8
FRC (liter)	2.9	2.6	2.2
RV (liter)	1.9	1.4	1.1
TLC (liter)	5.7	5.7	5.2
$DL_{CO}SB$ (ml/min/mm Hg)	29.0	—	29.0
$\dot{V}_E Max_{50}$	1.0	1.5	4.3
$\Delta\dot{V}_E Max_{50}$ (%)	33.0	36.0	> 20.0
Viso$\dot{V}$ (% VC)	19.0	10.0	> 26.5

maldistribution of ventilation and/or high residual volume require longer periods of breathing HeO_2 in order to replace 95% of the alveolar N_2 with helium.[5] Because maldistribution of ventilation and/or enlarged residual volume are often present in smokers, early detection of airways disease is facilitated by determining Viso$\dot{V}$ after one breath of HeO_2.[9] Otherwise, HeO_2 MEFV maneuvers should be obtained after breathing helium long enough to replace at least 95% of the alveolar N_2.

(4)   Lung volume changes after bronchodilators. In some individuals, large reductions in TLC occur postbronchodilator. Flow rates are usually compared isovolumetrically in these subjects (at the same absolute lung volume prebronchodilator and postbronchodilator). Similarly, $\Delta\dot{V}_E Max_{50}$ values are usually determined in bronchodilator studies at the same absolute lung volume prebronchodilator and postbronchodilator.[7] If large volume changes preclude isovolumetric comparisons at 50% of VC, density dependence may be compared at lower lung volumes.[7]

CONTROVERSIES

(1)   Although measurements of Viso$\dot{V}$ are generally considered the most sensitive physiologic tests for detection of early obstructive airways disease,[5,6,18] Lam and associates have recently suggested that HeO_2 MEFV maneuvers studies may actually not be very sensitive at detecting early obstructive lung disease.[22] Lam et al. explain the apparent lack of sensitivity of Viso$\dot{V}$ and $\Delta\dot{V}_E Max_{50}$ in their subjects on the basis of high coefficients of variation. Berend and colleagues have also found Viso$\dot{V}$ and $\Delta\dot{V}_E Max_{50}$ to be highly variable.[23]

(2)   Although current information suggests that Pel is a relatively important determinant of Viso$\dot{V}$ but not $\Delta\dot{V}_E Max_{50}$,[6] there are some patients in whom Viso$\dot{V}$ occurs exactly at 50% of VC. In these individuals, it is difficult to understand how Pel could be an important determinant of Viso$\dot{V}$ but not $\Delta\dot{V}_E Max_{50}$.

(3)   Although density-dependence data are often used to evaluate peripheral or central airways flow limitation, interpretation of results without knowledge of baseline data (which are usually not available) may be misleading. For example, the patient in case 4, ($\Delta\dot{V}_E Max_{50}$–33%, Viso$\dot{V}$–19%) has predominantly central flow limitation. Yet, if this patient's $\Delta\dot{V}_E Max_{50}$ and Viso$\dot{V}$ were 50% and 10% prior to the onset of asthma, it would be reasonable to suggest that asthma caused increased peripheral resistance in this individual even though flow limitation remained predominantly central. Density-dependence studies reflect the relative contributions of viscous, convective, and turbulent pressure losses. Predominant flow limitation in one segment of the airway does not exclude obstruction at another level of the airway.

(4)   Analyses of density dependence have generally assumed similar air-

way geometries during air and HeO_2 maximal expiratory flow. Recently, Mink and associates used retrograde catheter techniques to investigate the density dependence of resistance during $\dot{V}_E Max$.[12] In most cases, they found that CP were similarly located during air and HeO_2 maximal expiratory flow, but that airway geometry upstream from CP was different on the two gases. Furthermore, Mink et al. suggested that viscous pressure losses are not necessarily limited to the peripheral airways and that reduced density dependence does not specifically distinguish between central and peripheral obstruction.[12] Knudson has also indicated that density-dependence measurements are of questionable value for detecting peripheral airways dysfunction.[24]

REFERENCES

1. Dean RB, Visscher MB: Kinetics of lung ventilation; evaluation of viscous and elastic resistance to lung ventilation with particular reference to effects of turbulence and therapeutic use of helium. *Am J Physiol* 134:450–468, 1941.
2. Grape B, Channin E, Tyler JM: The effect of helium and oxygen mixtures on pulmonary resistance in emphysema. *Am Rev Respir Dis* 81:823–829, 1960.
3. Schilder DP, Roberts A, Fry DL: Effect of gas density and viscosity on the maximal expiratory flow volume relationships. *J Clin Invest* 42:1705–1713, 1963.
4. Despas PJ, Leroux M, Macklem PT: Site of airway obstruction in asthma as determined by measuring maximal expiratory flow breathing air and a helium-oxygen mixture. *J Clin Invest* 51:3235–3243, 1972.
5. Hutcheon M, Griffin P, Levinson H, et al.: Volume of isoflow. A new test in detection of mild abnormalities of lung mechanics. *Am Rev Respir Dis* 110:458–465, 1974.
6. Dosman J, Bode F, Urbanetti J, et al.: The use of a helium-oxygen mixture during maximum expiratory flow to demonstrate obstruction in small airways in smokers. *J Clin Invest* 55:1090–1099, 1975.
7. Ingram RH Jr, Wellmann JJ, McFadden ER Jr, et al.: Relative contributions of large and small airways to flow limitation in normal subjects before and after atropine and isoproterenol. *J Clin Invest* 59:696–703, 1977.
8. Benatar SR, Clark TJH, Cochrane GM: Clinical relevance of the flow rate response to low density gas breathing in asthmatics. *Am Rev Respir Dis* 111:126–134, 1975.
9. Fairshter RD, Wilson AF: Volume of isoflow: effect of distribution of ventilation. *J Appl Physiol* 43:807–811, 1977
10. Fairshter RD, Wilson AF: Relationship between the site of airflow limitation and localization of the bronchodilator response in asthma. *Am Rev Respir Dis* 122:27–32, 1980.
11. Meadows JA III, Rodarte JR, Hyatt RE: Density-dependence of maximal expiratory flow in chronic obstructive pulmonary disease. *Am Rev Respir Dis* 121:47–53, 1980.
12. Mink S, Ziesmann M, Wood LDH: Mechanisms of increased maximum expiratory flow during He-O_2 breathing in dogs. *J Appl Physiol* 47:490–502, 1970.

13. Ingram RH Jr, Schilder DP: Effect of thoracic gas compression on the flow-volume curve of the forced vital capacity. *Am Rev Respir Dis* 94:56–63, 1966.
14. Mead J, Turner JM, Macklem PT, et al.: Significance of the relationship between lung recoil and maximum expiratory flow. *J Appl Physiol* 22:95–108, 1967.
15. Pride NB, Permutt S, Riley RL, et al.: Determinants of maximal expiratory flow from the lung. *J Appl Physiol* 22:95–108, 1967.
16. Dawson SV, Elliott EA: Wave speed limitation on expiratory flow—a unifying concept. *J Appl Physiol* 43:498–515, 1977.
17. Castile RG, Hyatt RE, Rodarte JR: Determinants of maximal expiratory flow and density-dependence in normal humans. *J Appl Physiol* 49:897–904, 1980
18. Gelb AF, Molony PA, Klein E, et al.: Sensitivity of volume of isoflow in the detection of mild airway obstruction. *Am Rev Respir Dis* 112:401–405, 1975.
19. Macklem PT: Workshop on screening programs for early diagnosis of airway limitation and severity of chronic airflow obstruction. *Am Rev Respir Dis* 109:567–571, 1974.
20. Fairshter RD, Wilson AF: Relationship between sites of airflow limitation and severity of chronic airflow obstruction. *Am Rev Respir Dis* 123:3–7, 1981.
21. Gelb AF, Gold WM, Wright RR, et al.: Physiologic diagnosis of subclinical emphysema. *Am Rev Respir Dis* 107:50–63, 1973.
22. Lam S, Abboud RT, Chan-Yeung M, et al.: Use of maximal expiratory flow-volume curves with air and helium-oxygen in the detection of ventilatory abnormalities in population surveys. *Am Rev Respir Dis* 123:234–237, 1981.
23. Berend N, Nelson NA, Rutland H, et al.: The maximum expiratory flow-volume curve with air and a low-density gas. *Chest* 80:23–30, 1981.
24. Knudson RJ, Schroter: A consideration of density-dependence of maximum expiratory flow. *Respir Physiol* 52:125–136, 1983.

CHAPTER 4

Response to Bronchodilators

RONALD D. FAIRSHTER

HISTORIC DEVELOPMENT

A detailed history of the use of bronchodilators is provided in the review by Paterson and colleagues.[1] Briefly, ephedrine-containing plants were used by the Chinese 5000 years ago. Antimuscarinic compounds have been used to treat asthma for at least several centuries. On the other hand, epinephrine and theophylline were first used as bronchodilators in the 20th century,[1-3] and, syntheses of relatively selective beta-2 adrenergic agonists are comparatively recent events.

METHODS

The laboratory response to bronchodilators is assessed by performing pulmonary function tests before and after administration of a bronchodilator. Although physiologic testing can be done using any bronchodilator, the studies are usually performed using inhaled sympathomimetic amines such as isoproterenol or metaproterenol. The inhaled sympathomimetics have the advantages of rapid onset of action and, in some cases, short duration of action (isoproterenol). The bronchodilator can be inhaled from metered-dose, freon-propelled cannisters, rubber-bulb–type nebulizers, or compressed-air–powered nebulizers.

The timing of the postbronchodilator tests should coincide with the time of peak response to the drug (5 to 30 minutes postinhalation with isoproterenol and 10 to 45 minutes with metaproterenol).[4,5] Controversial issues relating to bronchodilator testing include (1) dosage; (2) pattern of inhalation of the drug; (3) use of spacer devices; (4) tests utilized; and, (5) criteria for a significant response.

PULMONARY FUNCTION TESTING
INDICATIONS AND INTERPRETATIONS

DOSAGE

The dose of inhaled bronchodilator given for bronchodilator testing is usually the same as the recommended therapeutic dose. However, Williams and Kane suggested that 0.02 mg of inhaled isoproterenol (25% of the usual dose) was the fully effective dose.[6] On the other hand, there are data suggesting that higher doses of bronchodilators facilitate identification of significant responses.[7-9] Popa and Werner, in fact, found no limit of bronchodilator responsiveness in subjects given 0.65 to 2.60 mg of metaproterenol sulfate (half to double the usual dose).[8]

PATTERN OF INHALATION

Shim and Williams have suggested that many patients do not inhale their nebulized bronchodilator medications correctly;[10] other investigators have reached the same conclusion.[11] Yet, the best method to inhale nebulized bronchodilators remains unclear.[12] Shim and Williams teach their patients to initiate inhalation from residual volume, inhale deeply (presumably to total lung capacity [TLC]), hold their breath for a few seconds, and then exhale.[10] On the other hand, Riley and associates found that bronchodilator responses were better when the medications were inhaled at high rather than low lung volumes.[13,14] However, Riley's methodology required a very slow, relatively constant flow rate throughout inspiration.[13,14] This pattern of breathing is probably different from that utilized by most patients. Hence, Riley's data may not apply to most clinical situations. Although there are theoretical reasons favoring initiation of bronchodilator inhalation from higher lung volumes (such as functional residual capacity [FRC]),[12-14] additional data are needed to establish the validity of these theoretical concepts. In our laboratory, bronchodilator inhalation is initiated during a slow inspiration between FRC and TLC.[15] This is consistent with recommendations by Dolovich et al.[16] Those investigators recently suggested that maximum airway delivery of aerosol from metered dose inhalers could be achieved by holding the inhaler approximately 4 cm from the wide open mouth, inhaling very slowly from FRC, and breath-holding for ten seconds at TLC.[16]

USE OF SPACER DEVICES

Delivery of bronchodilators from metered-dose inhalers can also be modified by placing a spacer (chamber) between the lips and the orifice of the inhaler. Theoretically, by suspending the drug in the chamber, improved delivery of bronchodilator might result.[17] In particular, the need for good hand–lung coordination for activating the device and simultaneously inhaling would be reduced. Although the expectation of improved drug delivery was confirmed in some studies,[18,19] Epstein and associates recently found in asthmatics that bronchodilator responsiveness was not improved by the use of a spacer.[17] Currently, it appears that spacer devices would be advantageous for patients with poor hand–lung coordination or other handicaps that limit the use of metered-dose inhalers. Further study will presumably clarify the role of spacer devices in nonphysically handicapped patients with obstructive airways disease.

PHYSIOLOGIC TESTS

Significant bronchodilator responses can be detected using a variety of pulmonary function maneuvers. In practice, measurements of forced expiratory flow (FEF) with a spirometer are usually utilized; however, plethysmographic measurements of lung volumes and specific conductance (SGAW) provide additional useful data. Some studies have indicated that bronchodilator responsiveness is best assessed by measurements of SGAW.[7,8] On the other hand, in other studies, measurements of FEF (especially FEV_1) have been considered the best indices of bronchodilatation.[20,21] At this time, there is a lack of unanimity regarding the best physiologic method for detecting bronchodilatation. It has been recommended that significant improvement on at least two of three spirometric parameters (FEV_1, $FEF_{25-75\%}$ FVC) is indicative of "reversibility";[22] however, as previously noted,[15] data substantiating this recommendation were not published. Concordance between FEV_1 and $FEF_{25-75\%}$ measurements [23] would be another problem with the recommendation.

CRITERIA FOR A SIGNIFICANT RESPONSE

Response to bronchodilators may be quantitated as absolute changes, changes as a percentage of the predicted or maximum possible value for a particular variable, or as a percentage change from the prebronchodilator value. Because the latter method is most sensitive, percentage of change from baseline (prebronchodilator value) is usually used to quantitate bronchodilator responses. It has been recommended that a 15–25% improvement from baseline can be considered slight reversibility whereas 25–50% changes and greater than 50% changes constitute moderate and marked reversibility (for FEV_1, $FEF_{25-75\%}$, or FVC).[22]

Lorber and colleagues defined levels of pulmonary function above which no mean change occurred following inhalation of isoproterenol by normal subjects (zero mean change group).[21] Because there was no mean change after isoprotenenol, the individual changes can be considered variability or noise in the measurement. Lorber and associates suggested that for a given test improvements larger than those observed in 95% of the individual subjects from the zero mean change group were significant.[17] Using their criteria for a significant bronchodilator response (7.7%, 10.7%, and 20.2% change from baseline for FEV_1, FVC, and $\dot{V}_E Max_{x50}$), a high percentage of a group of potential bronchodilator responders did show significant improvements in pulmonary function after inhalation of isoproterenol.[21]

We studied 40 normal subjects before and after inhalation of isoproterenol or metaproterenol.[7] Our study differed from Lorber's because we did not define a zero mean change group (mean results improved postbronchodilator). Thus, the postbronchodilator results in our study were determined both by variability and by true physiologic changes. Ninety-five percent of our normal subjects had percent improvements from baseline $\leq 23\%$ for FEV_1 and $\leq 39\%$ for $\dot{V}_EMax_{50}$. Bronchodilator responses exceeding these limits could be considered significant.

Based upon a review of available literature as well as clinical experience, Ries recommended the following criteria for a significant expiratory flow rate response to bronchodilator administration:[15] (1) a percentage increase in FEV_1 $\geq 15\%$ accompanied by an absolute FEV_1 response ≥ 200 ml; (2) a percentage increase in $FEF_{25-75\%}$ or $\dot{V}_EMax_{50} \geq 20\%$; and (3) a percentage increase in isovolumetrically measured (see section on artifacts) $FEF_{25-75\%}$ or $\dot{V}_EMax_{50} \geq 30\%$. There have been multiple studies of bronchodilator responsiveness. Nevertheless, there are no uniformly accepted criteria for a significant response.[15] The criteria noted previously can be utilized;[7,15,21] however, a 15–20% improvement in FEV_1 may well be the most commonly utilized criterion for a significant response. Because the amount of improvement in normal subjects varies for different physiologic tests,[7,15,21] criteria for a significant response for a particular maneuver will not necessarily be valid for another test method.

PATHOPHYSIOLOGIC RATIONALE

At lung volumes below 70% of TLC, $\dot{V}_EMax$ for a particular gas is a function of the cross-sectional area and compliance of the airways at the flow-limiting segment (choke point [CP]), lung elastic recoil (Pel), and lateral pressure losses in airways between the alveoli and the choke point.[24-26] In many patients, lateral pressure losses are increased due to abnormally high airway resistance upstream (toward the alveoli) from the choke point; as a result, flow is limited at lower than normal values. In diseases such as asthma and chronic obstructive bronchitis, bronchospasm (increased smooth muscle tone) is often a major cause of the increased airway resistance. Although the mechanism(s) of increased bronchial smooth muscle tone are complex and incompletely understood, administration of drugs that ameliorate bronchospasm usually increases $\dot{V}_EMax$ and benefits the patient.

Measurement of pulmonary function tests before and after bronchodilators provides an objective means of assessing the reversibility of airflow obstruction and the potential benefits of bronchodilators. Although $\dot{V}_EMax$ may be reduced by factors other than bronchospasm, a rapid improvement in $\dot{V}_EMax$, airways resistance, or lung volumes following bronchodilator administration is considered evidence of a reduction in smooth muscle tone and an increase in airway caliber. Bronchodilators may also alter the pressure—volume characteristics of the lungs.[27-30] However, the effects of the drugs ordinarily used to evaluate bronchodilator responsiveness (sympathomimetics) on lung recoil have been small and/or inconsistent.[27-30] Therefore, alterations in lung elastic recoil are usually not considered in the routine evaluation of bronchodilator responsiveness.

Current evidence suggests that most bronchodilator agents are capable of dilating both central and peripheral airways.[30,31] Sites of action of bronchodilators are often investigated by comparing flow rates and density dependence before and after administration of the drug.[7,30,31] Although this type of testing gives information relative to the site of bronchodilator action, there is no current evidence that HeO_2 pulmonary function tests are more sensitive than other physiologic maneuvers in detecting significant bronchodilator responses.[7]

Although a significant bronchodilator response documents reversibility, the absence of a significant response does not exclude reversibility because: (1) some patients are relatively refractory to bronchodilator therapy in the early phases of an acute asthmatic attack.[32] Days of therapy may be required before significant bronchodilator responsiveness is evident;[32] (2) a bronchodilator response may be present on tests other than those utilized; (3) the bronchodilator drug may be delivered improperly; (4) in some patients, $\dot{V}_E$Max may be limited by mechanisms (such as collapse of central airways)[33] which are not bronchodilator responsive. Because these mechanisms of flow limitation may not be important at submaximal flow rates, it is still possible that bronchodilator responsiveness would be present during tidal breathing. For these reasons, it is currently recommended that a trial of bronchodilator therapy may be indicated in patients with airflow obstruction despite the absence of laboratory evidence of a significant bronchodilator response.[15,22]

INDICATIONS

Indications for bronchodilator testing include the following:

1. Assessment of the physiologic response to bronchodilator.

2. Assessment of the need for additional medication. Patients are generally tested for bronchodilator responsiveness after withholding regularly prescribed bronchodilators for 6 to 12 hours or longer. However, the potential benefits of additional medication may be evaluated by performing prebronchodilator and postbronchodilator studies without stopping the regularly scheduled medications.

3. Diagnosis of asthma. Pulmonary function tests including tests of bronchodilator responsiveness may be helpful in differentiating asthma from other types of airflow obstruction.

4.   Localization of the predominant site of bronchodilatation. Performance of pre and postbronchodilator maximal expiratory flow-volume maneuvers using air and HeO_2 mixtures may be helpful for localizing the major site of bronchodilator response.[8,30,31] These maneuvers are used frequently for research investigations. Currently, however, there are no established clinical indications for prebronchodilator and postbronchodilator HeO_2 flow-volume measurements.

EXAMPLES

CASE 1

A 34-year-old asthmatic is referred for pulmonary function tests as shown in Table 4-1.

Interpretation and discussion.   Following bronchodilator administration, a 43% increase is noted in FEV_1 compared to the baseline value. Other pulmonary function tests, including $FEF_{25-75\%}$ and R_{aw}, also show substantial improvement; these studies demonstrate significant reversibility of airflow obstruction following bronchodilator inhalation.

CASE 2

A 48-year-old man with a 50-pack-year smoking history is referred for pulmonary function tests. The patient is dyspneic and complains of wheezing. Tests are depicted in Table 4-2.

Interpretation and discussion.   The pulmonary function tests document substantial airflow obstruction with modest reversibility. The $DL_{CO}SB$ is also

Table 4-1   Case 1

| | Observed | | |
	Prebronchodilator	Postbronchodilator	Predicted
FEV_1 (liter)	2.1	3.0	2.6
FVC (liter)	3.6	3.9	3.2
$FEV_1/FVC\%$	58.0	77.0	81.0
$FEF_{25-75\%}$ (liter/sec)	1.5	2.9	3.3
R_{aw} (cm/liter/sec)	4.3	1.3	<2.7
FRC (liter)	2.8	2.2	2.5
RV (liter)	1.7	1.4	1.5
TLC (liter)	5.3	5.3	4.7
$DL_{CO}SB$	33.0	—	25.6
(ml/min/mm Hg)			

Table 4-2 Case 2

| | Observed | | |
	Prebronchodilator	Postbronchodilator	Predicted
FEV_1 (liter)	2.0	2.3	3.9
FVC (liter)	4.7	5.0	5.2
$FEV_1/FVC\%$	43.0	46.0	75.0
$FEF_{25-75\%}$ (liter/sec)	1.2	1.3	4.0
R_{aw} (cm/liter/sec)	5.8	4.7	<2.4
FRC (liter)	4.2	3.8	3.1
RV (liter)	3.2	2.6	1.9
TLC (liter)	7.9	7.6	7.1
$DL_{CO}SB$ (ml/min/mm Hg)	17.0	—	33.0

reduced. These results are consistent with chronic airflow obstruction (chronic obstructive bronchitis and emphysema) rather than with asthma. Differential features are the relatively weak response to bronchodilator and the reduced $DL_{CO}SB$, neither of which are characteristic of asthma.

CASE 3

A 62-year-old man with a long history of chronic airflow obstruction secondary to cigarette smoking is referred for pulmonary function tests as shown in Table 4-3.

Interpretation and Discussion

There is no significant flow rate response to bronchodilator. The increase in FEV_1 of 0.1 liter is within the range of variability of the method.[21] However,

Table 4-3 Case 3

| | Observed | | |
	Prebronchodilator	Postbronchodilator	Predicted
FEV_1 (liter)	0.8	0.9	2.9
FVC (liter)	2.5	3.2	4.2
$FEV_1/FVC\%$	32.0	28.0	69.0
R_{aw} (cm/liter/sec)	7.8	5.6	<2.0
FRC (liter)	4.4	3.8	2.7
RV (liter)	5.5	4.9	1.8
TLC (liter)	8.0	8.1	6.0
$DL_{CO}SB$ (ml/min/mm Hg)	8.0	—	27.0

because of the low baseline FEV_1, the 0.1 liter change represents a 12.5% increase from baseline. This patient's small absolute increment in FEV_1 is actually reasonably close on a percentage basis to values considered to be significant (15–20% change from baseline). This example illustrates a problem with analyses of bronchodilator responsiveness as a percent change from baseline; small absolute changes indistinguishable from variability may represent relatively large percentage changes if baseline values are very low. This example also illustrates that analysis of parameters besides FEV_1 can be helpful. The 28% increment in FVC is a significant bronchodilator response.

CASE 4

A 26-year-old asthmatic was referred for pulmonary function tests before and after inhalation of 1.3 mg of metaproterenol (Table 4-4). The patient had taken his regularly scheduled medications two hours previously.

Interpretation and discussion.   Following inhalation of metaproterenol, there is an increase in FVC which is borderline in significance (16%). However, FEV_1 increases substantially (33%). These results suggest that bronchodilatation from the patient's regularly prescribed medication is not maximal and that the patient might benefit from additional treatment.

ARTIFACTS

If the forced vital capacity (FVC) increases following bronchodilator administration, flow rates measured at fixed percentages of the FVC ($FEF_{25-75\%}$, $\dot{V}_EMax_{50}$, $\dot{V}_EMax_{25}$) will not be calculated at the same absolute lung volumes as the prebronchodilator determinations (Table 4-5).[15,34] Consequently, the postbronchodilator flow rates are underestimated;[15,34] Sherter and colleagues found that FEV_1 and FVC increased substantially after administration of ephedrine whereas $FEF_{25-75\%}$ changed very little.[34] Isovolumetric measurements of $FEF_{25-75\%}$ (measurements at the same absolute prebronchodilator and postbronchodilator lung volumes) eliminated the artifact. If $FEF_{25-75\%}$ or $\dot{V}_EMax_{50}$ are used to assess bronchodilator responsiveness, the determinations should be made

Table 4-4   Case 4

| | Observed | | |
	Prebronchodilator	Postbronchodilator	Predicted
FEV_1 (liter)	1.8	2.4	3.5
FVC (liter)	3.7	4.3	4.2
FEV_1/FVC%	49.0	56.0	83.0

Table 4-5 Test Results

	Prebronchodilator	Postbronchodilator
FEV_1 (liter)	0.73	1.24
$FEF_{25-75\%}$ (liter/sec)	0.38	0.47 (1.32)
FVC (liter)	1.78	2.79
$FEV_1/FVC\%$	41	44
RV (liter)	5.31	4.10
TLC (liter)	7.09	6.89

isovolumetrically. Ideally, this requires determination of TLC with a body plethysmograph. Although some studies have shown that TLC may not change significantly from the prebronchodilator value,[34,35] this is not always the case.[28,36]

Postbronchodilator changes in lung volumes may also influence the ratio $FEV_1/FVC\%$.[37] Although both parameters may increase after bronchodilator administration, the $FEV_1/FVC\%$ ratio may change very little or diminish depending upon the relative increments in FEV_1 and FVC. In this regard, Ramsdell found that 46/129 patients with airflow obstruction had no improvement in $FEV_1/FVC\%$ after inhalation of isoproterenol.[37] Because FVC increased by an average of 15% in these subjects, it is evident that FEV_1 must have increased by a comparable amount. Large changes in static lung volumes have been documented in subjects with airflow obstruction following bronchodilator administration.[36-38] The following example provides data from a patient with significant flow and volume responses to inhaled metaproterenol (Table 4-5).

Interpretations and discussion. This patient had similar percentage increases in FEV_1 and FVC. Therefore, there was little change in the ratio FEV_1/FVC. Without correction for changes in lung volume, $FEF_{25-75\%}$ improved from 0.38 liter/sec to 0.47 liter/sec; the improvement in $FEF_{25-75\%}$ was much more impressive when measured isovolumetrically (0.38 liter/sec to 1.32 liter/sec).

REFERENCES

1. Paterson JW, Woolcock AJ, Shenfield GM: Bronchodilator drugs. *Am Rev Respir Dis* 120:1149–1188, 1979.
2. Solis-Cohen S: The use of adrenal substance in the treatment of asthma. *JAMA* 34:1164–1166, 1900.
3. Herrmann G, Aynesworth MB: Successful treatment of persistent extreme dyspnea "status asthmaticus". *J Lab Clin Med* 23:135–148, 1937.
4. Roth M, Wilson AF, Novey HS: A comparative study of the aerosolized bronchodilators, isoproterenol, metaproterenol and terbutaline in asthma. *Ann Allergy* 38:16–21, 1977.

5. Freedman BJ, Meisner P, Hill GB: A comparison of the actions of different broncho-dilators in asthma. *Thorax* 23:590–597, 1968.

6. Williams MH Jr, Kane C: Dose response of patients with asthma to inhaled isopro-tenenol. *Am Rev Respir Dis* 111:321–324, 1975.

7. Fairshter RD, Wilson AF: Response to inhaled metaproterenol and isoproterenol in asthmatic and normal subjects. *Chest* 78:44–50, 1980.

8. Popa VT, Werner P: Dose-related dilatation of airways after inhalation of metapro-terenol sulfate. *Chest* 70:205–211, 1976.

9. Shenfield GM, Paterson JW: Clinical assessment of bronchodilator drugs delivered by aerosol. *Thorax* 28:124–132, 1973.

10. Shim C, Williams MH Jr: The adequacy of inhalation of aerosol from canister nebulizers. *Am J Med* 69:891–894, 1980.

11. Orehek L, Gayrard P, Grimaud C, et al.: Patient error in use of bronchodilator metered aerosols. *Br Med J* 1:76, 1976.

12. Popa VT: How to inhale a whiff of pressurized bronchodilator. *Chest* 76:496–498, 1979.

13. Riley DJ, Liu RT, Edelman NH: Enhanced responses to aerosolized bronchodilator therapy in asthma using respiratory maneuvers. *Chest* 76:501–507, 1979.

14. Riley DJ, Weitz BW, Edelman NH: The responses of asthmatic subjects to isopro-terenol inhaled at differing lung volumes. *Am Rev Respir Dis* 114:509–515, 1976.

15. Ries AL: *Response to Bronchodilators. Pulmonary Function Testing Guidelines and Controversies*, Clausen JL, (ed). New York, Academic Press, 1982.

16. Dolovich M, Ruffin RE, Roberts R, et al.: Optimal delivery of aerosols from metered dose inhalers. *Chest* 80 (Suppl): 911–915, 1981.

17. Epstein SW, Parsons JE, Corey PN, et al.: A comparison of three means of pressur-ized aerosol inhaler use. *Am Rev Respir Dis* 128:253–255, 1983.

18. Newman SP, Moren JF, Pavia D, et al.: Deposition of pressurized aerosols inhaled through extension devices. *Am Rev Respir Dis* 124:317–320, 1981.

19. Bloomfield P, Crompton GK: A tube spacer to improve inhalation of drugs from pressurized aerosols. *Br Med J* 2:1479, 1979.

20. Light RW, Conrad SA, George RB: The one best test for evaluating the effects of bronchodilator therapy. Chest 72:512–516, 1977.

21. Lorber DB, Kaltenborn W, Burrows B: Responses to isoproterenol in a general population sample. *Am Rev Respir Dis* 118:855–856, 1978.

22. Report of the Committee on Emphysema, American College of Chest Physicians. Criteria for the assessment of reversibility in airway obstruction. *Chest* 65:552–553, 1974.

23. Kuperman AS, Riker JB: The predicted normal maximal midexpiratory flow. *Am Rev Respir Dis* 107:231–238, 1973.

24. Mead J, Turner JM, Macklem PT, et al.: Significance of the relationship between lung recoil and maximum expiratory flow. *J Appl Physiol* 22:95–108, 1967.

25. Pride NB, Permutt S, Riley RL, et al.: Determinants of maximal expiratory flow from the lung. *J Appl Physiol* 23:646–662, 1967.

26. Dawson SV, Elliott EA: Wave-speed limitation on expiratory flow—a unifying concept. *J Appl Physiol* 43:498–515, 1977.

27. McFadden ER Jr, Newton-Howes J, Pride NB: Acute effects of inhaled isopro-terenol on the mechanical characteristics of the lungs in normal man. *J Clin Invest* 49:779–790, 1970.

28. Peress L, Sybrect G, Macklem PT: The mechanism of increase in total lung capacity during acute asthma. *Am J Med* 61:165–169, 1976.
29. Bouhuys A, van de Woestijne KP: Mechanical consequences of airway smooth muscle relaxation. *J Appl Physiol* 30:670–676, 1971.
30. Ingram RH Jr, Wellman JJ, McFadden ER Jr, et al.: Relative contributions of large and small airways to flow limitation in normal subjects before and after atropine and isoproterenol. *J Clin Invest* 59:696–703, 1977.
31. Fairshter RD, Wilson AF: Relationship between the site of airflow limitation and localization of the bronchodilator response in asthma. *Am Rev Respir Dis* 120:27–32, 1980.
32. Rebuck AS, Read J: Assessment and management of severe asthma. *Am J Med* 51:788–798, 1971.
33. Macklem PT, Fraser RG, Bates DV: Bronchial pressures and dimensions in health and obstructive airway disease. *J Appl Physiol* 18:699–706, 1963.
34. Sherter CB, Connolly JJ, Schilder DP: The significance of volume adjusting the maximal midexpiratory flow in assessing the response to a bronchodilator drug. *Chest* 73:568–571, 1978.
35. McFadden ER Jr, Kiker R, DeGroot WJ: Acute bronchial asthma: Relations between clinical and physiologic manifestations. *N Engl J Med* 288:221–226, 1973.
36. Fairshter RD, Novey HS, Wilson AF: Site and duration of bronchodilatation in asthmatic patients after oral administration of terbutaline. *Chest* 79:50–57, 1981.
37. Ramsdell JW, Tisi GM: Determination of bronchodilatation in the clinical pulmonary function laboratory. Role of changes in static lung volumes. *Chest* 76:622–628, 1979.
38. Ayres SM, Griesbach SJ, Reimold F, et al.: Bronchial component in chronic obstructive lung disease. *Am J Med* 57:183–191, 1974.

CHAPTER 5

Bronchial Challenge

WILLIAM MICHAEL ALBERTS
JOE W. RAMSDELL

HISTORIC DEVELOPMENT

The ability of certain substances to provoke bronchospasm when inhaled by susceptible individuals was recognized in the late 1940s[1] when researchers and clinicians began testing various agents in hopes of diagnosing asthma in patients with normal lung function. Currently, bronchial provocation testing is promoted as being useful not only for diagnosis of asthma, but also for identification of specific allergens, for screening individuals at risk of developing certain types of occupational lung disease, and as a laboratory model of reversible airways obstruction.

The clinical value of provocation testing is still being defined and its use as a research model has led to often contradictory views about the pathophysiology of bronchospasm. This has been due in part to the lack of a universally accepted method of performing the test and reporting the results. In response to this problem, a group of investigators interested in the standardization of inhalation techniques was selected by the program directors of the Asthma and Allergic Disease Centers. Assisted by the National Institutes of Health, this group proposed criteria for procedures and materials in order to standardize bronchial inhalation challenges.[2] Although these standard methods have not been definitively validated or universally adopted and variations on the original method constantly appear, this attempt at standardization does provide a guideline to laboratories that wish to perform bronchial challenges. Recently, a position paper was presented under the auspices of the American Thoracic Society that served to update and re-emphasize the initial standardization suggestions.[3]

PULMONARY FUNCTION TESTING
INDICATIONS AND INTERPRETATIONS

REVIEW OF METHODS

PATHOPHYSIOLOGIC RATIONALE

Bronchial hyperreactivity is a nearly universal finding in patients with asthma and may be a frequent feature of such respiratory diseases as chronic bronchitis, allergic rhinitis, cystic fibrosis, sarcoidosis, and hypersensitivity pneumonitis. Whether this hyperreactivity represents an increased sensitivity of sensory neuroreceptors, decreased stability of mast cells, and/or increased sensitivity of airway smooth muscle is unknown. Bronchial provocation testing has evolved from the assumption that bronchial hyperreactivity could be detected in the laboratory.

Simply stated, bronchial provocation testing is accomplished by administering progressively larger doses of the testing material while monitoring respiratory function. Individuals with bronchial hyperreactivity develop increased airway resistance and expiratory airflow obstruction at a dose of the test material that is well tolerated by normal individuals. Such testing requires a mechanism for delivering a reproducible amount of provocative material to the airways and a method of recognizing a response.

There are three types of provocative materials: (1) nonspecific pharmacologic (generally, histamine, or methacholine);(2) nonspecific irritant (e.g.,SO_2, smoke, or citric acid); and(3) specific (individual allergens or occupational inhalants). Various systems have been used for delivery of nonspecific pharmacological and allergenic provocative materials to the airways. Most rely on a nebulizer from which the substance being utilized is aerosolized in the vicinity of the patient's mouth. The initial standardization report recommended a timed, breath-activated dosimeter system. Others have utilized a Wright nebulizer to generate an aerosol that is either stored in a reservoir (spirometer bell or bag-and-box system) from which the patient inspires through a one-way valve or is constantly being added to the patient's inspired air.[4] Comparison of these two methods suggest that, with some exceptions, they provide similar information.[5] Specific occupational inhalants or nonspecific irritants are best delivered in a manner that mimics the "natural" or occupational exposure as closely as possible. For this reason, methods of delivery are usually individualized.

Respiratory function may be monitored by any spirometric system that allows rapid and accurate determinations of FEFs and volumes. Measurement of airways resistance and conductance are desirable in some situations.

Bronchial provocation testing begins with a prechallenge evaluation. Patients with preexisting airways obstruction may be tested for bronchospasm by response to sympathomimetic bronchodilators. Patients who demonstrate a response to bronchodilators are likely to have bronchial hyperreactivity; however, the converse is not necessarily true.[6] If baseline respiratory function is markedly depressed, then evaluation for specific bronchial hyperreactivity is usually better deferred until the patient exhibits less physiologic impairment.

Standard bronchodilators (methylxanthines, beta-agonists, and anticholinergics) should be withheld prior to any type of bronchial provocation, and cromolyn sodium and corticosteroids should be withheld prior to testing for responses to antigens. Several factors including recent viral infections, level of ambient allergens, and recent influenza immunizations have been shown to increase bronchial reactivity in susceptible individuals; these factors should be taken into consideration when scheduling and interpreting bronchial provocation tests.

Following determination of baseline function the patient either initiates a series of five inhalations (from Functional Residual Capacity [FRC] to Total Lung Capacity [TLC]) of the test material from an intermittently driven nebulizer, or breathes tidally for two minutes inspiring the test material from a continuously driven nebulizer. Diluent alone is given first; if no significant change is seen in respiratory function, then the challenge begins with inhalation of the lowest concentration of the test material chosen. Respiratory function is evaluated after each successive dose of the test material. Progressively more concentrated material is inhaled until a positive endpoint is reached and the test is terminated.[2]

INDICATIONS FOR TESTING

In the vast majority of patients, a careful history and physical examination coupled with simple spirometry and, perhaps, a therapeutic trial with bronchodilators, will obviate the need for bronchial provocation testing. This is not always the case, however, and although the indications for bronchial provocation testing are continually evolving, at this time they can be grouped in the following three areas.

1. To identify patients with hypersensitive or hyperreactive airways, nonspecific pharmacologic bronchial challenge tests can be used to confirm a clinical suspicion of hyperreactive airways. The test is especially useful in diagnosing asthma in remission and cough-variant asthma. Additionally, the severity of asthma seems to correlate positively with the degree of responsiveness to methacholine challenges.[7]

2. To identify specific provocative factors, bronchial provocation testing utilizing inhalation of specific stimuli may help to identify environmental factors that may be contributing to respiratory difficulty. Often, clinical history, skin tests, and/or in vitro tests will allow a presumptive diagnosis and identification of the offending agent. In this case, specific bronchial provocation testing is not necessary. There are however, instances when specific bronchial provocation testing is useful. Testing with specific agents is especially helpful in determining cause-and-effect relationships between occupational and environmental factors and patient symptoms. This may be critical in instances of alleged occupational lung disease or in instances when avoidance of suspected allergies may be expensive or difficult for patients.[8]

3.   To study the pathophysiology of acute reversible bronchospasm, bronchial provocation testing can be a valuable research tool to examine the mechanisms surrounding acute reversible airways narrowing and to evaluate the effectiveness of pharmacologic agents in prevention of induced bronchospasm.

DISCUSSION OF ABNORMALITIES:
INTERPRETATION, LIMITATIONS, AND
QUANTIFICATION OF IMPAIRMENT

There are differences in the nature of the response of susceptible individuals to various stimuli. Nonspecific pharmacologic agents seem capable of initiating an immediate (2–5 minutes) bronchospastic response in susceptible individuals once a critical-dose threshold is reached. This reaction is short-lived, responding to bronchodilators or returning to baseline spontaneously in less than 90 minutes; it is the only type of response to these agents. Specific allergens, however, have the potential of causing not only a typical immediate reaction but may also cause a delayed response (at 4–12 hours and sometimes longer) following challenge. This response develops slowly over several hours and is poorly responsive to bronchodilators. However, it can be terminated with corticosteroids and may be blocked with cromolyn, if the latter is administered prior to the initial challenge. Fever, myalgias, and other systemic complaints often accompany the delayed response. Allergen inhalation challenge may lead to only immediate, delayed, or a compound immediate and delayed response.[9] The nature of responses to nonspecific irritants and specific occupational inhalants is varied. While an immediate response is the norm for nonspecific irritants, occupational inhalants may cause immediate or delayed responses. The mechanisms responsible for these reactions are not completely understood.

Changes in respiratory function in response to bronchial provocation can be recognized by any of several measures of airways obstruction. The most commonly used parameters are those derived from FEF tracings. The forced expired volume in one second (FEV_1), forced expiratory flow rates between 25-75% of vital capacity ($FEF_{25-75\%}$), maximum expiratory flow at 50% vital capacity (FEF_{50}), and peak expiratory flow (PEF) have all been shown to be useful parameters. Specific conductance (SGAW), vital capacity (VC), and functional residual capacity (FRC) have also been used to monitor change. Suggested guidelines for identifying a significant change in each of the monitored parameters have been delineated, but these values have not been validated (Table 5-1).[2,3]

The measurement of FEV_1 is the most widely applied test because it is easily performed and highly reproducible. The addition of measuring SGAW by body plethysmography increases the likelihood of detecting a significant response.

Table 5-1 Guidelines for a Significant Response to
Bronchial Provocation

Parameter	Change (%)	Parameter	Change (%)
FEV_1	20	SG_{AW}	35
$FEF_{25-75\%}$	25	VC	10
FEF_{50}	30	FRC	25*
PEFR	20		

Suggested fall from baseline that implies a significant response to
bronchial challenge (change $= \dfrac{\text{baseline} - \text{measured}}{\text{baseline}} \times 100$;
*—increase from baseline).

The magnitude of change in respiratory function parameters suggested as representing a biologically significant response have undergone limited experimental scrutiny. As a result, definition of a positive response to bronchial challenge is not always clear-cut. If a significant change in respiratory function parameters occurs and the patient reports reproduction of symptoms, there is strong evidence for a positive test. If, however, borderline change in pulmonary function occurs without symptoms or clinical complaints, then the results of the test are, at best, equivocal. In the absence of definite criteria for a positive test, clinical judgement plays an important factor in interpreting equivocal tests.

Reports of the results of bronchial provocation testing should include the testing system and technique used, the material tested, the cumulative dose or lowest actual dose at which a positive response occurred, the magnitude of that response (compared to baseline), and the nature of the response when antigen material is tested (i.e., immediate or delayed). The respiratory function parameter or parameters evaluated should also be clearly stated. The term recommended for expression of most of these parameters is the provocative dose (PD), followed by percent change and type of parameter tested expressed as either the lowest actual dose following which a positive response occurs, sometimes referred to as the provocative concentration (PC), or as cumulative units over the time following exposure that the positive response occurred (Fig. 5-1). For example, PD_{20} $FEV_1 = X$ mg/ml with X being the lowest concentration of the test material (e.g., methacholine) producing a positive response of a drop of 20% FEV. Alternatively, PD_{35} SGAW $= Y$ units/Z minutes signifies Y as the cumulative units of the test material (e.g., *Alternaria* extract) that produces a significant response and Z as the time at which a 35% fall in SGAW was noted. The latter method is more often applied to specific antigen challenge.[2] The provocative dose reflects the level of bronchial sensitivity to inhaled substances. It has also been shown that the slope of the cumulative dose response curve, said to be a

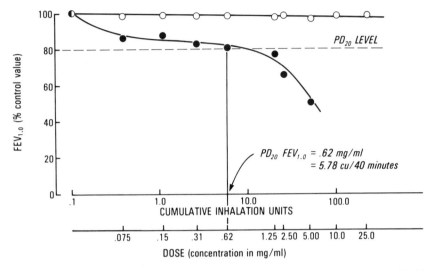

Fig. 5-1.   Results of methacholine bronchial provocation test (cases 1 and 2, pgs. 64–66) plotted on four-cycle semilogarithmic paper.

measure of bronchial reactivity, is steeper in asthmatics than in normals.[10] One may choose, therefore, to report these parameters also.

Interpretation of bronchial provocation testing is aided by viewing asthma as a disease process composed of both clinical symptoms and a physiologic abnormality. In the presence of appropriate symptoms, bronchial provocation testing documents bronchial hyperreactivity confirming the diagnosis of asthma. A positive provocation testing in the absence of clinical symptoms of asthma is occasionally seen in patients with allergic rhinitis and various types of pulmonary disease. In such situations, the presence of hyperreactive airways may not be synonymous with a diagnosis of asthma. The absence of a positive reaction in symptomatic individuals suggests that hyperreactive airways leading to bronchospasm may not be the cause of the patient's disability.

ARTIFACTS/QUALITY CONTROL

Basic issues of quality control in measuring respiratory function are discussed elsewhere.[11] Certain issues are unique to bronchial provocation testing and include the difficulty of quantitating the dose of the provocative agent that is actually delivered to the tracheobronchial tree, which depends on the concentration of material added to the nebulizer; the delivery system used; and the volume, rate, and, in some systems, frequency of inhalation. Even with a highly standardized system such as the dosimeter, malfunction can occur, for example, due to excessive moisture on the thermister (obviously, nebulizers should be thoroughly cleaned prior to use). Methacholine is very hygrophilic and should be carefully dessicated prior to diluting for use.[12] Finally, the act of deep inspiration and forced expiration associated with measuring the response to a provocative agent may precipitate bronchospasm in some asthmatics.[13] This phenomenon should be watched for and reported by those performing the test.

CONTROVERSIES

In asthma, there are varying degrees of obstruction of both large and small airways. Depending on the etiology and resultant pathophysiology of the individual attack of asthma, various amounts of obstruction are contributed by the various pulmonary compartments.

The test material to be used may affect the choice of pulmonary function test. Cholinergic agents may affect the large central airways more than the small airways. Antigenic challenge may affect both large and smaller airways.[14] It would appear advantageous, therefore, to monitor at least two parameters of pulmonary function during bronchial provocation testing, one to follow changes in the central airways and one to monitor the smaller airways. It has been shown that combining the FEV_1 with the $FEF_{25-75\%}$, which is theoretically more sensitive to changes in small airways, will identify a larger proportion of positive reactions than either test alone.[15] On occasion, patients will respond to the provocative test material with a significant change in airway resistance (R_{aw}), SGAW, or PEF without a similar change in FEF_{50} or $FEF_{25-75\%}$. This positive response would be overlooked, if one of the former function tests was not being monitored. This pattern is occasionally seen in patients with allergic rhinitis and cough asthma (case 3).

New indications for bronchial provocation testing need to be carefully studied prior to wide clinical use. Nonspecific pharmacologic inhalation provocations have been suggested to select workers at risk for developing occupational asthma.[8] It remains to be proven, however, whether or not cholinergic hyperreactivity is an industrial risk factor. Likewise, bronchial hyperreactivity has been suggested as a risk factor for developing chronic obstructive pulmonary disease.[16] Again, the clinical implications of this observation are not clear. Bronchial provocation testing may be useful for assessing response to therapy. Either specific or nonspecific bronchial provocation testing can be utilized to assess the efficacy of a treatment modality. A shift in the PD_{20} FEV_1 after specific hyposensitization has been shown in a patient with bronchial reactivity to cat dander.[9] A change in bronchial reactivity or sensitivity following an intervention would seem to suggest efficacy; however, it is difficult to directly extrapolate this finding in experimentally induced bronchospasm to spontaneously occurring asthma. It is obvious that pathophysiologic processes other than bronchospasm are operative in clinical asthma and the use of bronchial provocation testing for assessing response to therapy is most properly reserved for research studies when controlled trials allow for the effects of limited spontaneous fluctuation. Making judgements based upon limited observations in individuals may be hazardous, unless changes in sensitivity are dramatic, because of spontaneous day-to-day and week-to-week variations that, for example, even in the absence of specific confounding influence, amount to as much as a tenfold difference in provocation concentration for antigen-induced bronchospasm.

Finally, it has been suggested that nonpharmacological tests of bronchial reactivity may be preferable to more traditional modes of assessing airway reactivity. Inhalation of aerosolized water,[17] isocapnic hyperventilation (with and without the use of subfreezing air),[18,19] and exercise testing have, among others, been suggested as indicators of nonspecific bronchial hyperreactivity. Three preliminary reports suggest good correlation between methacholine challenge and voluntary hyperventilation,[19] bronchoconstriction due to aerosolized distilled water and the diagnosis of asthma,[18] and positive voluntary hyperventilation and positive exercise-induced bronchospasm.[20] The sensitivity and specificity of these tests remains to be established. The ultimate usefulness of the broad application of these nonspecific methods await further information.

EXAMPLES

Case 1

A 32-year-old man was referred from his personal physician who wondered if bronchial hyperreactivity was playing a role in the patient's symptoms. The patient was completely healthy until he began his current job as an auto painter 6 months previously. He complained of episodic shortness of breath and wheezing. These attacks occurred only at work, lasted one to two hours, occurred three to four times per week, and usually caused him to leave work early. The last attack occurred the day before testing. Baseline pulmonary function was normal. The results of a methacholine bronchial provocation test are displayed in Table 5-2.

Discussion. The patient completed the entire methacholine bronchoprovocation test protocol without developing symptoms or objective evidence of airways obstruction. Reactive airways disease is unlikely to be the cause of this patient's disability. Note the normal variability of the pulmonary function tests.

Case 2

A 28-year-old woman presented with a 4-month history of episodic chest tightness, shortness of breath, and rapid heart beat. These attacks occurred three

Table 5-2   Case 1

Dose (mg/ml)		CU*	FVC	FEV$_1$	PEFR	FEF$_{50}$	V$_{TG}$	SG$_{AW}$
Baseline	(1)		4.91	4.05	10.00	4.21	4.20	0.30
Saline	(2)		4.74	4.00	9.76	4.28	3.90	0.33
0.075	(3)	0.375	4.81	3.96	10.76	4.18	4.31	0.30
0.15	(4)	1.125	4.82	3.95	10.08	4.35	4.31	0.28
0.31	(5)	2.680	4.73	3.97	9.62	4.28	4.15	0.38
0.62	(6)	5.780	4.78	3.96	9.77	4.17	4.13	0.39
1.25	(7)	12.00	4.81	3.98	8.94	4.37	3.45	0.40
2.50	(8)	24.50	4.86	4.00	10.22	4.15	3.92	0.36
5.00	(9)	49.50	4.88	3.95	10.13	4.06	3.92	0.27
10.0	(10)	99.50	4.65	3.86	9.61	4.19	3.49	0.34
25.0	(11)	225.0	4.77	3.83	8.94	3.98	4.15	0.33
†B.D.	(12)	ISOPRO	4.88	4.00	9.88	4.00	4.10	0.36
Maximum change (%)			5.4			9.0		10.0

* Cumulative units/5 breaths.
† Bronchodilator (isoproterenol).

to five times a month, always began just before midnight, and lasted until morning. Symptomatic treatment with inhaled metaproterenol was only partially effective. The patient was referred for evaluation of occupational asthma. She had been employed for 2 years injecting insulation foam into the shells of refrigerators. On location, pulmonary function obtained before and after a work shift revealed no significant change in function.

A two-stage diagnostic approach was adopted: (a) is airway hyperreactivity present; and (b) is industrial exposure implicated? Results of a methacholine bronchial provocation test are displayed in Table 5-3.

Discussion.   The patient noted shortness of breath after inhaling five breaths of the 0.31 mg/ml concentration and was audibly wheezing after the 5.0 mg/ml concentration at which time the test was terminated. Two inhalations of isoproterenol resolved all symptoms in several minutes. The patient has bronchial hyperreactivity compatible with occupational asthma.

Following the provocation test, a simulated work environment was designed. The patient was exposed to the insulation foam (a mixture of toluene di-isocyanate and resin) for 15 minutes per hour for four hours. The patient was then admitted to the hospital and followed with serial pulmonary studies. Results are shown in Table 5-4.

Discussion.   The patient noted no symptoms until 12 hours after the initial exposure when she developed nasal congestion, chest tightness, and audible wheezing. By 24 hours, all symptoms had disappeared. The pattern is consistent

Table 5-3   Case 2

Dose	DU	FEV_1	FEF_{50}	SG_{AW}
Baseline		2.45	2.22	0.38
Saline		2.37	2.18	0.32
0.075	0.375	2.08	2.12	0.15
0.15	1.125	2.14	1.80	0.13
0.31	2.680	2.03	1.60	0.18
0.62	5.780	1.95	1.30	0.09
1.25	12.000	1.90	1.10	0.10
2.50	24.500	1.60	1.00	0.09
5.00	49.500	1.490	.90	0.08
Maximum change (5)		34.7	55.0	76.3

$PD_{20}FEV_1 = .62$ mg/ml or 5.78 cu/40 m; $PD_{30}FEF_{50} = 0.15$ mg/ml of 1.125 cu/20 m; $PD_{35}SG_{AW} = 0.075$ mg/ml or 0.375 cu/10 m. See Figure 5-1, pg. 62.

with a mixed-immediate (significant decrement in function at one hour) and delayed (change at 12 and 16 hours) reaction to the chemicals used during the test. This is typical of toluene di-isocyanate (TDI) asthma. It was suggested that the patient be removed from the work environment that contains isocyanates.

CASE 3

A 49-year-old woman presented with a 9-month history of annoying and, on occasion, disabling cough. Numerous antitussive preparations and several

Table 5-4   Case 2 Serial Pulmonary Studies (after exposure to insulation foam)

Hour	FVC	FEV_1	FEF_{50}	SG_{AW}
Baseline	3.0	2.37	2.80	0.21
1	2.85	1.67	1.70	0.11
2	2.78	1.94	1.82	0.13
3	2.75	1.84	1.68	0.16
4	2.81	1.77	1.88	0.14
5	2.86	2.37	2.20	0.18
6	2.81	2.21	2.68	0.20
8	2.91	2.26	2.72	0.20
10	2.89	2.28	2.58	0.24
12	2.76	1.42	1.65	0.12
16	2.80	1.56	1.68	0.08
20	2.96	1.86	2.00	0.16
24	3.06	2.10	2.20	0.20

Table 5-5   Case 3

Dose (mg/ml)	CU	FVC	FEV$_1$	FEF$_{50}$	SG$_{AW}$
Baseline		3.34	2.69	4.27	0.33
1.25*	12.00	3.28	2.39	4.05	0.11
% change		2%	11%	5%	66%

* = " + " dose; patient is unable to continue because of cough.

courses of antibiotics had failed to alleviate her symptoms. She was otherwise completely healthy, a nonsmoker with no history of respiratory problems. She was referred for evaluation of possible "cough asthma." Baseline pulmonary function was normal, as was her chest roentgenogram. Results of a methacholine bronchial provocation test are displayed in Table 5-5.

Discussion. The patient developed incessive cough after inhalations of the 1.25 mg/ml concentration of methacholine. A significant fall in specific conductance is noted with little change in the FEV$_1$, FVC, or FEF$_{50}$. The positive objective response would have been missed had the body plethysmograph not been used. The patient's symptoms, however, would suggest a positive response. On the basis of this test, a diagnosis of cough asthma is likely and a trial of therapy is warranted.

REFERENCES

1. Curry JJ: The action of histamine on the respiratory tract in normal and asthmatic subjects. *J Clin Invest* 25:785–791, 1945.
2. Chai H, Farr RS, Froehlich LA, et al: Standardization of bronchial inhalation challenge procedures. *J Allergy Clin Immunol* 56:323–327, 1975.
3. Guidelines for bronchial inhalation challenges with pharmacologic and antigenic agents. *Am Thorac Soc News* Spring, 1980.
4. Cockcroft DW, Killian DN, Mellon JJA, et al.: Bronchial reactivity to inhaled histamine: a method and clinical survey. *Clin Allergy* 7:235–243, 1977.
5. Ryan G, Dolovich MB, Roberts RS, et al.: Standardization of inhalation provocation tests: two techniques of aerosol generation and inhalation compared. *Am Rev Respir Dis* 123:195–199, 1981.
6. Benson MK: Bronchial responsiveness to inhaled histamine and isoprenaline in patients with airway obstruction. *Thorax* 33:211–215, 1978.
7. Townley RG, Bewtra AK, Nair NM, et al.: Methacholine inhalation challenge studies. *J Allergy Clin Immunol* 64:569–573, 1979.
8. Chester EH, Schwartz HJ: Study session on occupational asthma. *J Allergy Clin Immunol* 64:665–671, 1979.
9. Taylor WW, Ohman JL, Lowell FC: Immunotherapy in cat-induced asthma. *J Allergy Clin Immunol* 61:283–287, 1978.

10. Orehek J, Gayrard P, Smith AP, et al.: Airway response to carbachol in normal and asthmatic subjects: distinction between bronchial sensitivity and reactivity. *Am Rev Respir Dis* 115:937–943, 1977.

11. Ramsdell J, Hauer D, Nachtwey F: Bronchial provocation testing, in *Guidelines and Controversies in Pulmonary Function Testing*: New York, Academic Press, 1982.

12. Alberts WM, Ferguson P, Ramsdell J: Preparation and handling of methacholine chloride testing solutions: Effect of the hygroscopic properties of methacholine. *Am Rev Respir Dis* 127(Suppl 3):350–351, 1983.

13. Orehek J, Nicholi MM, Delpierre S, et al.: Influence of the previous deep inspiration on the spirometric measurement of provoked bronchoconstriction in asthma. *Am Rev Respir Dis* 123:269–272, 1981.

14. Oligiati R, Buck S, Rao A, et al.: Differential effects of methacholine and antigen challenge on gas exchange in allergic subjects. J Allergy Clin Immunol 67:325–329, 1981.

15. Murray AB, Ferguson AC: A comparison of spirometric measurements in allergen bronchial challenge testing. *Clin Allergy* 11:87–93, 1981.

16. Britt J, Cohen B, Menkes H, et al.: Airways reactivity and functional deterioration in relatives of chronic obstructive pulmonary patients. *Chest* 77(Suppl): 260–261, 1980.

17. Allegra L, Bianco S: Nonspecific broncho-reactivity obtained with an ultrasonic aerosol of distilled water. *Eur J Respir Dis* 106(Suppl):41–49, 1980.

18. Kivity S, Souhrada JF: A new diagnostic test to assess airway reactivity in asthmatics. *Bull Europ Physiopath Resp* 17:243–254, 1981.

19. Deal EC, McFadden ER, Ingram RH, et al.: Airway responsiveness to cold air and hyperpnea in normal subjects and in those with hay fever and asthma. *Am Rev Respir Dis* 121:621–628, 1980.

20. Kivity S, Souhrada JF: Hyperpnea: The common stimulus for bronchospasm in asthma during exercise and voluntary isocapnic hyperpnea. Respiration 40:169–177, 1980.

CHAPTER 6

Lung Volumes

ANDREW L. RIES
JACK L. CLAUSEN

Absolute lung volumes, also called static lung volumes, are parameters that include residual volume (RV), the amount of air remaining in the lungs after maximal exhalation; total lung capacity (TLC), the lung volume after maximal inspiration; and functional residual capacity (FRC), the amount of air in the lungs at the resting end-expiratory level.

An understanding of the determinants of each of the absolute lung volumes is important in interpreting changes of disease. Determinants of TLC include the elastic recoil of the lung, inspiratory muscle strength, and elastic recoil of the chest wall. FRC reflects a balance between the static recoil properties of the lung and chest wall. RV is determined by the elastic recoil of the chest wall, expiratory muscle strength, elastic recoil of the lung (a minor factor), and airway closure (particularly in older adults).[1,2]

There are three basic techniques for measuring absolute lung volumes.[3] Consideration of the fundamental differences in the volumes measured by each method is important for accurate interpretation and clinical decision making from these measurements. Multiple-breath, steady-state gas dilution techniques require patients to breathe continuously while a tracer gas is either equilibrated within (closed circuit helium dilution) or eliminated (open circuit nitrogen washout) from the lungs. Single-breath gas dilution methods may also be used;[4] this approach is usually included in the single-breath technique for measurement of pulmonary diffusing capacity (DL_{CO}).[5] Gas dilution methods measure the *communicating gas volume* which reflects the volume of air communicating with the airways and, therefore, is available for mixing with the inspired gas. Body plethysmography, the second basic technique, has been used increasingly in

PULMONARY FUNCTION TESTING
INDICATIONS AND INTERPRETATIONS

clinical laboratories in recent years and is considered to be the most accurate method for measuring absolute lung volumes. This technique measures the *compressible gas volume*, the total intrathoracic volume that is compressed during the panting maneuver. Radiographic techniques (either ellipsoid [6,7] or planimetric [8] methods) estimate lung volumes from standard chest radiographs. These techniques measure intrathoracic volume, the total volume contained within the perimeter of the thoracic cage, diaphragm, and mediastinum.

In groups of normal subjects, these three different approaches to measuring lung volumes have been shown to give mean values for TLC measurements that are virtually equal.[6-10] For the single-breath gas dilution technique, mean values for TLC measurements were 400 m lower than TLC measurements by plethysmography in one study of normal subjects [11] although smaller differences have been reported in other studies.[4,12,13] In individual subjects, a number of studies comparing plethysmographic and radiographic TLC measurements have noted significant differences between the two TLC measurements (differences are sometimes more than 25% in some subjects).[6,11,14] Calculations of radiographic techniques are based on the assumption that the shape of the thoracic cage can be approximated by an ellipse or are based on equations empirically derived from samples of normal subjects. Due to these limitations, it is assumed that in these subjects it is the radiographic measurements which are erroneous. It is our conclusion that these occasional erroneous radiographic measurements limit the usefulness of radiographic TLC measurements in individual patients; the technique, however, may still be valid and useful for comparing mean values from groups of subjects in research studies.

In patients with pulmonary disease these three basic techniques may differ significantly in the results of TLC measurements. In patients with obstructive airway or bullous disease, areas of the lung may either not communicate or communicate poorly with the central airways; this may result in significant underestimation of absolute lung volumes measured by the gas dilution techniques when compared with either plethysmographic or radiographic measurements of TLC.[4,9,10] In some patients with very severe obstructive disease, the plethysmographic measurements may overestimate TLC, but usually only in patients with severe obstruction (e.g., acute bronchospasm) and if the measurements are made during panting rather than tidal breathing.[15,16] In patients with intrathoracic space-occupying disease (e.g., pneumonia, interstitial fibrosis, or pleural effusion), in which gas is replaced by tissue or fluid, the radiographic TLC may be larger than the TLCs measured by plethysmography or gas dilution techniques.[9,17] Crapo et al.[18] have demonstrated in a group of young adult males that radiographs made after the normal instructions ("Take a deep breath and hold it.") averaged 95% of the TLC values measured from repeat radiographs taken after specific instructions to achieve maximal inspiration. Only 1 out of 19 subjects had an uncoaxed radiographic TLC that was less than 90% of the maximal effort measurement. Conversely, Wade and Gibson concluded that significant underestimation of TLC would occur if the measurements were made from routine radiographs.[19] As is the case with any physiologic measurement requiring subject cooperation, the results of such studies are critically dependent upon the particular instructions given to patients during routine chest radiographs.

The reproducibility of repeat measurements is important to consider when comparing techniques. We are not aware of published studies that have defined the reproducibility of duplicate measurements of TLC from repeat chest radiographs; mean values for interobserver differences in TLC measurements on the same radiograph have varied from 1.1–4.8%.[11,18] The coefficient of variation for plethysmographic measurements (each calculated from two panting maneuvers) was reported by Viljanen et al. to be 4.0% for TLC and 6.7% for FRC.[20] Similar coefficients of variation of 4.8% have been reported for duplicate measurements of TLC by multiple-breath helium dilution.[11] Some loss in accuracy and precision may occur if the absolute lung volume parameters are calculated from summing direct measurement of FRC with the inspiratory capacity (IC) measured during a separate spirometric maneuver. With gas dilution systems (and some plethysmographs) these problems can be avoided by making measurements of RV, FRC, and TLC directly during one continuous maneuver. Bohadana et al. have published data that showed that there were minimal differences of less than 0.3 liter between mean TLC values when different methods of summing FRC and VC measurements were used.[21]

INDICATIONS

RESTRICTIVE LUNG DISEASE

Restrictive lung diseases (RLD) are a heterogeneous group of disorders which result generally in reduction of lung volumes. The physiologic mechanisms that can reduce lung volumes include space-occupying abnormalities within the thoracic cage (e.g., pleural effusion, pneumonia, tumor), increased recoil of the lung (e.g., interstitial fibrosis), weakness of the respiratory muscles, or abnormal recoil or deformity of the chest wall (e.g., ankylosing spondilitis). Restrictive disease can be suspected from spirometry when the VC is reduced and expiratory flow rates are normal or supernormal. In this situation, absolute lung volume measurements may be useful for: (1) confirming a diagnosis of RLD; (2) establishing a baseline and quantitating the level of impairment; (3) evaluating serially the course of disease or response to therapy; and (4) suggesting the physiological type of disease from the pattern of lung volume alterations.

All RLDs may lead to a reduction in VC. However, because of the large variability between subjects in a reference population, a reduced VC for an individual may be within normal limits. If prior testing results are not available for comparison, the fact that a patient's VC is reduced may be missed. In this situation, measurement of the absolute lung volumes may help detect, confirm, or exclude a suspected diagnosis. However, published data to support the usefulness of absolute lung volumes as a supplement to VC in detecting RLD are lacking. In patients with interstitial pneumonia studies have concluded that TLC is less sensitive than VC in detecting patients with proven disease and is frequently normal.[22,23] In patients with RLD due to congestive heart failure, TLC has been found to be reduced below the diagnostic lower limits of normal only in patients with more severe disease.[24]

Evaluating the significance of a low VC in a patient with combined restrictive and obstructive disease processes can be difficult because both can reduce VC. In such cases, absolute lung volumes that are reduced (or lower than expected considering the degree of expiratory airflow obstruction present) may be an important clue that the patient has a significant restrictive process. This clue may be very helpful clinically in indicating that worsening of dyspnea in a patient with COPD may be due to another process rather than to an exacerbation of airway disease. In addition, measurements of TLC may potentially be important in cases in which a restrictive process is dominant because reductions in lung volumes can also cause decreases in expiratory flow rates and a misleading interpretation of obstructive disease if testing is limited to spirometry alone. Because of the potential underestimation of TLC measurements by the gas dilution techniques in obstructive air disease, measurements made by these techniques are of use only in ruling against the presence of a restrictive process. A reduced gas dilution TLC in this situation may be secondary to a significant amount of noncommunicating space rather than to a restrictive process. However, we were unable to find studies in the literature that have investigated the potential value of lung volume measurements for the recognition of restrictive disorders in patients with obstructive airway disease. Currently, the conclusion that TLC measurements are useful in this setting can only be based on our clinical experience and that reported anecdotally by others.

Because of the difficulty in establishing a diagnosis of RLD in patients with mild disease from lung volumes measured at one point in time, serial measurements of lung volumes may have greater usefulness in a single patient. The sensitivity of detecting changes in lung volumes in one individual is greater than sensitivity that depends upon measurements being outside the range of normalcy of a reference population with large intersubject variability. Used in a serial fashion, absolute lung volume measurements may help to confirm a suspected diagnosis and follow the course of disease or response to therapy. We are unaware of studies that support (or disprove) the assumption that serial measurements of TLC may be clinically useful for evaluating patients who develop or have an exacerbation of a restrictive disease.

Although often relatively nonspecific, the pattern of changes in absolute lung volumes may be useful in suggesting the type of process causing the restrictive disease. All restrictive processes, if sufficiently severe, will cause reduction of both VC and TLC; most commonly (but not always) VC will fall below the lower limits of normal before TLC is reduced below the lower limits of reference values. FRC should be (1) reduced by diseases affecting the lung parenchyma (alveolar filling or interstitial process) or by certain thoracic cage processes (e.g., kyphoscoliosis)[25]; (2) unaffected by neuromuscular diseases [25,26] in which the lung parenchyma is not affected (e.g., by scarring or atelectasis); and (3) may be increased in other thoracic cage disorders (e.g., ankylosing spondylitis)[25]. Similarly, RV may be (1) significantly reduced by space occupying processes or lung resection; (2) less affected by processes that predominantly decrease the compliance of the lung (because of the relatively minor contribution of lung recoil to RV);[27-29] (3) increased by diseases with expiratory muscle weakness; [25] and (4) variably affected by thoracic cage diseases.[25,30] Reduction of TLC, FRC, and RV as measured by plethysmography has been recently reported in 30–50% of a series of patients with precapillary pulmonary hypertension (either primary pulmonary hypertension or chronic thromboemboli). The other patients in this series had normal lung volumes.[31] The pathophysiologic mechanisms resulting in these findings and the clinical significance of these observations are currently under investigation. These points are summarized in Table 6-1. However, it should be emphasized that considerable variations occur in the pattern of changes in lung volumes observed in different patients and the presence of a particular

Table 6-1 Patterns of Lung Volume Changes in Restrictive Lung Disease

	VC	TLC	FRC	RV
Alveolar filling/loss diseases	↓	↓	↓	↓
Interstitial diseases (↓ compliance)	↓	↓	↘	N/↘
Neuromuscular* Selective inspiratory	↓	↓	N	N
Selective expiratory	↓	N	N	↑
Both	↓	↓	N	↑
Thoracic Cage e.g., kyphoscoliosis	↓	↓	↓	↘
e.g., ankylosing spondylitis	↓	↓	↑	↑
Pleural disease	↓	↓	↓	↓
Pulmonary vascular disease	N/↓	N/↓	N/↓	N/↓

N Normal; ↓ Decreased; ↘ Slightly decreased; ↑ Increased; * These patterns are for pure neuromuscular disease. Associated complications such as atelectasis and pneumonia will produce concomitant reduction in lung volumes related to alveolar filling.

pattern of lung volume changes can not be used to exclude disease processes with a high degree of certainty.

OBSTRUCTIVE LUNG DISEASE

At some stage, all obstructive lung diseases (OLD) cause reductions in expiratory flow rates. Asthma, chronic bronchitis, and emphysema are the most common types of these diseases. In all three of these conditions, RV and FRC are often elevated. Elevation of RV in OLD is primarily due to airway closure or narrowing. The pathophysiologic determinants of the elevation of FRC are more complex and controversial, but include an increase in inspiratory muscle tone, prolonged expiratory time secondary to expiratory airflow limitation, and decrease in lung elastic recoil.[32-36] The mechanisms for the remarkable increase in TLC observed in some patients with OLD are also incompletely understood; they include decrease in lung recoil, increase in inspiratory muscle force or strength, and possibly, change in chest wall recoil.[32-36] The recent observations that plethysmographic measurements of lung volumes may overestimate the degree of hyperinflation in some patients with severe obstruction [15,16] add further confusion to the interpretation of a number of previous studies on the mechanisms of hyperinflation.

The potential indications for absolute lung volume measurements in addition to spirometry for evaluating patients with known or suspected OLD include (1) differentiating types of OLD; (2) assessing the severity of disease; (3) assessing the clinical course and response to therapy or bronchial challenge; (4) detecting mild airways disease; and (5) detecting a noncommunicating space.

Applications for distinguishing asthma, chronic bronchitis and emphysema

In emphysema, TLC is characteristically increased.[32,37-39] Increased TLC may also be observed in patients with asthma, although it is often within normal limits.[33,40] Many of the earlier classic studies of patients with chronic bronchitis using gas dilution techniques concluded that in pure chronic bronchitis TLC measurements are normal or only moderately elevated, whereas in the more common patient with combined bronchitis and emphysema, the TLC may be as high as observed in pure emphysema.[38] In a retrospective review of absolute lung volumes measured by gas dilution techniques in over 8000 patients categorized as having chronic bronchitis or emphysema based primarily on the presence or absence of a history of productive cough of more than 3 months duration, Gaensler concluded that the mean values for VC, RV, FRC, and TLC did not differ significantly in these two groups of patients.[38a] Whether or not these conclusions reflect the inherent limitations of the gas dilution technique, the clinical criteria by which the patients were classified, or limitations in the usefulness of TLC measurements for separating patients with relatively pure emphysema and chronic bronchitis remains an issue of controversy. Other studies that used pathologic assessments of the extent of emphysema have reported significant correlations between measurements of TLC and the presence and severity of emphysema.[32,39] Clearly, however, one cannot use measurements of TLC as the sole criterion for placing a patient in a clinical category of chronic bronchitis or emphysema; rather, TLC measurements need to be interrelated with a number of other clinical parameters (sputum production, radiographic findings, DL_{CO} etc.).

Whether or not it is clinically important to differentiate between asthma, chronic bronchitis, and emphysema in an individual patient is another controversial issue. Many clinicians feel that treatment should be based on the identification of other characteristics (e.g., atopic history, clinical response to bronchodilators) rather than the type of OLD that the patient is thought to have.

Assessment of severity of OLD

Because of the beliefs that hyperinflation of FRC and TLC represent adaptive responses to airflow limitations and that inspiratory muscle function may be less effective at high lung volumes, it is often concluded that measurement of FRC and TLC gives clinicians useful information for assessing the severity of OLD. Whether or not this information can be used to answer specific questions of clinical importance (e.g., prognosis, risk of surgery, predicted response to therapy) is controversial. Most studies on prognostic factors in OLD with absolute lung volume measurements used gas dilution techniques. In such studies, appropriate statistical testing to evaluate the discriminative potential of absolute lung volume measurements in individual patients was not done; nevertheless, the general conclusion is that the simpler measurement of $FEV_{1.0}$ is more useful than measurements of RV, FRC, and TLC for predicting a patient's life expectancy.[41,42] For assessment of risk of surgery, few studies have routinely included measurement of absolute lung volumes. Although some studies have shown significant correlations between RV or TLC and surgical morbidity and mortality,[43,44] the general conclusion is that for standard screening purposes, measurements of RV and TLC add little to simpler spirometric measurements.[43-46] However, in individual patients with abnormal spirometry, measurements of TLC may be useful for detecting the presence of restrictive lung disease. In addressing the issue of how to determine impairment for disability conditions, Epler et al. observed that although the TLC expressed as percent predicted did show a significant correlation with the severity of dyspnea reported during exercise testing in patients with diffuse infiltrative lung disease, a significant correlation was not noted between those parameters in patients with chronic OLD.[47]

Usefulness for assessing the clinical course and response to bronchodilator therapy or bronchial challenge.

We are unaware of studies that have assessed the clinical usefulness of serial measurements of absolute lung volumes in the management of patients with

OLD. As discussed in previous sections, measurement of TLC may be a useful supplement to spirometry for detecting the development of a restrictive disorder in patients with OLD.

For evaluating the response to bronchodilators, measurements of absolute lung volumes rarely increase the sensitivity of testing with spirometry alone. Although some patients may respond to bronchodilators with partial or complete reversal of hyperinflation without changes in standard maximal expiratory flow parameters,[48,49] such patients usually have significant increases in VC, indicating a response to bronchodilation.[48]

Recognition that a patient's FRC decreases appreciably after bronchodilators may improve understanding of why such patients often describe a greater reduction in dyspnea than expected from the observed improvement in maximal inspiratory or expiratory flow rates. However, this probably only rarely would change the approach to therapy.

Relating the observed changes in maximal expiratory flow rates to absolute lung volumes may improve the sensitivity for detecting responses to bronchodilators, but for clinical purposes, adequate increases in sensitivity can probably be achieved by calculating isovolume flow rates referenced to maximal inspiratory volumes measured during baseline spirometry studies.[50,51]

There are no reports in the literature that establish that measurements of absolute lung volumes increase the sensitivity of bronchial provocation testing over and above the use of spirometry. However, the observations that patients with hypersensitivity pneumonitis often have low TLC [52] and the report of apparently acute reductions in TLC as part of a disease process, which otherwise simulates asthma,[53] raise the possibility that bronchial challenge to specific antigens in some patients may cause restrictive dysfunction while, in others, may cause obstructive airway changes. In both cases, spirometry alone would detect decreases in VC or flow rates indicating a need for cessation of chronic exposure to the agents being tested. For research purposes, it may be important to differentiate between these two processes; hence, arguments can be made for the current clinical importance of having such information. However, the clinical usefulness of TLC measurements in such cases is not established.

Usefulness as a sensitive test for early airway disease

Although it is the impression of a number of clinicans that RV is the only abnormal pulmonary function test in a number of patients with early airway disease or resolving reversible airway dysfunction, there are relatively few reports documenting such cases.[54,56] Vulterini et al. [57] reported a series of 14 subjects with significant elevation of RV whose value for VC, $FEV_{1.0}$, and R_{aw} were within normal limits; most of these subjects also had $FEF_{50\%}$ within normal limits. Because of the high incidence of cigarette smoking and high frequency of decreased lung recoil in this sample, it was concluded that these findings represent a group of patients with airway disease and isolated elevation in RV.

Another possibility that has been raised but neither established nor rejected by published studies is the potential usefulness of noting high-normal values for RV in combination with low-normal values for $FEF_{25-75\%}$ (values well below the predicted value but within the lower limits of normal at the 5 percentile level) as signs of early disease. In order for such multivariate analyses to be useful, it is necessary to define the frequency with which such suspicious combinations of borderline abnormal results occur in a disease-free normal population.

Measurements of the noncommunicating space

The difference between the communicating volume measured by gas dilution techniques and the compressible intrathoracic gas volume measured by plethysmography is often called the *noncommunicating volume*. In normal subjects, most studies have concluded that this volume is negligible or small.[4,11-13] In a large study of 512 nonsmoking adults, Viljanen et al. [20] noted that noncommunicating volumes were age dependent, increasing from a volume of less than 100 ml in an average 30-year-old subject to 300 ml at age 70 years. We have observed an almost identical relationship to age in normal subjects in a study in progress.

The physiologic changes responsible for the development of a noncommunicating space with aging or with disease are multifactorial. In most cases, this space probably represents a summation of a large number of spaces in which gas equilibration is slow secondary to airway narrowing rather than single or multiple areas that are totally noncommunicating with the central airways.

In most patients with obstructive airway disease, measurement of the noncommunicating volume is probably of limited clinical usefulness. When appreciable noncommunicating volume is noted, patients most often have abnormal spirometry diagnostic of OLD. Whether or not measuring this volume adds clinically useful information in some patients has not been substantiated. We have seen occasional cases (and have heard of similar cases from other laboratories) in which an abnormally large difference between gas dilution and plethysmographic measurements of FRC (often in conjunction with a widened A-a0₂ gradient) was the sole abnormality noted on conventional pulmonary function testing of pulmonary mechanics. Because of the relatively low frequency of such cases, it is probably not cost-effective to do routine measurements of both gas dilution and plethysmographic lung volumes. This should be considered only in selected cases in which the etiology or pathophysiologic basis of symptoms is not recognized from simpler evaluation.

INTERPRETATION

NORMAL VALUES AND LIMITS OF NORMALCY

Considerable differences in normal predictive values for absolute lung volumes are noted when published studies are compared. For instance, comparing several commonly used reference studies [58-61] in predicting lung volumes for a 60-year-old male (height = 178 cm weight = 73 kg, BSA = 1.9 m²) reveals a range of 1.83 [60] to 2.69 [61] for RV, 2.76 [60] to 3.90 [58] for FRC, and 6.58 [60] to 9.25 [61] for TLC. As is the case for many PFT parameters, these discrepancies emphasize the need for laboratories to test the reference studies selected for use by studying at least ten normal subjects and confirming that the predictive values are indeed appropriate for the methods of testing used in each laboratory and the population of patients being served.

Upper and lower limits of normalcy

Because of the considerable differences in upper and lower limits of normal predictive values reported in different studies of normal populations, it is probably best to use the limits defined by the particular study selected for use. Crapo et al.[62] concluded that it was most appropriate to use a single value for the 95% confidence intervals (e.g., ± 1.077L for TLC in females, ± 0.76L for RV in males) and warned that in the population they studied, the use of limits of normalcy defined by single values expressed as percent predicted (e.g., ± 20% for TLC) was not valid. Viljanen et al. noted 95% confidence limits for TLC in males and females of 80–125% and limits for RV of 60–160% in males and 65–155% for females, and presented data that allow for more precise computations of limits of normalcy in specific subjects.[20]

INTERPRETATION OF PATTERNS OF LUNG VOLUME ABNORMALITIES

When using the term *hyperinflation*, it is best to specify which lung volumes are elevated. Some physicians cite hyperinflation only when TLC is above the upper limits of normal. Others describe hyperinflation when the RV is elevated. The patterns of lung volume abnormalities associated with obstructive airway disease range from an isolated elevation of RV (which, however, can also occur with neuromuscular disease involving expiratory muscles in the absence of COPD), elevation of both RV and FRC, and elevations of RV, FRC, and TLC.

When the term *restriction* is used, it most commonly refers to abnormally low values of TLC. Reductions in FRC alone occur most frequently with obesity or processes in which the abdominal contents are increased (e.g., pregnancy, ascites). Isolated reductions in RV usually reflect inadequacies in the normal values and are not recognized to be associated with specific disease processes.

ASSESSING SEVERITY OF ABNORMALITIES

Because of the wide variety of physiologic abnormalities present in populations of patients, it is often of limited clinical usefulness to assign specific assessments of severity to isolated physiologic parameters. A TLC of 70% of predicted may be noted postpneumonectomy in a patient with minimal exercise limitation, but may also be noted in a patient in the terminal phase of diffuse interstitial fibrosis with severe exercise limitation. Nevertheless, for rough guides of severity the following very approximate ranges can arbitrarily be assigned (Table 6-2).

PITFALLS

SUBJECT COOPERATION

As is the case with many pulmonary function measurements, accurate and clinically meaningful measurements require cooperation and understanding by the patient and an adequate effort. The FRC can be artificially elevated if the measurement is inadvertently made at lung volumes higher than the relaxed resting end-tidal point or if for some reason (e.g., anxiety, chest wall pain) the patient is breathing above the relaxed tidal volume range.

DIFFERENCES IN VOLUMES MEASURED BY THE THREE TECHNIQUES.

As discussed earlier, each of the three techniques discussed measures different theoretical absolute lung volumes: communicating gas volume by gas dilution methods, compressible gas volume by body plethysmography, and intrathoracic volume by radiographic techniques. Because most laboratories measure volumes with only one technique, these differences should be considered in interpreting results in patients with suspected disease. In patients with OLD, gas dilution methods may underestimate lung volumes measured by plethysmographic or radiographic methods. This effect of noncommunication (or slowly communicating) gas space may be particularly accentuated by single-breath TLC measurements. In cases of relatively severe bronchial constriction, erroneously

Table 6-2 Arbitrary Assignments of Degrees of Severity for Lung Volumes*

Volume	Mild	Moderate	Severe
TLC	70–80%	60–70%	< 60%
	120–130%	130–150%	> 150%
FRC	55–65%	45–55%	< 45%
	135–150%	150–200%	> 200%
RV	55–65%	45–55%	< 45%
	135–150%	150–250%	> 250%

* Expressed as percent of predicted—upper and lower limits.

elevated plethysmographic measurements of lung volumes have been reported.[15,16] In patients with space-occupying restrictive disorders (e.g., severe pneumonia), radiographic estimates of thoracic volume may be significantly larger than either plethysmographic measurements of gas volume or gas dilution measurements of communicating gas volume.

CONTROVERSIES

In the preceeding text, a number of controversies were presented which cannot be currently resolved because of the scarcity of pertinent objective data. These controversies include

1. The basic question of the usefulness of absolute lung volume measurements as a supplement to spirometry for the diagnosis of pure restrictive lung diseases.
2. The sensitivity and specificity of lung volume measurements for recognition of restrictive disorders combined with obstructive airway disease.
3. The sensitivity of absolute lung volume measurements for the early detection of airway disease.
4. The most appropriate studies for defining normal values.

EXAMPLES

Case 1

A 30-year-old male nonsmoker with symptoms of chronic cough and mild epi-sodic dyspnea. PFTs were ordered to evaluate for possible asthma (Table 6-3).

Table 6-3 Case 1

	Predicted	Observed	% Predicted
a. **Spirometry**			
VC, L	4.63	4.86	105.0
FEV_1, L	3.76	3.70	98.0
FEV_1/FVC, %	81.0	76.0	—
$FEV_{25-75\%}$, Lps	4.22	3.14	74.0
b. **Lung volumes**			
FRC (plethys), L	2.62	3.22	123.0
RV, L	1.52	2.35	155.0
TLC, L	5.89	7.21	122.0
RV/TLC, %	26.0	33.0	—
FRC (He Dil), L	2.62	2.81	108.0

Interpretation. Spirometry remarkable only for $FEF_{25-75\%}$ in low-normal range. Lung volumes reveal high-normal FRC (by plethysmography), elevated RV, and slightly elevated TLC. These help to confirm diagnosis of obstructive lung disease. Note that helium dilution FRC is normal and hyperinflation would have been much less obvious if measured solely by this technique. Patient was treated with bronchodilators. Symptoms improved and repeat PFTs showed increase in flow rates with less hyperinflation in lung volumes. The differences between helium dilution and plethysmographic FRCs disappeared.

CASE 2

A 25-year-old male with symptoms of progressive dyspnea and a normal chest radiograph (Table 6-4).

Interpretation. Spirometry reveals low VC and low-normal expiratory flow rates. This may suggest either obstructive or restrictive disease. Lung volumes confirm definite restrictive disease. In other studies DL_{CO} and compliance were reduced. The patient underwent lung biopsy resulting in a diagnosis of interstitial pneumonia.

CASE 3

A 45-year-old male was referred for evaluation of dyspnea. He had a 30-pack year smoking history. The physical exam revealed a grade 2/6 low-pitched diastolic murmur, clear lung fields, and no edema. A chest radiograph showed mild cardiomegaly but no definite left heart failure. PFTs were ordered for further evaluation (Table 6-5).

Interpretation. Spirometry reveals low-normal VC and reduced flow rates suggesting obstructive lung disease. However, lung volumes are within

Table 6-4 Case 2

	Predicted	Observed	% Predicted
a. **Spirometry**			
VC, L	5.46	3.32	61.0
FEV_1, L	4.35	2.59	60.0
FEV_1/FVC, %	80.0	86.0	—
$FEF_{25-75\%}$, Lps	4.59	3.18	69.0
b. **Lung volumes**			
FRC (plethys), L	3.85	2.00	52.0
RV, L	1.78	1.16	65.0
TLC, L	7.19	4.49	62.0
RV/TLC	25.0	26.0	—

Table 6-5   Case 3

	Predicted	Observed	% Predicted
a. **Spirometry**			
VC, L	4.85	3.89	80.0
FEV_1, L	3.64	2.43	67.0
FEV_1/FVC, %	75.0	70.0	—
$FEF_{25-75\%}$, Lps	3.62	1.50	41.0
b. **Lung volumes**			
TLC (plethys), L	6.73	5.85	87.0
FRC, L	3.70	3.68	99.0
RV, L	2.10	1.96	93.0
RV/TLC, %	31.0	34.0	

normal limits without expected hyperinflation. This suggests combined obstructive and restrictive disease. The patient underwent cardiac catheterization for further evaluation. This showed normal LV function and mean Pulmonary artery wedge pressure of 25. On this basis, he was treated more aggressively for left heart failure and was not given bronchodilators. A repeat PFT was done 3 weeks later revealing results as shown in Table 6-6.

Interpretation.   Increase in VC, expiratory flow rates, and lung volumes and consistent with improvement in left heart failure. Heart failure may show features of both restrictive and obstructive disease. In this case, lung volumes measurements initially suggested that restrictive disease was present and helped direct therapy. Changes on repeat testing helped to confirm diagnosis. The patient was symptomatically improved. Serial PFT may be useful in following this patient's cardiac status noninvasively.

Table 6-6   Case 3 Repeat of PFT

	Predicted	Observed	% Predicted
a. **Spirometry**			
VC, L	4.85	4.45	92.0
FEV_1, L	3.64	4.01	110.0
FEV_1/FVC, %	75.0	90.0	—
$FEF_{25-75\%}$, Lps	3.62	2.18	78.0
b. **Lung volumes**			
TLC (plethys), L	6.73	6.41	95.0
FRC, L	3.70	3.92	106.0
RV, L	2.10	2.08	99.0
RV/TLC	31.0	32.0	

REFERENCES

1. Murray JF: *The Normal Lung.* Philadelphia, W.B. Saunders Co, 1976, p 87–88.
2. Leith DE, Mead J: Mechanisms determining residual volume of the lungs in normal subjects. *J Appl Physiol* 23:221–227; 1967
3. Zarins LP, Clausen JL: Pulmonary function testing: Guidelines and controversies, New York, Academic Press, 1982, Chaps. 13–15.
4. Mitchell MM, Renzetti AD Jr: Evaluations of a single breath method of measuring total lung capacity. *Am Rev Respir Dis* 97:571–580, 1968.
5. VanKessel AL: *In Pulmonary Function Testing: Guidelines and Controversies,* Clausen J (ed). New York, Academic Press, 1982, Chap. 16.
6. Barnhard HJ, Pierce JA, Joyce JW, et al.: Roentgenographic determination of total lung capacity. *Am J Med* 28:51–60, 1960
7. Barrett WA, Clayton PD, Lambson CR, et al.: Computerized roentgenographic determination of total lung capacity. *Am Rev Respir Dis* 113:239–244, 1976.
8. Harris TR, Pratt PC, Kilburn KH: Total lung capacity measured by roentgenograms. *Am J Med* 50:756–763, 1971.
9. Miller RD, Offord KP: Roentgenologic determination of total lung capacity. *Mayo Clin Proc* 55:694–699, 1980.
10. Nicklaus TM, Watanabe S, Mitchell MM, et al.: Roentgenologic, physiologic and structural estimations of the total lung capacity in normal and emphysematous subjects. *Am J Med* 42:547–553, 1967.
11. Ferris BG: Epidemiology standardization project. *Am Rev Resp Dis* 118:80 and appendix p. 104, 1978.
12. Sterk PJ, Quanjer PH, Vandermass LLJ, et al.: The validity of the single-breath nitrogen determination of residual volume. *Bull Europ Physiopath Resp* 16:195–213, 1980.
13. Rodarte JR, Hyatt RE, Westbrook PR: Determination of lung volume by single and multiple breath nitrogen washout. *Am Rev Resp Div* 114:131–136, 1976.
14. Lloyd HM, String TS, Dubois AB: Radiographic and plethysmographic determination of total lung capacity. *Radiology* 86:7–14, 1966.
15. Shore S, Milic-Emili J, Martin JG: Reassessment of body plethysmographic techniques for the measurement of thoracic gas volume in asthmatics. *Am Rev Resp Dis* 126:515–520, 1982.
16. Rodenstein DO, Staneson DC: Frequency dependance of plethysmographic volume in healthy and asthmatic subjects. *J Appl Physiol* 54:159–165, 1983.
17. Clausen JL, Zarins L, Ries A: Measurements of abnormal increases of pulmonary tissue in restrictive lung disease. *Am Rev Resp Dis* 117:322, 1978.
18. Crapo RO, Montague T, Armstrong J: Inspiratory lung volume achieved on routine chest films. *Invest Radiol* 14:137–140, 1979.
19. Wade OL, Gilson JC: The effect of posture on diaphragmatic movement and vital capacity in normal subjects with a note on spirometry as an aid in determining radiological chest volumes. *Thorax* 6:103–126, 1951.
20. Viljanen AA, Viljanen BC, Halttunen PK, et al.: Body plethysmographic studies in non-smoking healthy adults. *Scand J Clin Lab Invest* 41(Suppl 159):35–50, 1981.
21. Bohadena AB, Teculescu D, Peslin R, et al.: Comparison of four methods for calculating the total lung capacity measured by body plethysmography. *Bull Europ Physiopath Resp* 16:769–776, 1980.

22. Carrington CB, Gaensler EA, Coutu RE, et al.: Natural history and treated course of usual and desquamative interstitial pneumonia. *N Engl J Med* 298:801–810, 1978

23. Epler GR, McLoud TC, Gaensler EA, et al.: Normal chest roentgenograms in chronic diffuse infiltrative lung disease. *N Engl J Med* 298:934–939, 1978.

24. Richards DGB, Whitfield AGW, Arnott WM, et al.: The lung volume in low output cardiac syndromes. *Br Heart J* 13:381–386, 1951.

25. Bergofsky EH: Respiratory failure in disorders of the thoracic cage. *Am Rev Respir Dis* 119:643–669, 1979.

26. Haas A, Lowman EW, Bergofsky EH: Impairment of respiration after spinal cord injury. *Arch Physiol Med Rehab* 45:399–405, 1965.

27. Becklake MR: Asbestos-related disease of the lung and other organs: Their epidemiology and implications for clinical practice. *Am Rev Respir Dis* 114:187–227, 1976.

28. Murphy DMF, Hall DR, Peterson MR, et al.: The effect of diffuse pulmonary fibrosis on lung mechanics. *Bull Europ Physiopath Resp* 17:27–41, 1981.

29. Bates DV, Macklem PT, Christie RV: *Respiratory Function in Disease* (ed 2). Philadelphia, WB Saunders Co, 1971, p. 277.

30. Cotes JE: *Lung Function* (ed 4). Oxford, Blackwell Scientific Publication, 1979, pp. 388–456.

31. Horn M, Ries A, Neveu C, et al.: Restrictive ventilatory pattern in precapillary pulmonary hypertension. *Am Rev Respir Dis* 128:163–165, 1983.

32. Boushy SF, Aboumrad MH, North LB, et al.: Lung recoil pressure, airway resistance, and forced flows related to morphologic emphysema. *Am Rev Respir Dis* 104:551–561, 1971.

33. Finucane KS, Colebatch HJH: Elastic behavior of the lung in patients with airway obstruction. *J Appl Physiol* 26:330–338, 1969.

34. Woolcock AJ, Read J: Lung volumes in exacerbations of asthma. *Am J Med* 41:259–273, 1966.

35. Martin J, Powell J, Shore S, et al.: The role of respiratory muscles in the hyperinflation of bronchial asthma. *Am Rev Respir Dis* 121:441–447, 1980.

36. Peress L, Sybrecht G, Macklem PT: The mechanism of increase in total lung capacity during acute asthma. *Am J Med* 81:165–169, 1976.

37. Jones NL: Pulmonary gas exchange during exercise in patients with chronic airway obstruction. *Clin Sci* 31:39–50, 1966.

38. Duffell GM, Marcus JH, Ingram RH Jr: Limitation of expiratory flow in chronic obstructive pulmonary disease; relation of clinical characteristics, pathophysiological type and mechanisms. *Ann Int Med* 72:365–374, 1970.

38a. Gaensler EA: *Lung Volumes.* Monterey, CA, California Thoracic Society Conference on Pulmonary Function Abnormalities. March, 1982.

39. Pane PD, Brooks LA, Bates J, et al.: Exponential analysis of the lung pressure-volume curve as a predictor of pulmonary emphysema. *Am Rev Respir Dis* 126:54–61, 1982.

40. Schlueter DP, Immekus J, Stead WW: Relationship between maximal inspiratory pressure and total lung capacity (coefficient of retraction) in normal subjects and in patients with emphysema, asthma, and diffuse pulmonary infiltration. *Am Rev Respir Dis* 96:656–665, 1967.

41. Vandenberg E, Clement J, Van de Woestijne KP: Course and prognosis of patients with advanced chronic obstructive pulmonary disease. *Am J Med* 55:736–746, 1973.

42. Thurlbeck WM, Henderson JA, Fraser RG, et al.: Chronic obstructive lung disease:

A comparison between clinical, roentgenologic, functional and morphologic criteria in chronic bronchitis, emphysema, asthma and bronchiectasis. *Medicine* 49:81–144, 1970.

43. Lockwood P: The relationship between pre-operative lung function test results and post-operative complications in carcinoma of the bronchus. *Respiration* 30:105–116, 1973.

44. Mittman C: Assessment of operative risk in thoracic surgery. *Am Rev Respir Dis* 84:197–207, 1961.

45. Lockwood P, Lloyd MH, Williams GV: The value of a wide range of tests in the assessment of lung function in carcinoma of the bronchus. *Br J Dis Chest* 74:253–258, 1980.

46. Tisi GM: Pre-operative evaluation of pulmonary function. State-of-the-art. *Am Rev Respir Dis* 119:293–310, 1979.

47. Epler GR, Saber FA, Gaensler EA: Determination of severe impairment (disability) in interstitial lung disease. *Am Rev Respir Dis* 121:647–659, 1980.

48. Ramsdell JW, Tisi GM: Determination of bronchodilation in the pulmonary function lab; role of changes in static lung volumes. *Chest* 76:622–628, 1979.

49. Rebuck AS, Read J: Assessment and management of severe asthma. *Am J Med* 51:788–798, 1971.

50. Cockcroft DW, Berscheid BA: Volume adjustment of maximal mid-expiratory flow. *Chest* 78:595–600, 1980.

51. Saunders KB, Rudolf M: The interpretation of different measurements of airways obstruction in the presence of lung volume changes in bronchial asthma. *Clin Sci Mol Med* 54:313–321, 1978.

52. Schlueter DP, Fink JN, Hensley GT: Wood-pulp worker's disease: a hypersensitivity pneumonits caused by Alternaria. *Ann Int Med* 77:907–914, 1972.

53. Hudgell BW, Cooper D, Souhrada J: Reversible restrictive lung disease simulating asthma. *Ann Int Med* 85:328–332, 1976.

54. McFadden ER Jr, Kiser R, DeGroot WJ: Acute bronchial asthma: Relations between clinical and physiologic manifestations. *N Engl J Med* 288:221–225, 1973.

55. Gold WM, Kaufman HS, Nadel JA: Elastic recoil of the lungs in chronic asthmatic patients before and after therapy. *J Appl Physiol* 23:433–438, 1967.

56. Levine G, Housley E, MacLeod P, et al.: Gas exchange abnormalities in mild bronchitis and asymptomatic asthma. *N Engl J Med* 282:1277–1282, 1970.

57. Vulterini S, Bianco MR, Pellicciotti L, et al.: Lung mechanics in subjects showing increased residual volume without bronchial obstruction. *Thorax* 35:461–466, 1980.

58. Goldman HI, Becklake MR: Respiratory function tests: normal values at median altitudes and the prediction of normal results. *Am Rev Tuberc* 79:457–467, 1959.

59. Grimby G, Soderholm B: Spirometric studies in normal subjects; III. Static lung volumes and maximum voluntary ventilation in adults with a note on physical fitness. *Acta Med Scand* 173:199–206, 1963.

60. Boren HG, Kory RC, Syner JC: The Veteran's Administration-Army cooperative study of pulmonary function. The lung volume and its subdivisions in normal man. *Am J Med* 41:96–114, 1966.

61. Needham CD, Rogan MC, McDonald I: Normal standards for lung volumes, intrapulmonary gas-mixing, and maximum breathing capacity. *Thorax* 9:313–325, 1954.

62. Crapo RO, Morris AH, Clayton PD, et al.: Lung volumes in healthy non-smoking adults. *Bull Europ Physiopath Resp* 18:419–425, 1982.

CHAPTER 7

Distribution of Ventilation

ROBERT J. FALLAT
MICHAEL G. SNOW

The study of intrapulmonary gas distribution can be dated to 1799 when Davy[1] introduced hydrogen to measure residual volume and gas mixing in a lung-spirometer system. Early investigators realized that lungs were not evenly ventilated based on fractional analysis of exhaled breath.[2,3] A systematic study began early in 1940 with the pioneer work of Darling, Cournand, and Richards[4] who described the seven-minute nitrogen washout test. The development of rapid gas analyzers for helium (He) and nitrogen (N_2) introduced the closed-circuit He method[5] and the single-breath oxygen test.[6,7] The use of radioactive gases, xenon (Xe 133) and krypton (Kr 51) made regional measurements of lung ventilation possible.[8]

In the modern clinical pulmonary laboratory, one of three methods is generally available for testing distribution of ventilation: the single-breath oxygen test (SBO_2), the closed-circuit helium mixing time (HMT), and the open-circuit nitrogen washout method (N_2WO). The choice between the last two methods depends on which method is chosen for the measurement of lung volumes. The single-breath oxygen test (SBO_2) is frequently used in addition to the HMT and the N_2WO because it is specifically designed as a test of distribution of ventilation and offers some unique advantages. These three methods will be the primary focus of this chapter.

Many other estimates of maldistribution of ventilation are available; they are listed in Table 7-1 and will be briefly discussed here for completeness, but details are beyond the scope of this chapter.

Mapping of inhaled 133 Xe with a scintillation camera gives unique regional information, but this test is done in nuclear medicine rather than pulmonary laboratories.

PULMONARY FUNCTION TESTING
INDICATIONS AND INTERPRETATIONS

Table 7-1 Distribution of Ventilation Tests

Test	Equipment	Approximate Equipment Cost	Time	Advantage/Disadvantage
Single-breath oxygen	N_2, meter Volume-measuring device Flow monitor	$ 6,000	Less than 1 min per test	Noninvasive Inexpensive Sensitive/Nonspecific
He mixing time	He meter Spirometer Mixing pump CO_2 absorber	$ 3,500	3–5 min	Noninvasive Inexpensive Sensitive/Nonspecific
N_2 Washout	N_2 meter Volume-measuring device	$ 3,500	7 min	Noninvasive Inexpensive Sensitive/Non-Specific
Low-density spirometry	Spirometer	$ 2,500	5–10 min	Noninvasive Inexpensive Sensitive/Nonspecific
Frequency-dependent compliance	Esophageal balloon Pressure transducers Oscilloscope Multiple-channel recorder Volume-measuring device	$10,000	2 hr	Invasive Sensitive/Technically very difficult
Wagner-west 6-inert gas	2 Gas chromatographs IV infusion set Gas collection apparatus	$35,000	3 hr	Invasive Sensitive/Technically very difficult
Radioisotope Xe & krypton	Gamma camera Isotope source Xenon trap	$80,000	1 hr	Gives regional information/ Radiation exposure
Bronchospirometry	Bronchospirometer	$ 3,000	2 hr	Very invasive Gives regional information/ Outmoded by radioisotope Xe & krypton

Any measurement of residual volume (RV) and total lung capacity (TLC) gives an estimate of the efficiency of ventilation from the RV/TLC ratio. The differences between TLC values determined by alternative methods is yet another index of maldistribution. For example, TLC values determined from the SBO₂ and that are determined as a byproduct of the single-breath diffusing capacity (i.e., a ten-second helium dilution) are frequently lower in obstructive lung disease than those measured by several minutes of helium dilution or by a seven-minute nitrogen washout, and these, in turn, are usually lower than the TLC determined by body plethysmography or radiologic planimetry in subjects with severe lung disease. The difference in these TLC measurements becomes a gross estimate of maldistribution of ventilation.

Low-density spirometry may be used to estimate the uniformity of ventilation. Here, the maximal flow rates increase in proportion to the number of breaths of HeO_2 and the efficiency of the distribution of the He.[9]

Yet another method is that developed by Wagner and West.[10] During the continuous intravenous infusion of five gases of varying solubilities, the arterial-venous differences are used to derive distribution of both ventilation and perfusion. This method has important physiologic and research applications, but is not used as a routine clinical test.

The determination of the change in compliance with increasing respiratory rates, *frequency-dependent compliance*,[11] is another sensitive test of inequality of ventilation. It is a difficult test to perform, both technically and for the subject. It has been used in the research laboratory as a standard for mild abnormalities, but is not a practical test for clinical laboratories.

Bronchospirometry using a Carlen's double-lumen catheter to divide the ventilation of the two lungs has been used to define right–left differences in ventilation for special evaluations, e.g., before pneumonectomy. Xe 133 studies have generally replaced this invasive method.

PATHOPHYSIOLOGIC CORRELATIONS

The mechanical properties of the alveoli and airways associated with disease states can cause grossly uneven ventilation. Comroe[12] lists four regional causes: (1) decreased elasticity; (2) airway obstruction; (3) check valves; and (4) increased alveolar stiffness. Even in the normal lung, gas distribution is unequal. The major factor is interregional differences in ventilation. Radioactive gas studies of West,[13] Milic-Emili et al.,[14] and Anthonisen et al.[15] demonstrate gravity-dependent regional differences in ventilation in the normal lung. The vertical differences in the intrapleural pressure results in unequal size of the alveoli and airways which vary with lung volume (Fig. 7-1). The regional differences in lung expansion as explained in Figure 7-1 are essential to understanding the effects that lung volume, mode of ventilation, and body position have on the distribution of ventilation. A second factor is the intraregional differences in ventilation. These are due to diffusion into the periphery of the lung. The work of Rauwerda[16] in 1946 suggested that diffusion was not a factor in normal lungs, though it was recognized as a major factor in disease, particularly emphysema. Subsequent studies have shown that diffusion is a factor in normal lungs as well.[17] Finally, the concept of airway closure or closing volume (Fig. 7-1) has been emphasized in recent years as a limiting factor for the exhalation of gas in the normal, aging lung, and probably the earliest pathology in obstructive airways disease.

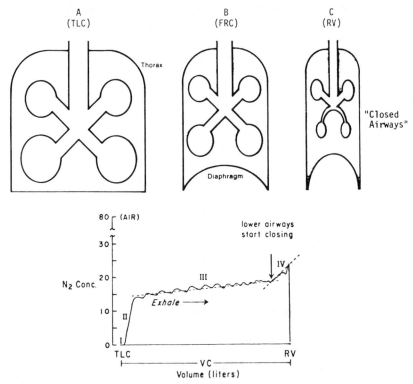

Fig. 7-1. Causes of uneven ventilation in normal lung. Due to vertical gravity factors, the air spaces are always smaller in the dependent part of the lung. At RV, airways may actually be closed in the bottom of the lung and a greater portion of the initial ventilation from RV may go to the less dependent or apical regions of the lung. At FRC, all airways should be open in normal lungs though this may not be true in older subjects. From FRC to TLC, there is a greater expansion of the dependent alveoli resulting in greater dilution of the resident gas. The apical region always maintains a larger volume and has considerably less ventilation per unit volume and therefore has the least dilution of resident gas by the inspired test gas.

On exhalation, the initial gas exhaled after a single breath of pure O_2 would have 0% N_2 as the anatomic dead space is cleared (Phase 1). There is a short rise (Phase 2) to the alveolar plateau (Phase 3) which has a low slope (less than 5%/liter). When airway narrowing or closure occurs in the basal units, emptying from the less diluted, (i.e., high concentration of N_2) apical regions predominates and results in a sharp increase in N_2 (Phase 4).

In the 1950s, McLean[18] published a series of articles on the pathogenesis of emphysema in which he stressed the importance of the abnormalities of the terminal airways as an early event. Machlem et al.[20] using retrograde airway catheters, and Hogg et al.,[21] using bronchograms and histologic studies, found peripheral airway abnormalities with little change in total airway resistance. These researchers emphasized the fact that the small airways make up only 5–20% of the total airway resistance, and therefore have minimal effect on maximal flow rates as measured by spirometric techniques. Yet abnormalities in these airways have major effects on the distribution of ventilation and gas exchange. The need for more effective means of estimating the pathology in this "silent zone" became apparent.

In a series of studies, the Montreal group[22-24] identified small airways disease in those individuals with normal spirometry, airway resistance, compliance, and chest roentgenograms, but with abnormalities of frequency-dependent compliance and A-a oxygen gradients. Studies with radioactive xenon showed regional abnormalities in ventilation, in particular, an increase in the volume at which airway closure occurred in the lung bases.[25] These tests were difficult to extend beyond the research laboratory. The similarity between the bolus Xe 133 studies and the SBO_2 test led to the suggestion that the phase 4 of the SBO_2 did represent the closing volume and would be a sensitive test for peripheral airways disease. This stimulated a number of epidemiologic studies in the early 1970s which showed that closing volumes were high in association with cigarette smoking and early lung disease.[26,27] Later studies, notably those by Knudson et al.[28] and Dosman et al.,[29] suggested that the slope of phase 3, or an analysis of the air flows at lower lung volumes such as $\dot{V}_{MAX}$ 50, are perhaps more sensitive and more specific than the phase 4 measurements. Hyatt, Okeson, and Rodarte,[30] and others[31] have demonstrated that phase 4 is grossly affected by flow rate and, in fact, is determined by the flow-volume relationships of the lung. Yet, more recent studies demonstrate that gas exchange ratio may also alter phases 3 and 4.[32a,32b]

Despite these differences and criticisms, it is clear that the SBO_2 and other tests of maldistribution of ventilation do provide physiologic information not only about ventilation, but also about the major function of the lung, gas exchange. The most common cause of hypoxemia is low ventilation to perfusion ($\dot{V}/\dot{Q}$) ratios. In fact, such low $\dot{V}/\dot{Q}$ areas are mostly due to decreased $\dot{V}$ rather than increased $\dot{Q}$. The earliest change in ventilation occurs in the small airways and is most sensitively detected by tests of maldistribution.

In summary, there is a pathophysiologic rationale for using tests of distribution of ventilation in several ways. (1) To quantitate gross defects in ventilation in diseased lungs; (2) To provide confirmatory evidence for ventilatory abnormalities in subjects with mild abnormalities in other function tests such as spirometry or blood gases; (3) To provide a screening test before doing more invasive studies of ventilation or gas exchange such as radioisotopic scans or arterial blood gas studies; (4) As a possible early indicator of small airways disease in subjects with otherwise normal lung function studies; (5) As a research tool for the better understanding of the physiology of ventilation.

METHODS

Details of the equipment and methodology for the SBO_2, N_2 washout and He dilution can be found in Chapters 11, 12, and 13, respectively, of *Pulmonary Function Testing: Guidelines and Controversies*.[33a,33b,33c] The salient features of these tests for evaluation of their clinical usefulness will be presented here.

The determination of phases 3 and 4 is usually done with a single breath of O_2 taken from residual volume using a fast responding N_2 analyzer to obtain a continuous N_2-versus-volume curve, as shown in Figure 7-1. The determination of the slopes of phases 3 and 4 is usually determined by hand, but computer automation has been reported.[34] The intersection of these two slopes determines the closing volume. As discussed later in this chapter, cardiac pulsations are superimposed on the curves and variations in expiratory flows can produce marked fluctuations in the contour of this curve, creating difficulties in reproducibility and interpretation. Many factors influence the test, but the emphasis should particularly be placed on (1) slow, uniform inhalation; (2) no breath holding; and (3) a controlled, slow exhalation at less than 0.5 liter/sec.

A bolus of another test gas such as He or Xe may be used to obtain comparable curves, but these tests are systematically different from the SBO_2 method.[35] The SBO_2 method has been standardized and used in multicenter trials by the National Heart-Lung and Blood Institute (NHLBI).[36] Even when all of the recommendations of this standardized method are followed, it is advisable to test a group of normals to determine the variability of the test and to find which of the predicted normal equations are best suited for one's own laboratory.

The He mixing time is obtained during the closed-circuit He dilution determination of FRC as described in Chapter 13 *Pulmonary Function Testing: Guidelines and Controversies*.[33c] The time is usually defined either as the time to equilibration or to 90% of equilibration. The equilibration point is defined as the time at which the He concentration remained unchanged for one minute, and did not drop by more than 0.05% after two vital capacity (VC) maneuvers. Several factors affect this time: (1) volume of the lungs; (2) volume of the circuit; (3) the respiratory rate and tidal volume; (4) the mixing pump; and (5) the efficiency or uniformity of ventilation. Factors 1, 2, and 3 are readily measured; factor 4 is kept constant, leaving factor 5 which is the measurement desired.

The time to equilibration, including the time lag of the system, has been used as the index of distribution. The use of such a simple time index has been criticized because of the great variation in the volume of the circuit, size of the mixing pump, minute ventilation, (VE), respiratory rate, (RR), forced residual capacity (FRC), and deadspace V_D. A mixing index including many of these factors was defined as the ratio of the expected number of breaths to reach 90% of equilibration.[37] Values of this index between 0.45 and 0.80 have been found for normal subjects.[37] Becklake defined a *lung clearance index* as the volume required to reach the 90% of the equilibration point divided by 90% of FRC.[38] Normal values of 7.0 $\pm$ 1.7 were reported to give better separation of normals from diseased subjects. Attempts have been made to develop an index with better sensitivity or specificity, but such is unlikely, based on the theoretical analysis of the inherent errors in closed-circuit techniques, as has been shown by Nye.[39]

The open-circuit N_2 washout technique as originally described simply measured the percent increase in N_2 during a forced exhalation after seven minutes of breathing O_2 at a resting minute ventilation.[6,7] Several investigators[6,7,40] found less than 2.5% increase in N_2 in normal subjects under the age of 60 years. As with the He mixing time, this test can be markedly affected by the tidal volume, respiratory rate, and FRC. A lung clearance index was defined by Bouhuys[41] as the volume required to lower the concentration of N_2 in the end-tidal gas to 2% divided by the FRC. In healthy young adults, the normal range of this lung clearance index is 5 to 9.[42]

Because the washout of N_2 is an exponential function, it is possible to derive many indices of efficiency of ventilation by the analysis of the washout curve. The analysis may take the form of dividing the curve into two compartments, a fast and a slow space, as popularized by Briscoe.[43] More sophisticated mathematical analysis allows determination of a distribution of ventilation into multiple compartments.[41,44] The scope of this chapter does not permit detailed descriptions of these tests, but the reader is encouraged to review the references cited.

INDICATIONS

Indications for a single-breath oxygen test or other tests for distribution of ventilation may be divided into four general categories: (1) specialized physiologic studies; (2) epidemiologic studies; (3) occupational and disability evaluations; and (4) clinical uses. Each of these areas is briefly discussed, but only the fourth is emphasized in this chapter.

As discussed in the pathophysiologic correlations, the single-breath oxygen test has provided a noninvasive means of seeing into the small airways and of perhaps defining parenchymal pathology and gas exchange. Recent studies have shown that phases 3 and 4 can be affected by the gas exchange ratio.[32a,32b] These effects are of physiologic interest, but are too small to be useful for clinical evaluation. Several investigators have used the single-breath oxygen test as a sensitive indicator of increased pulmonary artery wedge pressures and pulmonary edema.[45,46] At present, single-breath oxygen studies are not readily available at the bedside and cannot be considered as a clinical test of pulmonary edema or acute gas exchange problems. In the future, as computerized bedside physiologic monitoring becomes more common, such applications of SBO_2 tests may move from the experimental to the clinical realm. Already, two groups have proposed using N_2 washout or O_2 washin studies as a measure of pulmonary abnormalities in mechanically ventilated patients in intensive care units.[47,48]

Epidemiologic studies have been the most prominent use of the single-breath oxygen studies in recent years. The early studies by Buist and Ross in 1973[40] in a largely symptomatic group of cigarette smokers, showed that 44% had abnormal closing volume, while only 20% had abnormal MMFs, and only 11% had abnormal FEV_1. Similarly, Martin et al.,[49] showed that most smokers over age 40 years had abnormal closing volumes. Later studies by Abboud and Morton[50] show that in mild obstructive airways disease, the MMF was more often abnormal than the closing volume. In 1977, Knudson and collaborators[28] in a population study of more than 700 subjects found that only 12% had abnormal phases 3 or 4 while 17% had abnormal flow parameters; another 16% were abnormal by both criteria. These authors suggested that the single-breath oxygen study defined abnormalities different from simple small airways disease, and that its meaning and usefulness either as an epidemiologic predictor of disease or in the clinical setting was limited. In another (more recent) large population community study, Dosman and colleagues[29] found that phase 4 was not a sensitive test at all, being abnormal in 18% of smokers, and in addition, phase 3 had both good specificity (65%) and sensitivity (76%) in identifying smokers who may have early airways disease. These conflicting studies emphasize the uncertainty regarding the use of closing volume as an early diagnostic test, but do indicate the sensitivity of SBO_2 tests in epidemiologic studies.

The role of the single-breath oxygen or other distribution of ventilation studies in disability evaluation is limited. The recent American Thoracic Society (ATS) statement on disability evaluation[51] clearly states that the "miscellaneous tests of flow and volume, the FEF 25–75, closing volume, closing capacity, and volume of isoflow are not recommended for the assessment of impairment." Nevertheless, in occupational health studies the sensitivity of these tests might play a useful role in detecting the effects of occupational hazards early. The basis for this derives primarily from the epidemiologic studies discussed previously. However, the usefulness of these tests as a component of occupational screening tests remains to be established.

The clinical indications for tests of distribution of ventilation has a long and established history. In the original paper by Comroe and Fowler,[7] 77 patients were studied by both the single-breath oxygen and the seven-minute N_2 washout technique. Almost all of the patients showed abnormal results, including six of nine cases of sarcoid and over 50% of patients with congestive heart failure (Table 7-1). The current vogue is to use the single-breath oxygen test only with obstructive airways disease, but these original studies indicate that it is a sensitive test in conditions generally considered as restrictive. A later study by Renzetti and colleagues[52a] (Table 7-2) found 26% of those with pure restrictive lung disease had abnormal phase 3 results. As with the later epidemiologic studies described previously, these earlier workers showed that the slope of phase 3 is a sensitive test; it is abnormal in 26% of patients with normal spirometry and 40% of those with mild airway obstruction. The slope of phase 3 is almost always abnormal when moderate or severe obstructive airways disease is present (Table 7-2).

Why then is a test indicated in patients with known airways disease? There are two main indications. In mild disease, when spirometry and other clinical evidence are equivocal, distribution tests may give confirmatory evidence (see Case 1). When pulmonary disease is definitely present, the SBO_2 oxygen test or other tests of distribution of ventilation may provide a more sensitive indicator of response to treatment or challenges. For example, the single-breath oxygen test may provide a basis for response to bronchodilators, as shown by a decrease in phase 4 volume or an increase in phase 4 height[52b] (see Cases 2 and 4). These authors point out that phase 4 may be altered in both directions by isoproterenol because it may increase the vertical gradient of N_2 in the lung (increasing phase

Table 7-2   Test Results

	Total Number Subjects	Slope of Phase 3 > 3.0%/liter	7-Min N_2 > 2.5%
Comroe & Fowler, 1951[7]		Percent Abnormal	
Asthma	22	82	41
Emphysema	12	100	75
Bronchiectasis	9	89	33
Sarcoid	9	67	0
Congestive heart failure	7	56	14
Miscellaneous	18	65	16
			% He Mixing Time > 3 Min
Hathirat, Renzetti, & Mitchell, 1970[52]			
Normal	43	0	0
Patients with normal spirometry	62	26	19
Pure restrictive lung disease	19	26	16
Mild obstructive airways diease	53	40	53
Moderate to severe obstructive airways disease	182	98	98

Comparison of the seven-minute nitrogen test with the single-breath oxygen test, where only slope of phase 3 was measured, was done in an extensive group of patients by Comroe and Fowler, published in 1951 (7). The slope of phase 3 was a very sensitive test, detecting abnormalities in 100% of patients with emphysema and in over 80% of patients with asthma and brochiectasis. Of particular note is the fact that many restrictive lung diseases, namely sarcoid and congestive heart failure, showed a very high percentage of abnormalities, though the seven-minute nitrogen was seldom abnormal. Comparison of the helium mixing time with the single-breath oxygen study was done by Hathirat et al. in 1970 (52a). Once again, all the patients with obstructive airways disease show abnormalities by both tests, but in their series only 26% of the patients with pure restrictive lung disease showed abnormalities of phase 3.

3) while at the same time it may decrease the intraregional inhomogenities that would decrease phase 3. Several studies[53a,53b,53c] have shown effects on phase 3 and 4 from acute cigarette smoking, but spirometry was equally or, in two studies,[53c,53d] more sensitive than the SBO$_2$ test. Nevertheless, it is yet another indicator of the change.

How widely should single-breath oxygen or other tests of distribution of ventilation be applied in a clinically oriented pulmonary function laboratory? Any laboratory doing more than simple spirometry will probably have available some method for estimating distribution of ventilation. If either the He dilution or the N$_2$ washout method is used for determining TLC, then a distribution test is available from these methods. If the laboratory performs a single-breath diffusing capacity and uses body plethysmography as the prime mode for determining TLC rather than N$_2$ or He methods, then the difference in the TLC values and the RV/TLC ratio are an estimate of distribution of ventilation. One study[53e] suggests that the difference in TLC determined during the SBO$_2$ test and from the seven-minute N$_2$ washout test may be present even in the face of a normal phase 3. The difference in TLC correlates with increases in phase 3. Is it then reasonable to have a single-breath oxygen test as well? The data cited in Table 7-2 comparing SBO$_2$ with HMT and N$_2$ washout indicate that the phase 3 test is more sensitive, but the information obtained is usually complementary rather than essential for diagnosis and management. Therefore, unless the pulmonary laboratory is a referral center or involved in occupational epidemiologic or research studies, the SBO$_2$ test is likely to be underutilized and of questionable necessity.

The use of radioactive xenon to determine regional ventilation is usually not the domain of a pulmonary function laboratory, but in many situations such studies are indicated because of abnormal pulmonary tests and are an essential part of pulmonary diagnosis and management. When pulmonary vascular disease or pulmonary emboli are suspected from the history or lung function studies, a $\dot{V}/\dot{Q}$ scan is indicated. When bronchiectasis is suspected or known, regional ventilation studies can show the extent and severity of the disease. Bullous lung disease likewise may be quantitated much more precisely and the anatomic extent of the bullae can be determined by radioactive xenon studies (see Case 4). The decision for surgery in bronchiectasis and bullous lung disease probably should not be made without preoperative evaluation by Xe 133. When focal disease is suggested by history or examination, such as localized wheeze or rhonchi or a nonspecific finding such as a persistent cough, focal abnormalities such as cancer, foreign bodies, or other airway masses may be present and localized using ventilation scans. Such studies will also help to guide subsequent studies such as bronchoscopy or bronchograms.

INTERPRETATIONS

The beginning of interpretation of any test is to establish a range of normal. The test of distribution of ventilation and particularly the SBO$_2$ test, has considerably more variation than other tests of lung function. Predicted formulas for phase III and IV were given in Chapter 10 of *Pulmonary Function Testing: Guidelines and Controversies*,[33a] and are shown graphically in Figures 7-2A and 2B. It is recommended that each laboratory test use at least 10–30 healthy, nonsmoking subjects to determine the best prediction formula to use.

The slope of phase 3 is not as variable or difficult to measure as phase 4. The original description by Fowler and Comroe[6,7] found the percent N_2 change from 750–1250 ml expired volume was between .5 and 1.5% N_2 (a slope then of 1–3% N_2 liter) in young subjects, ages 18–38 years. In subjects over 50 years old, the upper limit has been reported as high as 9.0% N_2/liter.[54] Later studies by Buist and Ross[55] and Knudson[56] where phase 4 was also measured showed a lesser age effect on phase 3. There does not appear to be a significant variability with size of the subject for either phase 3 or 4.

In interpreting the meaning of these tests of distribution of ventilation, the wide variability within an individual must be recognized even when the test is rigorously done. Several studies of variability have been done that show much higher coefficient of variation in all of the tests of distribution compared to volume and flow measurements.[57] Unlike peak flow measurements where the highest value has been shown to be the most useful with the least variation, Becklake et al.[58] have shown that the greatest sensitivity for the SBO_2 tests is obtained from a mean of three values. They found a within-individual standard deviation (SD) for phase 4 to be large, ranging from 2–6% of the VC. For phase 3, the standard deviation is less than 0.45%/liter and is usually below 0.2%.

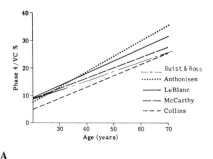 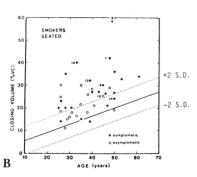

A   B

Fig. 7-2. (A) Predicted values for closing volumes. Five different predicted formulas for closing volume are shown for erect, healthy subjects. In general, there is good agreement between the various studies. All studies show considerable increase in closing volume with age.

(B) Distribution of closing volumes in symptomatic asymptomatic cigarette smokers. Many symptomatic and asymptomatic cigarette smokers have closing volumes beyond two SDs above the predicted value. Only two of the subjects had FEV_1/FVC ratios less than 50%. One of these had a closing volume greater than 5 SDs above the predicted. It is suggested that six SDs be used as the criteria for severe abnormalities. The predicted range is taken from McCarthy et al.[26]

Despite the large variations within normal individuals, these tests have considerable sensitivity and increase dramatically with disease. Because disease always increases the test variable, the 95% confidence limits in one-tailed direction can be set at 1.64 SDs. Figure 7-2B shows the range of normal values for each of these tests. From 1.64 to 2.0 SD might be considered a minimal abnormality if found in association with other evidence for disease. Based on the variations noted in smokers (see Fig. 2B), mild, moderate, and severe abnormalities could be defined as 2.0 to 4.0 SD, 4.0 to 6.0 SD, and over 6.0 SD, but there is no agreement on such divisions even with the most frequently used variables, FEV_1 and FVC.

PATTERNS OF DISEASE

Under the section on indications, two major clinical pictures or patterns are mentioned. First is the early airway obstruction or small airways disease pattern, where the SBO_2 test which may be the only clearly abnormal function test (Case 1). When obstructive airways disease is established, tests of maldistribution give yet another dimension of abnormality and may provide evidence of change not found in other tests such as evaluating the response to bronchodilators (Case 3).

Yet another major pattern could be that seen with restrictive lung disease. The degree of abnormality (or normalcy) in the SBO_2 test may give some clue relative to the difficulties in gas exchange to be expected (Case 2). When closing volume is high, above the FRC, some have suggested this is a clue to expect more atelectasis and hypoxia, particularly when sedation or narcosis is present, such as postoperatively.

PITFALLS AND LIMITATIONS

The major pitfall in the SBO_2 test is in the methodology. The wide coefficient of variation already noted can be even more exaggerated if careful attention is not paid to inspiratory or expiratory flow rates and breath holding. Phase 4 may be absent in young individuals and may not be evident in some subjects with severe obstructive airways disease when phase 3 is already so high. Perhaps the major pitfall is to expect a high phase 3 and 4 in all patients with obstructive airways disease. In a series of 202 patients, we found a surprising lack of correlation between airway obstruction and phase 4, but a good correlation with phase 3, as shown in Figure 7-3. Many patients with significant airway obstruction (e.g., $FEF_{25-75\%}$ less than 2 liter/sec) still had normal closing volumes (Fig. 7-3).

CONTROVERSIES

Major controversies in this field concern the usefulness and meaning of phase 4. Does it really represent a closed airway? Is it solely affected by airway disease or are other factors of equal or greater importance? Most important, does it really indicate the beginning of a progressive disease process? The study of Knudson and Lebowitz[28] found poor concordance between phase 4 and low

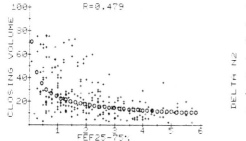 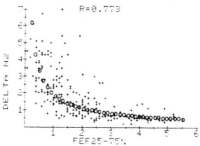

Fig. 7-3. Correlation of closing volume and slope of Phase 3 (Delta N_2) with MMF ($FEF_{25-75\%}$). In a series of 38 normal subjects and 202 patients done in our clinical pulmonary function laboratory, we found a relatively good geometric correlation ($r = .773$) between the slope of phase 3 and MMF, and a poorer correlation ($r = 0.479$) between closing volume and MMF. A number of subjects with clearly abnormal MMF have normal closing volumes.

flow rates; these authors suggested that phase 4 is "an answer in search of a question."

As stated in the NHLI workshop,[36] "although CV and CC are sensitive tests, they are probably of low specificity and moderate precision, and their validity as a diagnostic test is unknown." Little has changed since 1973 to alter this conclusion.

CASE 1 (FIGURE 7-4)

A 54-year-old female smoker (65 packs a year) presents normal volumes and normal FEV_1, but a curved flow-volume loop, a borderline abnormal $FEF_{25-75\%}$ and a distinctly low $F_{75\%}$. Confirmation of the airways disease is seen in the distribution of ventilation studies. The helium mixing time is prolonged at 3.5 minutes; closing volume is increased at 28.5% of the VC; and the slope of phase 3 is markedly elevated at 4.8%/liter. Despite the definite presence of small airway obstruction, the TLCs measured by the various methods agree quite well.

CASE 2 (FIGURE 7-5)

A 52-year-old male with a minimal smoking history, but with industrial exposure presents. The VC is definitely reduced and the TLC, though normal, is low, suggesting restrictive lung disease. Mild but definite airway obstruction is indicated by the low FEV_1/FVC ratio and more markedly reduced $FEF_{25-75\%}$ and $F_{75\%}$. Distribution of ventilation studies confirm that there is a response to bronchodilators, as seen by the marked decrease in the closing volume that is high prebronchodilator. The slope of phase 3 declines somewhat, though this may go in either direction following bronchodilators. Note also the difference in the TLCs, the highest being from the body plethysmograph at 5.3 liters; by neon

Fig. 7-4   Volumes for patient discussed in case 1. Age: 54; Height: 166 Cm; Weight: 66.2 Kg; Sex: F; Smoking history: 65 Pk Yrs

		Predicted	Observed	% Pred
Vital Capacity	L	3.1	2.9	(93)
Residual Volume	L	2.1	2.3	(109)
Total Lung Cap (Pleth)	L	5.2	5.2	(100)
RV/TLC	%	40.0	44.0	
Forced Exp Vol (FEV$_1$)	L	2.6	2.2	(83)
Forced Vital Cap (FVC)	L	3.1	2.9	(93)
FEV$_1$/FVC	%	75.0	75.0	
Forced Exp Flow (FEF$_{max}$)	L/S	7.2	5.4	(74)
Forced Exp Flow (FEF$_{25-75\%}$)	L/S	2.4	1.6	(68)
Flow at 75% FVC (F$_{75\%}$)	L/S	1.1	0.5	(44)
Airway Resistance (TLC = 5.2)		<2.5	2.5	
Diffusing Capacity (TLC = 5.0)		25.0	21.7	(87)
Closing Volume (TLC = 5.0)		18.6%	28.5	(High)
Slope of Phase 3		<3.0%/liter	4.8	
Helium Mixing Time (TLC = 5.1)		<3.0 min	3.5	

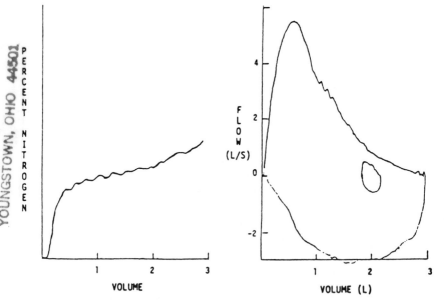

dilution during the diffusing capacity the TLC was 4.9 liters; and the single-breath oxygen study measured the TLC at 4.2 liters.

CASE 3 (FIGURE 7-6)

Severe restrictive lung disease is clearly indicated by the low volumes. No significant airway obstruction is present, as seen by the high FEV$_1$/FVC ratio, the high peak flow rate, and the lack of significant curvature to the flow volume loop. Despite the absence of airway obstruction and the seemingly pure restrictive disease, note that the distribution of ventilation studies show abnormalities.

Fig. 7-5 Volumes for patient discussed in case 2. Age: 52; Height: 175 Cm; Weight: 79.4 Kg; Sex: M; Smoking history: 2 Pk Yrs; Quit 7 Yrs

		Predicted	Obser	% Pred	Post Obser	Isoproterenol % Pred
Vital Capacity	L	4.4	2.9	(64)	3.2	(71)
Residual Volume	L	1.9	2.2	(114)	2.1	(110)
Total Lung Cap (Pleth)	L	6.3	5.3	(83)	5.3	(83)
RV/TLC	%	30.0	41.0		40.0	
Forced Exp Vol (FEV₁)	L	3.4	2.2	(63)	2.4	(71)
Forced Vital Cap (FVC)	L	4.4	3.1	(70)	3.2	(71)
FEV₁/FVC	%	79.0	70.0		77.0	
Forced Exp Flow (FEF$_{max}$)	L/S	8.6	5.5	(64)	5.1	(59)
Forced Exp Flow (FEF$_{25-75\%}$)	L/S	3.5	1.5	(42)	2.3	(65)
Flow at 75% FVC (F$_{75\%}$)	L/S	1.4	0.5	(35)	0.8	(62)
Airway Resistance (TLC = 5.3)		<2.5	1.2		1.0	
Diffusing Capacity (TLC = 4.9)		25.0	22.8	(92)		
Closing Volume (TLC = 4.2)		19.0%	32.7		17.2	
Slope of Phase 3		<3.0%/l	2.5		2.2	

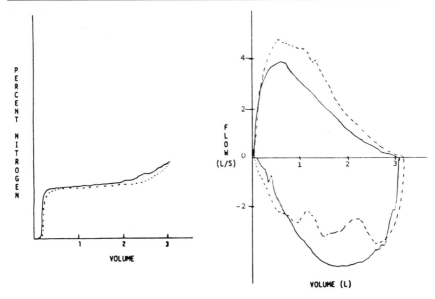

The helium mixing time is normal at 2.5 minutes, but in this patient it is probably due to her hyperventilation with a high respiratory rate and chronic hyperventilation, as indicated by the low PCO_2 and high pH. The single-breath oxygen tests indicate maldistribution of ventilation in that the slope of phase III is high; closing volume, however, is normal. Note that all of the TLCs were in good agreement for the TLC measured during the closing volume which was low; this is another indication for maldistribution of ventilation. Clinically significant ventilation abnormalities are indicated by the hypoxemia that occurred at a low level of exercise.

Fig. 7-6   Volumes for patient discussed in case 3. Age: 66; Height: 171 Cm; Weight: 65.3 Kg; Sex: F

		Predicted	Observed	% Pred
Vital Capacity	L	3.6	1.2	(33)
Residual Volume	L	2.4	1.4	(59)
Total Lung Cap (Pleth)	L	6.0	2.6	(43)
RV/TLC	%	40.0	54.0	
Forced Exp Vol (FEV$_1$)	L	2.6	0.9	(35)
Forced Vital Cap (FVC)	L	3.6	1.1	(30)
FEV$_1$/FVC	%	70.0	82.0	
Forced Exp Flow (FEF$_{max}$)	L/S	6.6	5.0	(66)
Forced Exp Flow (FEF$_{25-75\%}$)	L/S	1.9	1.6	(83)
Flow at 75% FVC (F$_{75\%}$)	L/S	0.9	0.3	(33)
Airway Resistance (TLC = 2.6)		<2.5	0.8	(32)
Diffusing Capacity (TLC = 2.5)		26.8	16.5	(56)
Closing Volume (TLC = 2.1)		22.1%	15.2	(69)
Slope of Phase 3		<3.0%/liter	3.3	
Helium Mixing Time (TLC = 2.6)		<3.0 min	2.5 min	

Arterial Blood Gases		PH	PCO$_2$	PQ$_2$	SAT %	HCO$_3$
Rest	Room Air	7.44	32	84	96.6%	21.9
Exercise	Room Air	7.37	40	56	88.5%	23.2

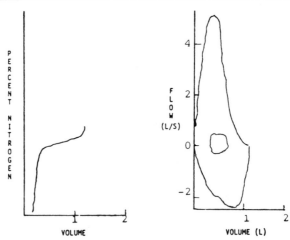

CASE 4 (FIGURE 7-7A and 7-7B)

A 50-year-old female has progressively enlarging bullous lung disease, as seen on the accompanying ventilation and perfusion scans, showing markedly diminished ventilation and perfusion to the left lower lobe. Characteristic reduction in VC associated with overinflated RV and TLC is present. There is severe airway obstruction, indicated by the low FEV$_1$/FVC ratio and low peak flow rates. Marked curvature of the flow-volume loop is seen and there is minimal flow response to bronchodilators, though the VC does improve by 300 cc. Airway resistance likewise is high and falls slightly following bronchodilators. Three different distributions of ventilation studies were performed. The helium

Fig. 7-7 (A) Volumes for patient discussed in case 4. (B) VP scan for patient discussed in Case 4. Age: 50; Height: 162 Cm; Weight: 63.1 Kg; Sex: F; Smoking history: 30 Pk Yrs; Quit 2 Yrs

		Predicted	Obser	% Pred	Post Obser	Dilation % Pred
Vital Capacity	L	2.9	2.1	(71)		
Residual Volume	L	1.7	2.2	(125)		
Func Resid Cap	L	2.7	4.4	(163)		
Total Lung Cap (Pleth)	L	4.7	6.8	(145)		
RV/TLC	%	38.0	52.0			
Forced Exp Vol (FEV$_1$)	L	2.5	0.9	(34)	1.1	(45)
Forced Vital Cap (FVC)	L	2.9	1.8	(61)	2.1	(72)
FEV$_1$/FVC	%	86.0	49.0		50.0	
Forced Exp Flow (FEF$_{max}$)	L/S	4.2-6.2	1.4	(low)	0.8	(low)
Forced Exp Flow (FEF$_{25-75\%}$)	L/S	2.9-6.6	3.3		5.1	
Flow at 75% FVC (F$_{75\%}$)			0.2		0.2	
Airway Resistance (TLC = 6.8)		<2.5	3.1		2.7	
Diffusing Capacity (TLC = 4.8)		24.7	19.7	(79)		
Closing Volume (TLC = 3.8)		12.6-22.4%	17.1		15.2	
Slope of Phase 3		<3.0%/1	3.4		3.2	
Helium Mixing Time (TLC = 4.4)		<3.0 min	3.0			
7 Minute Nitrogen (TLC = 6.1)		<2.5%	4.0			
Lung Clearance Index		<10.0	15.3			

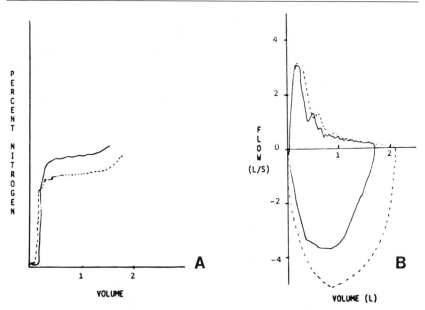

mixing time was normal in this patient, only three minutes, presumably because the bullous communicated so little with the airways. Likewise, the single-breath oxygen study showed a normal closing volume and the slope of phase III was only slightly above normal. The seven-minute N$_2$ washout study, however, showed a distinctly abnormal seven-minute expired nitrogen of 4% because the

9/76 BEFORE BULLECTOMY

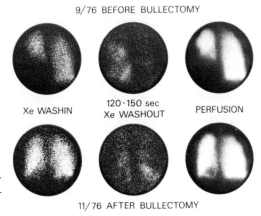

Xe WASHIN   120-150 sec   PERFUSION
                   Xe WASHOUT

Fig. 7-8. Ventilation and perfusion scans before and after bullectomy.

11/76 AFTER BULLECTOMY

poorly ventilated bullous did contribute nitrogen done on forced exhalation. The lung clearance index calculated from the minute volume required to reach an end tidal nitrogen of 2% divided by the FRC (method of Bouhuys[41]) was abnormally increased. Note the marked differences in the TLCs by the several methodologies: body plethysmography the TLC was 6.8 liters; the prolonged N_2 washout gave a TLC of 6.2 liters; whereas the diffusing capacity and helium mixing time gave TLCs of 4.8 and 4.4 liters; and finally, the single-breath oxygen gave only 3.8 liters. Note also that the closing volume is normal despite the severity of the airway obstruction. Postbronchodilators, the closing volume, and slope of phase 3 decreased slightly.

REFERENCES

1. Davy H: *Researches Chemical and Philosophical, Chiefly Concerning Nitrous Oxide, or Nephlogisticated Nitrous Air, and its Respiration*. London, Johnson, 1800.
2. Krogh A, Lindhard J: The volume of the dead space in breathing and the mixing of gases in the lungs of man. *J Physiol* (Lond) 51:59–90, 1917.
3. Roelsen E: Fractional analysis of alveolar air after inspiration of hydrogen as a method for the determination of the distribution of inspired air in the lungs. *Acta Med Scand* 95:452–482, 1938.
4. Darling RC, Cournand A, Richards DW: Studies on intrapulmonary mixture of gases. V. Forms of inadequate ventilation in normal and emphysematous lungs, analyzed by means of breathing pure oxygen. *J Clin Invest* 23-55–67, 1944.
5. Meneely GR, Kaltreider NL: The volume of the lung determined by helium dilution: Description of the method and comparison with other procedures. *J Clin Invest* 28:129–139, 1949.
6. Fowler WS: Lung function studies. III. Uneven pulmonary ventilation in normal subjects and in patients with pulmonary disease. *J Appl Physiol* 2:283–299, 1949.

7. Comroe JH Jr, Fowler WS: Lung function studies: IV Detection of uneven alveolar ventilation during a single breath of oxygen. *Am J Med* 10:408–413, 1951.

8. Ball WC Jr, Stewart PB, Newsham LGS, et al.: Regional pulmonary function studied with Xe[133]. *J Clin Invest* 41:519–531, 1962.

9. Fairshter RD, Wilson AF: Volume of isoflow: effect of distribution of ventilation. *J Appl Physiol* 43:807–811, 1977.

10. Wagner P, Saltzman H, West J: Measurements of continuous distribution of ventilation-perfusion ratios. *J Appl Physiol* 36:588–605, 1974.

11. Woolcock AJ, Vincent NJ, Macklem PT: Frequency dependence of compliance as a test for obstruction in the small airways. *J Clin Invest* 48:1097–1106, 1969.

12. Comroe JH Jr, Forster RE, Dubois AB, et al.: *The Lung*. New York, Year Book Medical Publishers, Inc, 1962.

13. Zardini R, West JB: Topographical distribution of ventilation in isolated lung. *J Appl Physiol* 21:794–802, 1966.

14. Milic-Emili J, Henderson JAM, Dolovich MB, et al.: Regional distribution of inspired gas in the lung. *J Appl Physiol* 21:749–759, 1966.

15. Anthonisen NR, Milic-Emili J: Distribution of pulmonary perfusion in erect man. *J Appl Physiol* 21:760–766, 1966.

16. Rauwerda PE: Unequal ventilation of different parts of the lung and the determination of cardiac output (thesis). Groningen, The Netherlands, Univ of Groningen, 1946.

17. George J, Lassen NA, Mellemgaard K, et al.: Diffusion in the gas phase of the lungs in normal and emphysematous subjects. *Clin Sci* 29:525–532, 1965.

18. Mc Lean KH: The pathogenesis of pulmonary emphysema. *Am J Med* 25:62–74, 1958.

19. Weibel ER: Morphometry of the Human Lung. New York, Academic Press, 1963.

20. Macklem PT, Mead J: Resistance of central and peripheral airways measured by a retrograde catheter. *J Appl Physiol* 22:395–401, 1967.

21. Hogg JC, Macklem PT, Thurlbeck WM: Site and nature of airway obstruction in chronic obstructive lung disease. *N Engl J Med* 278:1355–1360, 1968.

22. Antonisen NR, Bass H, Oriol A, et al: Regional lung function in patients with chronic bronchitis. *Clin Sci* 35:495–511, 1968.

23. Brown R, Woolcock AJ, Vincent NJ, et al: Physiological effects of experimental airway obstruction with beads. *J Appl Physiol* 27:328–335, 1969.

24. Levine GE, Housley E, MacLeod PT: Gas exchange abnormalities in mild bronchitis and asymptomatic asthma. *N Eng J Med* 282:1277–1282, 1970.

25. Dollfuss RE, Milic-Emili J, Bates DV: Regional ventilation of the lung, studied with boluses of [133]xenon. *Respir Physiol* 2:234–246, 1967.

26. McCarthy DS, Spenser R, Greene R, et al.: Measurement of "closing volume" as a simple and sensitive test for early detection of small airway disease. *Am J Med* 52:747–753, 1972.

27. Buist AS, Van Fleet DL, Ross BB: A comparison of conventional spirometric tests and the test of closing volume in an emphysema screening center. *Am Rev Respir Dis* 107:735–743, 1973.

28. Knudson RJ, Lebowitz MD: Comparison of flow-volume and closing volume variables in a random population. *Am Rev Respir Dis* 116:1039–1045, 1977.

29. Dosman JA, Cotton DJ, Graham BL, et al.: Sensitivity and specificity of early diagnostic tests of lung function in smokers. *Chest* 79:6–11, 1981.

30.   Hyatt RE, Okeson GC, Rodarte JR: Influence of expiratory flow limitation on the pattern of lung emptying in normal man. *J Appl Physiol* 35:411–419, 1973.

31.   Basoff MA, Ingram RH, Schilder DP: Effect of expiratory flow rate on N_2 concentration vs. volume relationship. *J Appl Physiol* 23:895–901, 1967.

32a.   Cormier Y, Belanger J: Contribution of gas exchange to slope of Phase III of the single breath N_2 test. *J Appl Physiol* 50:1156–1160, 1981.

32b.   Van Liew H, Arieli R: Exchanges of oxygen and carbon dioxide alter inert gas pattern in single-breath tests. *J Appl Physiol* 50:487–492, 1981.

33a.   Gold PM: Single breath nitrogen test for determination of closing volume and assessment of uniformity of alveolar ventilation, in Clausen J (ed): *Pulmonary Function Testing: Guidelines and Controversies.* New York, Academic Press, chapter 11, 1982.

33b.   Zarins LP: Closed circuit helium dilution method of lung volume measurement, in Clausen J (ed): *Pulmonary Function Testing: Guidelines and Controversies.* New York, Academic Press, chapter 13, 1982.

34.   Craven N, Sidwall G, West P, et al: Computer analysis of the single breath nitrogen washout curve. *Am Rev Resp Dis* 113:445–449, 1976.

35.   Kaneko L: Simultaneous helium and nitrogen single breath washout: Lung model simulation. *J Appl Physiol* 44:499–506, 1978.

36.   National Heart and Lung Institute. *Suggested Standardized Procedures for Closing Volume Determinations* (*Nitrogen Method*). Bethesda, Division of Lung Diseases, 1973.

37.   Bates DV, Christie RV: Intrapulmonary mixing in health and in emphysema. *Clin Sci* 9:17–29, 1950.

38.   Becklake MR: A new index of the intrapulmonary mixture of inspired air. *Thorax* 7:111–116, 1952.

39.   Nye RE Jr: Theoretical limits to measurement of uneven ventilation. *J Appl Physiol* 16:1115–1124, 1961.

40.   Buist AS, Ross BB: Quantitative analysis of the alveolar plateau in the diagnosis of early airway obstruction. *Am Rev Respir Dis* 108:1078–1087, 1973.

41.   Bouhuys A: *Distribution of Inspired Gas in the Lungs. Handbook of Physiology–Respiration.* chapter 29, pp. 715–733.

42.   Bouhuys A: Pulmonary nitrogen clearance in relation to age in healthy males. *J Appl Physiol* 18:297–300, 1963.

43.   Wiener F, Hatzfeld C, Briscoe W: Limits to arterial nitrogen tension in unevenly ventilated and perfused human lungs. *J Appl Physiol* 23:439–457, 1967.

44.   Fowler WS, Cornish ER, Kety SS: Lung function studies. VIII. Analysis of alveolar ventilation by pulmonary N_2 clearance curves. *J Clin Invest* 31:40–50, 1952.

45.   Rice D, Bedrossian C, Blair HT, et al.: Closing volumes with variations in pulmonary capillary wedge pressure. *Am Rev Respir Dis* 123:513–516, 1981.

46.   Hales CA, Kazemi H: Small airways function in myocardial infarction. *N Engl J Med* 290:761–765, 1974.

47.   Mitchell RR, Wilson RM, Hoczapfel L, et al.: The O_2 washing method for monitoring FRC. *Crit Care Med* 10:529–533, 1982.

48.   Paloski WH, Newell JC, Gisser DG, et al.: A system to measure FRC in critically ill patients. *Crit Care Med* 9:342–346, 1981.

49.   Martin RR, Lindsay D, Despas P, et al.: The early detection of airways obstruction. *Am Rev Respir Dis* 111:119–125, 1975.

50.   Abboud RT, Morton JW: Comparison of maximal mid-expiratory flow, flow volume curves, and nitrogen closing volumes in patients with mild airway obstruction. *Am Rev Resp Dis* 111:405–417, 1975.

51.   American Thoracic Society: Evaluation of impairment/disability secondary to respiratory disease. *ATS News*, 7:3, Summer, 1981.

52a. Hathirat S, Renzetti A Jr, Mitchell M: Intrapulmonary gas distribution. *Am Rev Resp Dis* 102:750–759, 1970.

52b. Siegler D, Fukuchi Y, Engel L: Influence of bronchomotor tone on ventilation distribution and airway closure in asymptomatic asthma. *Am Rev Resp Dis* 114:123–130, 1976.

53a. McCarthy D, Craig D, Cherniack R: Effect of modification of the smoking habit on lung function. *Am Rev Resp Dis* 114:103–113, 1976.

53b. Buist S, Sexton G, Nagy J, et al.: The effect of smoking cessation and modification on lung function. *Am Rev Resp Dis* 114:115–122, 1976.

53c. Bode F, Dosman G, Martin R, et al.: Reversibility of pulmonary function abnormalities in smokers: A prospective study of early diagnostic tests of small airways disease. *Am J Med* 59:43–52, 1975.

53d. Da Silva A, Hamosh P: Effect of smoking a single cigarette on the "small airways." *J Appl Physiol* 34:356–360, 1973.

53e. Rodarte J, Hyatt R, Westbrook P.: Determination of lung volume by single- and multiple-breath nitrogen washout. *Am Rev Resp Dis* 114:131–136, 1976.

54.   Sandovist L, Kjellmer I: Normal values for the single breath nitrogen elimination test in different age groups. *J Clin Lab Invest* 12:131–135, 1960.

55.   Buist AS, Ross BB: Predicted values for closing volumes using a modified single breath nitrogen test. *Am Rev Respir Dis* 107:744–752, 1973.

56.   Knudson RJ, Lebowitz MD, Burton AP, et al.: The closing volume test: evaluation of nitrogen and bolus methods in a random population. *Am Rev Respir Dis* 115:423–434, 1977.

57.   McCarthy D, Craig D, Cherniack R: Intraindividual variability in maximal expiratory flow-volume and closing volume in asymptomatic subjects. *Am Rev Resp Dis* 112:4-7–511, 1975.

58.   Becklake M, Leclerc M, Stroback H et al.: The N$_2$ closing volume test in population studies: Sources of variation and reproducibility. *Am Rev Resp Dis* 111:141–147, 1975.

CHAPTER 8

Airway Resistance

ANDREW L. RIES
JACK L. CLAUSEN

Airway resistance (R_{aw}) is a measure of the opposition to airflow provided by all of the airways between the atmosphere and the gas exchange units of the lung.[1] This pathway includes the mouth, nasopharynx, larynx, central airways, and peripheral airways. Total respiratory resistance (R Resp) is made up of chest wall resistance (R_{cw}) and pulmonary tissue resistance (Rti) in addition to airway resistance (R Resp = R_{aw} + R_{cw} + Rti).

R Resp can be measured by several methods. The forced oscillation technique [2-4] offers several advantages: portable equipment allows measurements to be made at the bedside, both inspiratory and expiratory resistance can be measured during normal tidal breathing as well as during abnormal breathing patterns such as panting, and resistance can be measured in unconscious patients. However, because of equipment limitations in some of the early studies and the relative paucity of studies that have evaluated the clinical usefulness of this technique, the forced oscillation method for measuring resistance is not widely used for clinical testing.

Pulmonary resistance (Raw + Rti) can be measured utilizing esophageal pressure measurements to estimate changes in transpulmonary pressure associated with measured airflow.[5] The discomfort of an esophageal balloon and the technical demands of such measurements, however, limit clinical application. Because of the limited clinical use of the forced oscillation and esophageal balloon techniques for measuring resistance, this chapter does not discuss these methods further and instead focuses primarily on airway resistance measurements made by body plethysmography.

With the plethysmographic technique, the subject breathes normally or

PULMONARY FUNCTION TESTING
INDICATIONS AND INTERPRETATIONS

pants lightly against the closed shutter and then through the open shutter and pneumotachograph. R_{aw} is measured as the ratio of alveolar pressure changes (ΔPalv) divided by airflow at the mouth ($\dot{V}$). With the shutter closed, changes in mouth pressure (ΔPmo) represent the changes in alveolar pressure during panting. The assumption is made that flow does not occur within the airways during closed-shutter panting. ΔPmo is graphically displayed on the Y axis versus the changes in box pressure (ΔP box) on the X axis (ΔP box relates to the changes in thoracic volume associated with compression and decompression during panting). When the shutter is then opened, flow at the mouth ($\dot{V}$) is plotted against ΔP box (Fig. 8-1). By recording these X–Y displays, these relationships can be represented by tangents of the closed-shutter and open-shutter angles, respectively. Dividing the closed angle tangent (ΔPmo/ΔP box) by the open-angle tangent ($\dot{V}/\Delta$P box) produces the measurement of R_{aw} after the resistance of the apparatus is subtracted from the overall resistance calculation.[1]

There are three reasons why plethysmographic resistance measurements are most commonly made with the subject panting. The first is that some plethysmographs do not have an adequate frequency response to permit accurate measurements at the low frequencies observed with normal tidal breathing. Second, by limiting the expired volumes with shallow panting, changes in plethysmographic chamber temperature that occur with expirations of larger volumes (e.g., tidal breathing) are avoided. These temperature changes can adversely affect the accuracy of measurements. Some systems can measure R_{aw} accurately during tidal breathing by making electronic BTPS corrections or by limiting the exchange of ventilation to a bag within the plethysmograph, which is maintained at body temperature. The third reason that resistance measurements are commonly made during panting is because the glottis remains open during panting. If one's primary interest is airway resistance of the lung, panting during the measurement will minimize the contributions of the glottis and larynx to the R_{aw} measured.

Measuring resistance during normal tidal breathing in systems in which such measurements are feasible offers several potential advantages: the measurements are often easier to achieve without special respiratory maneuvers, the measurements may accurately reflect the airway resistance which the patient normally experiences, and (as discussed later) erroneous estimates of lung volumes and R_{aw} that have been observed in some patients with severe obstruction can be minimized.

Because airway resistance measurement involves both inspiratory and expiratory airflow, the resultant loops can be used to measure either inspiratory or expiratory resistance. In normal subjects, these resistance values are equivalent (Fig. 8-1a). However, in certain patients with obstructive lung disease (OLD), they may not be equal (Fig. 8-1b).[6] In this situation, both inspiratory and expiratory resistance should be calculated and reported. If only one is reported, then the inspiratory value is usually reported.

In normal subjects, the airway resistance is constant within the range of flow rates encountered in normal panting, (Fig. 8-1a). In some subjects with obstructive airway disease, however, the resistance may increase at higher flow rates (presumably secondary to turbulence) resulting in curvilinear pressure-flow plethysmographic tracings (Fig. 8-1c). In order to achieve greater uniformity of test results, the flow rates at which resistance is measured is often standardized at 0.5 LPS (liters per second).

In some patients significant hysteresis of the pressure-flow plethysmo-

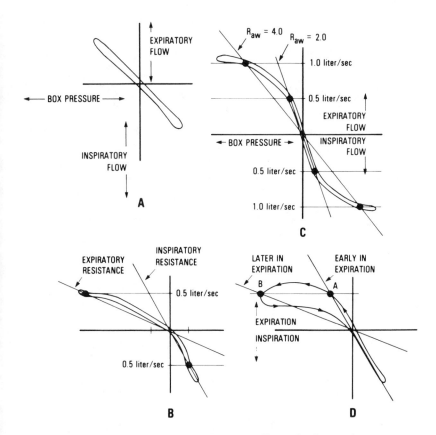

Figure 8-1. Plethysmographic pressure flow loops illustrating how resistance measurements that are measured from the slopes of the pressure-flow curves can vary when nonlinear loops are observed. (a) normal flow; (b) obstructive lung disease—low flow rate; (c) obstructive lung disease—high flow rate; (d) severe obstructive lung disease demonstrating hysteresis during expiration. (From Clausen J (ed): *Pulmonary Function Testing: Guidelines and Controversies*. New York, Academic Press, 1982. Modified with permission).

graphic tracings occurs resulting in a choice of different resistances that can be calculated. Most commonly, this hysteresis occurs during expiration as shown in Figure 8-1d, a plethysmographic tracing often seen in patients with severe emphysema. In the example shown, measurements made at 0.5 LPS early in expiration (point A) may differ significantly from resistances calculated at 0.5 LPS later in the expiratory phase of the panting maneuver (point B). One view-point is that the more elevated expiratory resistances calculated from point B represent the real increases in expiratory airway resistance secondary to collapsing airway and should be reported because such measurements will increase the sensitivity of airway resistance measurements for detecting disease. Another view is that the hysteresis represents either a technical artifact or is secondary to abnormal time constants of the relationship between pressure and flow, is not an accurate representation of the true resistance, and hence, should not be used for resistance measurements. Widespread consensus regarding the best method of measuring expiratory resistance in such patients is not available. The issues are of obvious importance when attempting to define the clinical usefulness or inter-pretation of results in such patients. Currently, however, in many labs these issues are circumvented and a single value for expiratory R_{aw} is reported which is calculated from the slope of a visually fitted best-fit linear line. These consider-ations usually do not affect measurement of inspiratory R_{aw}.

One of the potential advantages of resistance measurements for the evalua-tion of patients is that such measurements are largely independent of the extra efforts required for accurate and reproducible measurements of total lung capac-ity (TLC), RV (residual volume), DL_{CO} (diffusion capacity for carbon monox-ide) or maximal expiratory flow rates.

INDICATIONS

Measurement of R_{aw} currently requires a body plethysmograph. This is a relatively expensive instrument requiring a high level of technical sophistication for satisfactory operation. Most of the published experience regarding the useful-ness of R_{aw} measurements have come from research laboratory settings. How-ever, in recent years, the availability of plethysmographs suitable for clinical applications has greatly increased the number of plethysmographs currently in use in clinical laboratories. Based on available data and our experience, the following indications for R_{aw} measurements may be considered: (1) diagnosis or confirmation of obstructive lung disease; (2) detection of hyperreactive airway responsiveness to various challenges; (3) characterization of various types of OLD; (4) localization of the primary sites of flow limitation; and (5) evaluation of patients with localized airway obstruction.

DIAGNOSIS OF MILD ASTHMA OR COPD

Measurements of expiratory flow rates (e.g., FEV 1.0, FEF $_{25-75\%}$) using spirometry remain the standard laboratory approach for evaluating patients with OLD. However, some patients with suspected OLD have normal (or low-normal) expiratory flow rates and abnormal airway resistance. Some investigators suggest that this combination is an early indicator of OLD,[7] but this has not been a constant conclusion.[8] These findings may also represent obstructive airway disease in which the primary involvement is in more central airways as may occur in some patients with mild bronchospasm of acute onset. There is, however, a paucity of data on adequate numbers of patients regarding the frequency with which elevated resistances and normal maximal expiratory flows are observed coupled with adequate follow-up of these patients that defines the rates of subsequent development of clinically obvious OLD. McFadden et al.[9] reported that in asthmatics, normalization of R_{aw} correlated with relief of signs and symptoms of acute asthma despite the persistence of significant abnormalities in spirometric and lung volume measurements.

EVALUATION OF AIRWAY RESPONSIVENESS

Airway resistance (conductance) measurements have been proposed as important parameters in evaluating patients for hyperreactive airway responses to bronchodilators,[10] bronchial challenge,[11] or exercise.[12] However, because of the large variability of resistance measurements (discussed later in the section on interpretations), evaluation of hyperreactive airway responses to challenges using criteria of R_{aw} changes of less than 50% would tend to cause overestimation of true incidence (lack of test specificity).[13] Therefore, studies that have proposed R_{aw} measurements as sensitive indicators for detecting OLD after bronchodilator administration or bronchial provocation challenge with either exercise or chemical agents, need to be carefully scrutinized in relationship to the specificity of the tests using the proposed criteria.

CHARACTERIZATION OF VARIOUS TYPES OF OLD

Some investigators have used measurements of R_{aw} to help to separate those patients with emphysema (normal inspiratory resistance, low elastic recoil of the lung) from those with chronic bronchitis (elevated inspiratory resistance, normal elastic recoil).[14] Physiologic categorization of patients based solely on resistance measurements is of limited usefulness because elevations of resistance can occur in asthma, chronic bronchitis, or localized central airway obstruction. Conversely, many patients with chronic bronchitis proven from pathologic specimens have airway resistances that are within normal limits.

Although similar conclusions can often be made from comparisons of inspiratory and expiratory flow-volume loops, separation of resistances into inspiratory and expiratory components allows the recognization of high expiratory–low inspiratory resistance patterns so typical of advanced emphysema. Similar patterns are, however, occasionally seen in some patients with normal elastic recoil and a history consistent with asthma. The significance of these findings in asthmatic patients is not clear, but they may represent patients with abnormally high airway compliance. Although such a characterization may be useful for research purposes, it is unclear whether it currently would alter the choices of therapy.

LOCALIZATION OF THE PRIMARY SITES OF FLOW LIMITATION

Because most of R_{aw} in normal subjects is located in large, central airways, it has been suggested that R_{aw} could be useful in identifying the predominant site of flow limitation. Diseases that produce significant narrowing of the upper airway (e.g., vocal cord lesions) or flow obstruction in large airways (e.g., asthma) tend to elevate airway resistance more than diseases involving peripheral airways. Data to support the validity of this theoretical conclusion are not available; other techniques (e.g., spirometry with low density gases) may be more useful in separating large from small airway obstruction.

EVALUATION OF PATIENTS WITH LOCALIZED OBSTRUCTION

In theory, measurements of R_{aw} may be useful in the diagnostic or therapeutic evaluation of patients with localized obstruction involving the central and upper airways. If a single site of obstruction is localized in an airway distal to the right or left main stem bronchus, measurements of airway resistance will be of decreased sensitivity for detecting such lesions. Few studies have assessed the usefulness of R_{aw} measurements in patients with localized obstruction of central airways. Studies of patients with upper airway obstruction have reported elevated inspiratory and expiratory resistances,[15-19] but the diagnosis in most patients with these lesions can also be made from flow-volume loops. However, for flow-volume loops to show uniform reduction of flow rates (flattened flow-volume loop) typical of a fixed central airway obstruction, obstruction must be quite severe (e.g., tracheal lumen narrowed to 6–7 mm from the normal diameter of 25 mm.[15] Measurements of R_{aw} may offer a more sensitive test of early localized central airway obstruction than flow-volume loops and may be more reproducible for evaluating the response to therapy. Some investigators have suggested that comparison of inspiratory or expiratory obstruction on forced maneuvers (spirometry) with resistance measurements made with shallow panting may be useful in evaluating the dynamic nature of the airway obstruction.[15,19]

INTERPRETATIONS

NORMAL VALUES

Clearly, defining the upper limits of normal for R_{aw} is difficult because: (1) many of the studies that developed normal values studied small numbers of subjects and often did not exclude smokers;[1,20-22] (2) R_{aw} is inversely related to lung volume, both in the same subject at different volumes and in different subjects at functional residual capacity (FRC);[23,24] and (3) the distribution of the inverse of R_{aw}–airway conductance (G_{aw}) values within a population is not normal but skewed.[22] The upper limits of normal are particularly difficult to define with currently available data in subjects with small lung volumes.

Briscoe and Dubois[23] described the relationship of R_{aw} and lung volume according to the following equation:

$$R_{aw} \text{ (cmH}_2\text{O/LPS)} = \frac{4.0}{\text{Lung Vol (Liters)}}$$

The usefulness of the upper and lower limits of normal derived from this study ($R_{aw} = 7.7/\text{Vol}$ and $R_{aw} = 2.9/\text{Vol}$) are limited by the fact that only 26 subjects were studied and it was not stated whether or not smokers were excluded. Pelzer and Thompson[22] studied 82 adults, 35 of whom were smokers and noted the following limits of normalcy:

$$
\begin{aligned}
R_{aw} &= 0.6 &- 2.8 \\
G_{aw} &= .36 &- 1.7 \\
SG_{aw} &= 0.114 &- .404
\end{aligned}
$$

SGAW, or specific conductance, is equal to G_{aw} divided by FRC. Zapletal et al.[21] studied 65 children free of respiratory or cardiac disease, ages 6 to 18 years, and developed the following prediction equation:

$$G_{aw} \text{ at FRC} = 0.0623 + 0.138 \text{ (FRC)}$$

The lowest conductance observed in this group was approximately 0.18 LPS/cm H_2O.

In adults with FRC values greater than 2.0, the following arbitrary categorizations of severity may be used

R_{aw} (cm H_2O/LPS)	Severity
2.8 – 4.5	Mild
4.5 – 8.0	Moderate
> 8.0	Severe

These guidelines are based primarily on the anecdotal observations that subjects begin to sense dyspnea when R_{aw} is over 4.0 and that patients often have significant discomfort and intercostal retractions when R_{aw} is > 8.0.[9] Adequate data that relate R_{aw} to acute and chronic morbidity or mortality, exercise limitation, or postoperative morbidity and mortality were not found in this review.

Evaluation of the significance of serial changes in measurements of R_{aw} requires knowledge of the reproducibility of serial measurements in patients in whom significant changes in airway function are known not to have occurred. Obviously, it is difficult to collect such data; currently we have available primarily serial measurements of R_{aw} in normal subjects. Pelzer et al.[22] reported a mean coefficient of variation from four airway conductance measurements in a mixed group of trained and untrained subjects on the same day of 11.1% for G_{aw} and 10.2% for SG_{aw}. The variability that would include $\pm$ 2 SD (95% of the population) for repeat measurements of R_{aw}, G_{aw}, and SG_{aw} would be approximately 20%. For patients with airway collapse during expiration, the expiratory resistances may be more variable because they may be directly related to the intrathoracic pressures and amount of expiratory effort.

Evaluation of the change in a physiologic parameter before and after a therapeutic or diagnostic maneuver (such as testing the response to bronchodilators or bronchial challenge) usually is done for the purposes of separating subjects with disease (e.g., asthma) from normals. When used in this context, the definition of significant changes (i.e., indicating a nonnormal response) must be based on an appreciation of both the intrasubject reproducibility of the measurements and the expected response in normal subjects. Based on responses of normal subjects to bronchodilators, only changes in R_{aw} or G_{aw} over 75% of baseline should be considered significant; for subjects with baseline R_{aw} that are above normal limits, smaller changes in R_{aw} after bronchodilators may still be consistent with the diagnosis of asthma (or reactive airway disease).

Evaluation of the change in R_{aw} after bronchodilators is also used to assess the efficacy of drug therapy. Well-defined guidelines for a significant response in patients with elevated R_{aw} are not available. Changes of 50–75% from baseline are commonly accepted, but poorly substantiated, criteria for defining a significant response to bronchodilators.

The minimal acceptable change in SG_{aw} indicating a positive response to bronchial provocation testing has been suggested to be 40%.[11] Even greater responses have been reported in normals after testing the response to exercise.[25]

Although they are not well documented in the current literature, there are patterns of resistance measurements that may indicate specific disease categories. An elevation of inspiratory resistance that is much greater than expiratory resistance strongly suggests a variable extrathoracic upper airway obstruction (as seen in patients with bilateral vocal cord paralysis). Marked and equal elevations of both inspiratory and expiratory resistances may indicate a fixed localized obstruction such as tracheal stenosis, but they can also be observed in severe diffuse obstructive lung disease. Markedly elevated expiratory resistance with normal inspiratory resistance is commonly seen in patients with emphysema, but it has also been observed in asthmatic patients treated with bronchodilators. Sigmoid-shaped resistance loops (higher resistance at higher flow rates) may indicate obstructive disease (either localized or diffuse) even though the absolute measurements of resistance at low flow rates (e.g., 0.5 LPS) may be normal. Hysteresis observed during expiration (Fig. 8-1d) is, in our experience, most commonly observed in patients with emphysema but can be observed in patients with clinical presentations consistent with asthma.

ARTIFACTS AND PITFALLS

The primary factors to consider prior to interpreting R_{aw} measurements are the lung volume at which the resistance measurements were made, the phase of respiration (inspiratory or expiratory), and whether resistances were measured at defined flows (e.g., 0.5 LPS) using defined criteria in cases in which the resistance loop shows hysteresis. It is also important to assess patient cooperation during the panting maneuvers because voluntary glottal narrowing (grunting) or panting at lung volumes below FRC can artifactually elevate the measured R_{aw}.

EXAMPLES

CASE 1

A 62-year-old female presented with complaints of moderate dyspnea on exertion. Spirometry, body plethysmography, and an arterial blood gas (ABG) were ordered initially. The test results are shown in Table 8-1.

Table 8-1 Case 1

Parameter	Predicted	Observed	% Predicted
VC (liter)	2.46	2.31	94
FRC (liter)	2.38	2.37	100
RV (liter)	1.66	1.92	116
TLC (liter)	4.12	4.18	101
$FEV_{1.0}$ (liter)	2.04	2.01	99
$FEV_{1.0}$ (liter)	83.0	87.0	105
$FEV_{1.0}$/FVC (%)	2.48	2.0	81
R_{AW} (cm H_2O/LPS)	2.5	3.9	—
Resting ABG:			
pH	—	7.41	—
PO_2 (mm Hg)	—	69.0	—
PCO_2 (mm Hg)	—	41.0	—

Interpretation and discussion.   The tests were interpreted as showing normal spirometry, normal lung volumes (the RV was suggestive of hyperinflation but was well within normal limits), a clearly elevated R_{aw}, and mild hypoxemia. The shape of the flow-volume loop did not suggest localized stenosis. Because of the combination of an abnormal R_{aw}, mildly decreased PO_2, and a high normal RV, the presumptive diagnosis was chronic obstructive pulmonary disease (COPD) or asthma. Subsequent follow-up studies after a trial of bronchodilator therapy, confirmed the efficacy of bronchodilators with a decrease in RV to 98% of predicted, repeat R_{aw} of 2.4, resting ABG of pH = 7.45, PO_2 of 84, and a PCO_2 of 36 (but with minimal changes in spirometric flow rates).

CASE 2

A 21-year-old female presented with complaints of dyspnea weeks after a prolonged hospitalization for trauma, smoke inhalation, and ARDS. While in the ICU the patient had nasotracheal intubation for 11 days. Flow-volume loops, an R_{aw} and lung volumes were ordered. The results are shown in Table 8-2.

Interpretation and discussion.   The lung volumes were normal. Spirometry and the flow volume parameters were normal except for mildly reduced peak expiratory flow and FEF $_{25\%}$. Although in retrospect one could conclude that the shape of the flow-volume loop (Fig. 8-2) was consistent with localized central airway obstruction, the curve was also consistent with a variant of normal, mild diffuse obstructive airway disease, or less-than-maximal expiratory

Table 8-2   Case 2

Parameter	Predicted	Observed	% Predicted
VC (liter)	4.79	4.97	104
FRC (liter)	3.54	3.41	96
RV (liter)	2.08	1.80	87
TLC (liter)	6.64	6.50	98
$FEV_{1.0}$ (liter)	3.88	3.20	82
Peak Expiratory Flow (LPS)	7.0	5.1	73
$FEF_{25\%}$ (LPS)	6.7	5.0	75
$FEF_{50\%}$ (LPS)	4.8	4.3	90
$FEF_{75\%}$ (LPS)	2.1	1.9	90
Peak Inspiratory Flow (LPS)	5.0	4.8	96
$FEF_{25\%}$ (LPS)	5.2	4.6	88
$FEF_{50\%}$ (LPS)	4.9	4.4	90
$FEF_{75\%}$ (LPS)	4.4	4.2	95
R_{aw}, inspiratory (cm H_2O/LPS)	< 2.5	4.6	—
R_{aw}, expiratory (cm H_2O/LPS)	< 2.5	4.6	—

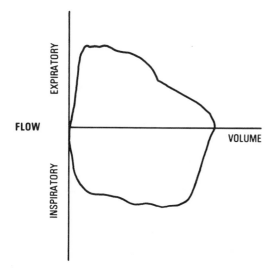

Figure 8-2. Flow-volume loop
for case 2.

effort. The disparity, however, between the normal FEF $_{50\%}$, FEF $_{75\%}$, and RV, with a significantly elevated R_{aw}, suggested a localized upper airway obstruction. Further evaluation showed a subglottic tracheal stenosis with a lumen of approximately 9 mm.

CONTROVERSIES

STANDARDIZATION OF MEASUREMENT TECHNIQUES

As discussed in the text (and in *Guidelines in Pulmonary Function Testing and Controversies*),[6] many patients with OLD have pressure volume plethysmographic tracings with alinearity or hysteresis. In such patients, calculated resistance may vary considerably depending upon the techniques of calculation. Uniformity or standardization of these measurement techniques has not been widely discussed. Lack of attention to these problems may make it difficult to compare studies from different laboratories, or from the same laboratory over time, and can thoroughly confuse attempts at on-line computer data reduction.

CLINICAL USEFULNESS OF MEASUREMENT CRITERIA RELATED TO ALINEARITY OR HYSTERESIS OF PLETHYSMOGRAPHIC LOOPS

As discussed in the text, recognition of hysteresis, alinearity, or significant differences between inspiratory and expiratory resistances may be of value in the evaluation of patients with OLD. However, adequate published studies confirming this potential usefulness are not available and such applications are not currently widely used in clinical practice. Some argue that the hysteresis observed is a technical artifact and, therefore, is not a valid representation of the patient's actual R_{aw}.

WHAT IS NORMAL?

More so than for most pulmonary function test parameters, there is a paucity of adequate studies defining the range of normal values for airways resistance, conductance, and specific conductance in nonsmoking subjects. Because of the apparent relationships of R_{aw} to lung volumes, appropriate predictive values for subjects with small lung volumes (children, adults of short stature) are particularly important and currently inadequate.

THE RELATIONSHIP OF R_{aw} TO THE MAGNITUDE OF FRC

A number of studies have demonstrated a curvilinear relationship between the lung volume and R_{aw} within individual subjects. This relationship is used in some laboratories to predict the R_{aw} expected at different FRC volumes in populations of different normal subjects although the few available studies of populations present conflicting conclusions.[20,24,26,27] Clinical experience has indicated that normal values for R_{aw} are quite high (4–6 cm H_2O/LPS) in children less than 8 years old. In small adults (e.g., a short, thin, Oriental woman) adequate data for relating predicted R_{aw} to the small FRC are not available. Availability of appropriate regression equations relating ranges of normalcy to lung volumes may increase the sensitivity and specificity of these measurements in these patients.

CLINICAL USEFULNESS OF R_{aw} MEASUREMENTS

Although R_{aw} is often elevated in patients with obstructive airway diseases, there are few studies that have evaluated the important question of whether R_{aw} measurements are useful supplements to the more simple measurements of spirometric inspiratory and expiratory flow rates for the diagnosis of airway obstruction. The anecdotal clinical experience of some centers indicates that there are patients in whom the physiologic diagnosis of obstructive airway disease would be missed if R_{aw} was not measured. Similarly, for evaluations of responses to either treatment (e.g., bronchodilators) or challenges (inhalation challenge, exercise induced asthma), currently available data do not conclusively establish whether R_{aw} measurements are useful in addition to spirometric evaluation. The magnitude of changes in R_{aw} in normal subjects may make resistance measurements more sensitive than spirometry for detecting changes, but less specific for identifying patients with OLD.

WHAT IS THE CLINICAL USEFULNESS OF R_{aw} MEASUREMENTS MADE DURING TIDAL BREATHING?

Some researchers claim that R_{aw} measurements made during tidal breathing are more useful than those made during panting maneuvers because they are more representative of the patient's normal breathing pattern.[28] Others argue that the panting maneuver is important because it opens the glottis, thus insuring that R_{aw} measurements will reflect lung airway function and not glottal resistance. In some patients (predominantly those with fairly severe obstructive airways), convincing evidence has been presented that establishes that plethysmography measurements of lung volumes are more accurate when done during tidal breathing than during panting;[29] these errors may also affect the measurements of R_{aw}, specific resistance, or SG_{aw}.

CLINICAL USEFULNESS OF RESPIRATORY RESISTANCE MEASUREMENT MADE BY THE FORCED OSCILLATION TECHNIQUE?

Although the forced oscillation techniques offer the distinct advantages of respiratory resistance measurements with portable compact equipment suitable for bedside and ICU applications, the clinical usefulness of such measurements has not been established. Areas of potential usefulness include continuous intraoperative and postoperative monitoring of patients with reactive airways (e.g., asthma or bronchospasm associated with COPD) without interruption of mechanical ventilation, and continuous evaluations of responses to inhaled challenges.

REFERENCES

1. Dubois AB, Botelho S, Comroe JH Jr: A new method for measuring airway resistance in man using a body plethysmograph. Values in normal subjects and in patients with respiratory disease. J Clin Invest 35:327–335; 1956.
2. Fisher AB, Dubois AB, Hyde RW: Evaluation of the forced oscillation technique for the determination of resistance to breathing. J Clin Invest 47:2045–2057; 1968.
3. Frank NR, Mead J, Whittenberger JL: Comparative sensitivity of four methods for measuring changes in respiratory flow resistance in man. J Appl Physiol 31:934–938; 1971.
4. Petro W, Nieding GR, Boll W, et al.: Determination of respiratory resistance by an oscillation method. Respiration 42:243–251, 1981.
5. Mead J, Whittenberger JL: Physical properties of human lung measured during spontaneous respiration. J Appl Physiol 5:779–796; 1955.
6. Zarins LP, Clausen J: Body plethysmography in *Pulmonary Function Testing:*

Guidelines and Controversies, Clausen J (ed). New York, Academic Press, 1982, p. 148.

7. Hutcheon M, Griffin P, Levison H, et al.: Volume of Isoflow. Am Rev Respir Dis 110:458–465; 1974.
8. Fairshter RD, Wilson AF: Relative sensitivities and specificities of tests for small airways obstruction. Respiration 37:301–308, 1979.
9. McFadden ER Jr, Kiser R, DeGroot WJ: Acute bronchial asthma. N Engl J Med 288:221–225; 1973.
10. Fairshter RD, Wilson AF: Response to inhaled metaproterenol and isoproterenol in asthmatic and normal subjects. Chest 78:44–50, 1980.
11. Cropp GJA, Bernstein IL, Boushey HA, et al.: Guidelines for bronchial inhalation challenges with pharmacologic and antigen agents. ATS News 11–19, 1980, (Spring).
12. Cropp GJA: Relative sensitivity of different pulmonary function tests in the evaluation of exercise-induced asthma. Pediatrics 56(Suppl):860–867, 1975.
13. Michoud MC, Ghezzo H, Amyot R: A comparison of pulmonary function tests used for bronchial challenges. Bull Europ Physiopathol Respir 18:609–621, 1982.
14. Duffell CM, Maraus JH, Ingram RH: Limitation of expiratory flow in chronic obstructive pulmonary disease. Ann Int Med 72:365–374, 1970.
15. Miller RD, Hyatt RE: Evaluation of obstructing lesions of the trachea and larynx by flow-volume loops. Am Rev Respir Dis 108:475–481; 1973.
16. Shim C, Corro P, Park SS, et al.: Pulmonary function studies in patients with upper airway obstruction. Am Rev Respir Dis 106:233–238, 1972.
17. Roncoroni AJ, Goldman E, Puy RJM: Respiratory mechanics in upper airway obstruction. Bull Physiopathol Respir 11:803–822, 1975.
18. Schiratzki J: Upper airway resistance during mouth breathing in patients with unilateral and bilateral paralysis of the recurrent laryngeal nerve. Acta Otolaryngol 59:475–496, 1965.
19. Cormier YF, Camus P, Desmeules MJ: Non-organig acute upper airway obstruction: Description and a diagnostic approach. Am Rev Respir Dis 121:147–150, 1980.
20. Butler J, Caro CG, Alcala R, et al.: Physiological factors affecting airway resistance in normal subjects and in patients with obstructive respiratory disease. J Clin Invest 39:584–591, 1960.
21. Zapletal A, Motoyama EK, Van de Woestigne KP, et al.: Maximum expiratory flow volume curves and airway conductance in children and adolescents. J Appl Physiol 26:308–316, 1969.
22. Pelzer AM, Thomson ML: Effect of age, sex, stature, and smoking habits on human airway conductance. J Appl Physiol 21:469–476, 1966.
23. Briscoe WA, Dubois AB: The relationship between airway resistance, airway conductance and lung volume in subjects of different age and body size. J Clin Invest 37:1279–1285, 1958.
24. Skoogh BE: Normal airways conductance at different lung volumes. Scand J Clin Lab Invest 31:429–441, 1973.
25. McNeill RS, Nairn JR, Millar JS, et al.: Exercise-induced asthma. Quart J Med 35:55–67, 1966.

26. Guyatt AR, Alpers JH: Factors affecting airways conductance: a study of 752 working men. J Appl Physiol 24:310–316, 1968.
27. Brunes L, Holmgren A: Total airway resistance and its relationship to body size and lung volumes in healthy young women. Scan J Clin Lab Invest 18:316–324, 1966.
28. Barter CE, Campbell AH: Comparison of airways resistance measurements during panting and quiet breathing. Respiration 30:1–11, 1973.
29. Rodenstein DO, Stanescu DC: Frequency dependence of plethysmographic volume in healthy and asthmatic subjects. J Appl Physiol 54:159–165, 1983.

CHAPTER 9

Elastic Recoil and Compliance

CLARENCE R. COLLIER

Elastic recoil and compliance of the lung are measures derived from the pressure-volume relationships of the lungs. Elastic recoil is commonly estimated from esophageal pressure[1] and is usually measured at several lung volumes ranging from functional residual capacity (FRC) to total lung capacity (TLC). Compliance is the relationship between elastic recoil (esophageal pressure) and lung volume.

It is important that elastic recoil and compliance be measured under conditions of no flow because otherwise additional pressure will be utilized to overcome airway resistance (R_{aw}). When measurements are made under flow conditions, dynamic compliance may be calculated. Static compliance may be estimated from dynamic data by subtracting a value proportional to flow from the pressure signal;[2] however, this technique is rarely used except under research conditions. Measurement of frequency dependence of dynamic compliance is another research procedure.[3] Compliance is measured under conditions of increasing frequency of respiration; in the presence of small airway obstruction, increasing frequency causes a marked decline of dynamic compliance because of the effects of uneven distribution of time constants (compliance × resistance).[3] Because a close estimate of mean intrapleural pressure can be easily obtained in the upright position by placing a small balloon in the esophagus, the pressure-volume (P-V) relations of the lung can be evaluated in patients with various types of parenchymal disease. The preferred method is to make static pressure and volume measurements during lung deflation after one or several maximal inhalations to provide a constant volume history and thereby avoid hysteresis.

Pressure-volume (P-V) curves are often interpreted as a direct measure of tissue elasticity; but surface tension forces, volume history of the lung, and the

PULMONARY FUNCTION TESTING
INDICATIONS AND INTERPRETATIONS

volume of the lung are usually more important determinants of P-V relations. In spite of this, measurement of the P-V curves is an important procedure that often assists in the understanding of the pathophysiology of many patients. It was demonstrated first by von Neergard in 1929[4] that about two thirds of the static lung recoil pressure (P_{st}) is due to surface tension forces. True tissue elastic forces can be measured only in an excised liquid-filled lung. It is commonly assumed that lung elastin is responsible for elastic recoil over most lung volumes and that the upper volume limit is set by collagen fibers causing the compliance to approach zero at high lung volumes. This concept has experimental support.[5,6] It has been pointed out, however,[7] that two observations make the collagen upper limit hypothesis untenable. First, the upper volume limit of liquid-filled lungs is greater than air-filled, and second, the upper volume limit can be remarkably but reversibly increased by an acute attack of asthma or in experimental airways obstruction. Therefore, it seems likely that surface tension force is the primary determinant of the upper volume limit, but the mechanism has not yet been explained.

Because the relationship of static elastic recoil of the lung (P_{st}) and lung volume (V) is curvilinear, compliance, the ratio of change of V to changes of P_{st} (V/P_{st}), may be difficult to define unless the range of lung volume change is carefully delineated. One method of overcoming this problem is to measure compliance over the range FRC to FRC plus 0.5 or 1.0 liters. Compliance is usually linear over this range, if it is not, chord compliance may be used. Chord compliance is obtained by drawing a straight line from FRC to FRC plus 0.5 or 1.0 liters. An even better method is to evaluate the entire P-V curve by comparing patient data with P_{st} values of a reference population, preferably nonsmokers, of the same age and gender (Fig. 9-1).

Reference values for P_{st} are in terms of percent of TLC. Patient data can be plotted as the percent predicted TLC and compared with the reference P_{st}. If patient TLC is not the same as predicted, it is then valuable to make another plot with ordinate as percent of actual TLC. These two reference curves may be combined with patient data into one plot with the volume on the ordinate. The reference curves are based either on predicted TLC (top curve, Figs. 9-1 and 9-2) or actual TLC (bottom curve, Figs. 9-1 and 9-2). Such a plot may be used to compare the entire curve with reference values using ± 2 SEE (Standard Error of Estimate) to define abnormality.

Another way to compare the entire curve with reference values is by exponential curve fitting. This was first proposed by Salazar and Knowles[8] and refined by Pengelly[9] as well as others.[10-12] The model that the data is fitted to is

$$V = V_{max} (1 - Ae^{-KP})$$

where P and V are the observed pressures and volumes, and V_{max} is an asymptotic volume above TLC that represents the extrapolation of *P* to infinity. *K* is a

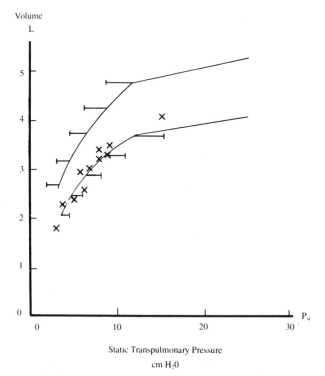

Figure 9-1. The patient points (x) were obtained during brief periods of obstructing the airway during deflation from TLC. Two reference curves are shown: The one marked P is based on predicted TLC and that marked A is based on actual TLC. The top of each curve is at TLC, each horizontal bar represents one standard error of the estimate of P_{st} at 90%, 80%, 70%, 60%, and 50% of TLC.

shape parameter that is independent of lung size and is proportional to the compliance throughout the full volume range. This model provides an economic description of the whole curve. It probably deserves further use. Pengelly[9] gives the simplest method for curve fitting. Only the points above 50% TLC can be used to fit his model.

Several references claim that smokers show no difference in P_{st} from non-smokers.[10,13,14] Turner et al.,[13] however, show a much larger change of P_{st} with age than Knudson et al.[15] who studied only a nonsmoking group. Inspection of Turner's subjects reveals that the smokers were mainly the older members of the study group. The loss of P_{st} with aging may be mainly a function of smoking history.

It may be of value to evaluate the maximum static recoil pressure (P_{st}max) at TLC. Similarly, the coefficient of retraction (also called lung recoil or coefficient of elasticity) can be calculated as the ratio of P_{st}max to V at TLC. Both of these

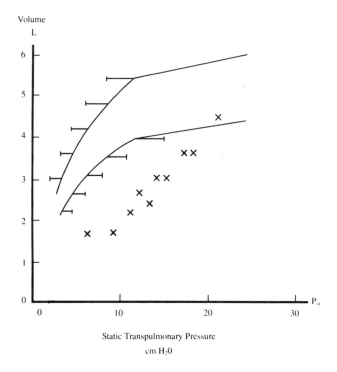

Figure 9-2.   See Fig. 9-1 for explanation.

measures are highly dependent on muscular strength and effort and, in question-able cases, maximal inspiratory pressure, MIP, should also be measured.

INDICATIONS

Measurements of lung elastic recoil and compliance are commonly used to evaluate patients with known or suspected parenchymal disease such as emphy-sema or interstitial lung disease. Measurement of the patient early in the course of the disease may provide an important baseline for evaluating changes in the future and may be indicated in all patients with markedly abnormal high or low TLC. In addition, consideration for the measurement of P-V relationships should be given in patients with abnormal flow-volume curves with decreased middle or late flow rates because the loss of lung recoil is one cause of this type of airflow. It has also been suggested that measurement of P-V curves may be useful in identification of those patients with bullous disease who will benefit from bullec-tomy by assisting in the diagnosis of emphysema.[16]

INTERPRETATION

Most individuals with clinical interstitial lung disease have a P-V curve that falls on the reference curve based on actual TLC as seen in Figure 9-1A. This type of change indicates primary lung shrinkage[17] with no change in distensibility of the ventilable lung tissue. Exponential analysis showed K to be normal in 12 of 14 patients with fibrosis.[14] Fine et al.,[18] showed that this situation could be produced experimentally by producing localized radiation fibrosis. A similar situation is seen in patients after pneumonectomy.

Only a few patients with interstitial disease show a P-V curve to the right of the reference curve based on actual TLC as in Figure 9-1B. This must represent abnormally reduced distensibility of ventilable lung. In only 2 of 14 patients with interstitial disease studied by Gibson et al.,[14] was the K value less than normal. Fine et al.,[18] reproduced this condition experimentally by producing diffuse fibrosis with injections of bleomycin. They point out the difficulties of interpretation of combination of localized and diffuse fibrosis. A progression of disease changing poorly inflatable lung into noninflatable tissue would result in an increase in specific compliance or K. Only a decrease in lung volume would indicate that the process was worsening.

Acute experimental pulmonary vascular congestion produces definite but small changes in the P-V curve with a decrease in compliance.[19] Pulmonary alveolar edema produces a marked change in compliance through volume effects. Although there are some opposite views, Hauge, Bo, and Aarseth[20] present convincing evidence that interstitial edema does not produce changes in lung recoil. The P-V curve in patients with heart failure sometimes shows a distinctive characteristic with high P_{st} at high lung volumes and normal or even low P_{st} at low lung volumes. This unusual effect is probably due to a displacement of air by blood at high lung volumes and due to an erectile effect with capillary turgor causing increased air at low lung volumes.[21]

Lung recoil is markedly abnormal in patients with emphysema. The P-V curve is displaced upward and to the left,[22] although in our laboratory it rarely is to the left of the reference curve based on actual TLC. Gibson et al.,[14] observed that K was elevated above the normal range in 10 of 12 patients with emphysema. Lung recoil can be used to differentiate COPD patients with emphysema from those without emphysema. Unfortunately, patients with asthma may also have P-V curves that are indistinguishable from those of emphysema.[23,24] However, the abnormal P-V curve of asthma can be reversed by proper therapy.[23]

QUANTITATION OF IMPAIRMENT

Quantitation of impairment is probably not possible beyond determining if the measure is normal or abnormal. This is done by comparison with values of a reference population using standard statistical methods.

Probably the best reference study is that of Knudson et al.[15] The subjects were nonsmokers that had been screened for alpha $_1$-antitrypsin deficiency. This population shows only small decreases of P_{st} with increasing age. As mentioned earlier, the data of Turner et al.[13] show a large age effect on P_{st} that may be due to smoking. Knudson[12] has recently done an exponential analysis of P-V curves and gives regression formulae for K and lnK.

CONTROVERSIAL ISSUES

There are those who believe that there is no clinical indication for measurement of elastic recoil. However, in our hands, the indications stated have provided data that is clinically useful. Especially in interstitial disease, the P-V curve has been observed to improve before other functional tests have improved.

A major problem in the determination of P_{st}max is stress relaxation. This was commented on at length by Dawson.[1]

There are a number of ways to evaluate the entire P-V curve. It would seem best to display two curves, one based on predicted TLC and one based on actual TLC or the equivalent as shown in Figures 9-1A and 9-1B. Whether exponential analysis can or will displace visual analysis is yet to be determined.

The esophageal pressure method to determine P_{st} is only applicable to erect humans. Esophageal pressure in the supine position has been shown to give a much higher P than simultaneous pleural pressures.[25] The prone position is suitable for P_{st} measures in dogs, but this has not been evaluated in humans.

The use of elastic recoil to differentiate emphysematous from nonemphysematous COPD has been questioned. In two articles,[26,27] elastic recoil and D_{LCO} (diffusing capacity for carbon monoxide) were compared with degree of emphysema. The correlation of the tests with degree of emphysema was comparable for both tests and one article[26] stated that both tests taken together gave better predictive value than either test alone. In these articles only the ratio of P_{st}max to TLC was used as a measure of lung recoil. Because Gibson et al.,[14] found that 10 out of 12 patients with emphysema had an abnormal K value, it may well be that analysis of the entire curve might be a much better discriminator of emphysema than D_{LCO}.

EXAMPLES

CASE 1

BR is a 56-year-old woman who had no respiratory complaints until 1 month before testing. Cough, fever, and shortness of breath began precipitously after she was given nitrofurantoin for a urinary infection. She had had an allergic reaction 7 years earlier when she was given a drug she believes was nitrofurantoin. The severe symptoms lasted only a few days, but her roentgenogram showed interstitial changes in the bases. There was a small loss of TLC due to a combination of minimal reduction of both VC and RV. The P(A-a)0_2 at rest was 43 mm Hg and the single-breath D_{LCO} was severely reduced to 6 ml/min/mm Hg. The P-V curve is shown in Figure 9-1B. Compared with the predicted TLC reference curve, all patient points are to the right. But all points are within 1 SEE of the reference curve based on the actual TLC. This indicates that the only change is a loss of lung volume and that the ventilable lung has normal recoil.

CASE 2

JT was a 57-year-old welder who had been short of breath for 5 years, accompanied by a severe cough with a small amount of sputum. He had worked in shipyards and in the Navy for 36 years as a pipe coverer and insulator. His chest roentgenogram demonstrated fine diffuse interstitial fibrosis in the lower third of both lungs, and there was extensive patchy pleural thickening bilaterally. The vital capacity (VC) was normal, but the residual volume (RV) and TLC were reduced. Diffusing capacity was normal. P-V curve is shown in Figure 9-2. The P_{st}max at TLC was 21 cm H_2O. All points except at TLC are significantly to the right of the reference curve based on actual TLC. This indicates a marked increased recoil above that due to loss of lung volume. This increased recoil could be due to interstitial fibrosis, pleural fibrosis, or both. The absence of a flattening of the P-V curve at high lung volumes may indicate muscular weakness, but this was not investigated further. In general, a patient with these findings would be expected to have a poorer prognosis than a patient with findings similar to patient 1 because increased P_{st} at all lung volumes is usually caused by diffuse parenchymal disease.

MAXIMAL INSPIRATORY AND EXPIRATORY PRESSURES

The measurement of maximal inspiratory pressure (MIP, P_{Imax}) and the measurement of maximal expiratory pressures (MEP, P_{Emax}) are simple, direct tests of respiratory muscle strength. They require very simple equipment and are not difficult for the technician to perform, but they require an all-out maximal effort on the part of the patient and may be uncomfortable. The test was devised by Rahn et al.,[28] and has been standardized by Black and Hyatt.[29] The MIP is commonly estimated from RV and the MEP from TLC.

INDICATIONS

The indications for measurement of MIP and MEP are to investigate any patient with neuromuscular disease that might involve the respiratory muscles,[30] to evaluate patients with unexplained dyspnea or respiratory failure, to evaluate patients before weaning from ventilators, to evaluate muscle dysfunction secondary to overinflation or chest deformities[31-35] and as a preoperative screening test.

The test is rarely done routinely in pulmonary function laboratories. Gilbert et al.,[36] report 236 measurements made as part of routine spirometry but do not demonstrate any clear-cut advantage over routine spirometry. However, Black and Hyatt[30] report several cases of neuromuscular disease that had normal spirometry but had abnormal MIP and MEP; only 2/10 patients had a clearly abnormal VC, but 8/10 had an abnormal MIP and MEP; the MIP changes were somewhat more pronounced. Maximal pressures are routinely measured in intensive care units as a means of following the progress of neuromuscular disease and to predict the likelihood of successful weaning from ventilatory support (see Chapter 18 this volume).

INTERPRETATION

True respiratory muscle force is equal to the MIP and MEP minus the elastic recoil of the lungs and thorax. This measurement can only be obtained by determining a relaxation pressure curve, which is difficult to perform except in a handful of exceptionally well-trained subjects. Luckily, such a correction is usually a small one and can and should be ignored lest a simple test be changed into an impossible test. Corrections for expansion or compression of volume during the test are also small and should be ignored.

The test is specific for inspiratory or expiratory muscles but cannot differentiate between muscle groups. Specifically, a low MIP could be due to either diaphragmatic or intercostal weakness or both. The only way to separate these two groups would be to measure maximal transdisphragmatic pressure, which is the pressure difference between the stomach and the pleural (esophageal) pressure during a maximal inspiratory maneuver against a closed shutter at RV. This measurement would specifically evaluate the diaphragm function.

Patients with generalized neuromuscular disease generally have a loss of both MIP and MEP. Quadriplegic patients have a larger loss of MEP which is sustained, but an initially low MIP improves considerably during therapy.[37]

The MEP has been found useful for evaluating the ability of a patient to cough and bring up secretions. An MEP > 40 cm H_2O is required for reasonable cough. Likewise, an MIP of > 20 cm H_2O is required for ability to breathe without a ventilator, especially in patients with neuromuscular disease.[38]

There is some correlation between MEP or MIP and spirometric pulmonary function tests. The MIP correlated better with MIF_1 than with FEV_1 or VC.[35] This is to be expected because sizable changes in MIP or MEP would be needed to affect VC sufficiently to detect abnormality. All expiratory flow rates at lung volumes less than 75% of VC are relatively independent of expiratory effort. The maximal voluntary ventilation (MVV) is also affected more by reduction of MIP than of MEP, for the same reason. Muscular fatigue and muscular weakness may be closely but not necessarily related.

Byrd and Hyatt[31] found that MEP was greater than normal in patients with COPD, and MIP was about the same as normal. When corrected for volume change, MIP was felt to be at least normal, if not greater than normal. This finding was verified recently by Decremer et al.[34] However, Sharp and others[32,33] and Rochester et al.,[35] both found decreased MIP that parallels the severe flattening of the diaphragm in advanced COPD. It is likely that the MIP measured in COPD represents mostly the contribution of rib cage muscles and accessory muscles. Druz et al. remark, "One of the intriguing mysteries of respiratory physiology is how a patient with a TLC of 120 to 150 percent of normal, breathing at an FRC greater than his predicted TLC can generate inspiratory pressures so effectively (or at all!)."[33]

QUANTIFICATION OF IMPAIRMENT

Quantification of impairment is difficult because marked nonlinearity certainly exists between MIP and MEP and other functional measures such as VC, MVV, and flow rates. If the lungs are hyperinflated, it is to be expected that MIP uncorrected for lung volume will be low.

The tests are very difficult to perform, so that one must be sure that maximal voluntary effort has been exerted before trying to interpret the results. A perforated eardrum could give false low results.

As with most other tests, the numbers are useful only to interpret the patient's physiologic state in light of clinical history and course and presence of other abnormalities.

CONTROVERSIES AND PROBLEMS

The standards of Black and Hyatt[30] often seem too high, especially for MEP. Part of this may be due to the use of a mouthpiece that cannot be held as tightly against the lips as Black and Hyatt originally designed.

Because MEP and MIP are a function of lung volume (and hence, of muscle length), it seems important to correct for abnormal TLC or RV. There is no accurate way to do this except in acute experiments in which maximal pressures can be used for correction. Some investigators prefer to measure MIP at FRC rather than at RV but adequate standards are not available.

Table 9-1   Case 1

	Observed	Predicted ± SD
MIP	68 cm H_2O	124 ± 22
MEP	100	233 ± 42

EXAMPLE

CASE 1

A 40-year-old welder, a former smoker, was seen after complaints of dyspnea on exertion for 6 months. His work for 3 years had been cutting bulkheads in remodelling the Queen Mary. The chest x-ray and physical exam were normal. He was 66 inches tall and weighed 167 lbs. Measurement of lung volume, forced flow rates, MVV, and gas exchange during rest and exercise were essentially normal except for a reduced expiratory flow at 50% of VC. The maximal pressures shown in Table 9-1 were observed.

After these data were obtained, the patient was suspected of having lead poisoning. This was confirmed by elevated lead levels in blood and urine.

REFERENCES

1. Dawson A: Elastic recoil and compliance, in Clausen J (ed): *Pulmonary Function Testing: Guidelines and Controversies* New York, Academic Press. 1–14, 1982.
2. Mead J, Whittenberger JL: Physical properties of human lungs measured during spontaneous respiration. J Appl Physiol 5:779–796, 1953.
3. Woolcock AJ, Vincent NJ, Macklem PT: Frequency dependence of compliance as a test of obstruction in the small airways. J Clin Invest 48:1097–1106, 1969.
4. v. Neergard K: New interpretations of basic concepts of respiratory mechanics, correlation of pulmonary recoil force with surface tension in the alveoli, in West J (ed): *Translations in Respiratory Physiology*. Pennsylvania, Dowden, Hutchinson & Ross, Inc., 1975, pp. 270–290.
5. Johanson WG, Pierce AK: Effects of elastase, collagenase, and papain on structure and function of rats lungs in vitro. J Clin Invest 51:288–293, 1972.
6. Karlinsky JB, Snyder GL, Franzblau C, et al.: In vitro effects of elastase and collagenase on mechanical properties of hamster lungs. Am Rev Respir Dis 113:769–777, 1976.
7. Hoppin FG, Hildebrandt J: Mechanical properties of the lung, in West J (ed): *Bioengineering Aspects of the Lung*. New York, Marcel Dekker, Inc., 1977, pp. 83–162.
8. Salazar E, Knowles JH: An analysis of pressure-volume characteristics of the lungs. J Appl Physiol 19:97–104, 1964.

9. Pengelly LD: Curve-fitting analysis of pressure-volume characteristics of the lungs. J Appl Physiol 42:111–116, 1977.

10. Yernault JC, Baran D, Englert M: Effect of growth and aging on the static mechanical lung properties. Bul Europ Physiopathol Respir 13:777–788, 1977.

11. Colebatch HJH, Greaves IA, Ng CKY: Exponential analysis of elastic recoil and aging in healthy males and females. J Appl Physiol 47:683–691, 1979.

12. Knudson RJ, Kaltenborn WT: Evaluation of lung elastic recoil by exponential curve analysis. Respir Physiol 46:29–42, 1981.

13. Turner JM, Mead J, Wohl ME: Elasticity of human lungs in relation to age. J Appl Physiol 26:644–671, 1968.

14. Gibson GJ, Pride NB, Davis J, et al.: Exponential description of the static pressure-volume curve of normal and diseased lungs. Am Rev Respir Dis 20:799–811, 1979.

15. Knudson RJ, Clark DF, Kennedy TC, et al.: Effect of aging alone on mechanical properties of the normal adult human lung. J Appl Physiol 43:1054, 1977.

16. Pride NB, Barter CE, Hugh-Jones P: The ventilation of bullae and their effect on thoracic gas volumes and tests of over-all pulmonary function. Am Rev Respir Dis 107:83–98, 1978.

17. Gibson GJ, Pride NB: Pulmonary mechanics in fibrosing alveolitis. Am Rev Respir Dis 116:637–647, 1977.

18. Fine R, McCullough B, Collins JF, et al.: Lung elasticity in regional and diffuse pulmonary fibrosis. J Appl Physiol 47:138–144, 1979.

19. Borst HG, Berglund E, Whittenberger JL, et al.: The effect of pulmonary vascular pressures on the mechanical properties of the lungs of anesthetized dogs. J Clin Invest 36:1708–1714, 1957.

20. Hauge A, Bo G, Aarseth P: Hydrostatic pulmonary edema in the cat. Effects on pulmonary blood and water volumes and on lung compliance. Acta Anaesth Scand 21:413–422, 1977.

21. Frank NR: Influence of acute pulmonary vascular congestion on recoiling force of excised cats' lung. J Appl Physiol 14:905-908, 1959.

22. Ebert RV: Elasticity of the lung in pulmonary emphysema. Ann Int Med 69:903–908, 1968.

23. Gold WM, Kaufman HS, Nadel JA: Elastic recoil of the lungs in chronic asthmatic patients before and after therapy. J Appl Physiol 23:433–438, 1967.

24. Colebatch HJH, Finucane KE, Smith MM: Pulmonary conductance and elastic recoil relationships in asthma and emphysema. J Appl Physiol 34:143–153, 1973.

25. Mead J, Gaensler EA: Comparison of intraesophageal and intrapleural pressures in subjects seated and supine. Fed Proc 15:127–128, 1956.

26. Boushy SF, Aboumrad MH, North LB, et al.: Lung recoil pressure, airway resistance, and forced flows related to morphologic emphysema. Am Rev Respir Dis 104:551–561, 1971.

27. Park SS, Janis M, Shim CS, et al.: Relationship of bronchitis and emphysema to altered pulmonary function. Am Rev Respir Dis 102:927–936, 1970.

28. Rahn H, Otis AB, Chadwick LE, et al.: The pressure-volume diagram of thorax and lung. Am J Physiol 146:161–178, 1946

29. Black LF, Hyatt RE: Maximal respiratory pressures: normal values and relationship to age and sex. Am Rev Respir Dis 99:696–702, 1969

30. Black LF, Hyatt RE: Maximal static respiratory pressures in generalized neuromuscular disease. Am Rev Respir Dis 103:641–650, 1971

31. Byrd RB, Hyatt RE: Maximal respiratory pressures in chronic obstructive lung disease. Am Rev Respir Dis 98:878–856, 1968

32. Sharp JG, Danon J, Druz WS, et al.: Respiratory muscle function in patients with chronic obstructive pulmonary disease. Am Rev Respir Dis 110:154–167, 1974

33. Druz WS, Danon J, Fishman HC, et al.: Approaches to assessing respiratory muscle function in respiratory disease. Am Rev Respir Dis 119:(Suppl)145–149, 1978

34. Decremer J, Demedts M, Rochette F, et al.: Maximal transrespiratory pressures in obstructive lung disease. Bull Europ Physiopathol Respir 16:479–490, 1980

35. Rochester DF, Braun NMT, Arora NS: Respiratory muscle strength in chronic obstructive pulmonary disease. Am Rev Respir Dis 119:(Suppl)151–154, 1979

36. Gilbert R, Auchincloss JH, Bleb S: Measurement of maximum inspiratory pressure during routine spirometry. Lung 155:23–32, 1978

37. McMichan JC, Michel L, Westbrook PR: Pulmonary dysfunction following traumatic quadriplegia. JAMA 243:528–531, 1980

38. O'Donohue WJ, Baker JP, Bell GM, et al.: Respiratory failure in neuromuscular disease. JAMA 235:733–735, 1976.

CHAPTER 10

Carbon Monoxide
Diffusing Capacity

LARRY N. AYERS

Measurement of CO diffusing capacity was developed by Krogh in the early 1900s to determine whether gas transport into the pulmonary capillary blood occurred by active secretion or diffusion. (As the name implies, the evidence strongly favored diffusion.) It was not until the 1950s that this measurement was modified by Forster, Ogilvie, and others for use as a clinically applicable single-breath technique.

Measurement of diffusing capacity gives information about the amount of functioning capillary bed in contact with ventilated alveoli and reflects the presence of certain types of pulmonary vascular and parenchymal diseases. Diffusing capacity may not be useful in the understanding of hypoxemia because diffusion limitation has a small role in producing clinically apparent abnormalities in gas exchange, at least under resting conditions.[1]

REVIEW OF METHODS

Diffusing capacity of the lung (DL) is defined as the rate at which gas enters the blood divided by the driving pressure of the gas, defined as partial pressure difference between alveoli and pulmonary capillaries. The units are ml/min/mm Hg. CO has several features that make this gas useful for measurement of DL. One feature is a great affinity for hemoglobin (Hb), about 210 times greater than that of oxygen. Thus, if CO is rapidly bound to Hb, it will not build up in plasma. Another useful feature is a very low concentration in blood prior to testing; hence, pulmonary capillary pressure may be taken to be zero.

PULMONARY FUNCTION TESTING
INDICATIONS AND INTERPRETATIONS

Resistance to diffusion is determined, in part, by resistance to transfer across the alveolar-capillary membrane (D_m) and by resistance to chemical combination with Hb (Θ and Vc [pulmonary capillary blood volume]) where Θ is the reaction rate of CO for Hb and Vc is the pulmonary capillary blood volume.[2,3] Increases in diffusion path caused by alveolar filling and edema, interstitial edema, capillary membrane thickening, and thickening as well as destruction of the membrane surface as in emphysema will result in a decrease in D_m. Reduction of the pulmonary capillary bed as in pulmonary vascular disease and in end-stage emphysema cause reduction of Vc (and DL_{CO}).

In both the single breath (DL_{SB}) and steady-state (DL_{SS}) tests for diffusion the drive for overcoming the resistance to gas movement and promoting gas uptake is the difference in partial pressure of CO in the alveolus compared to the pulmonary capillary blood. In the measurement of DL_{SB} the partial pressure of CO in the pulmonary capillaries may be regarded as zero because CO is firmly bound to Hb; thus, the pressure gradient for gas diffusion depends only on the alveolar partial pressure of CO.

Several techniques have been used to measure diffusing capacity including single-breath, steady-state, and rebreathing methods. For the purpose of this discussion only the single-breath and steady-state methods will be mentioned.

The DL_{SB} method has the advantages of being relatively easy to perform, less affected by uneven ventilation distribution, relatively insensitive to carboxy-hemoglobin back pressure, well standarized, and very useful in screening, especially in emphysema, interstitial, and chronic pulmonary vascular occlusive diseases. The disadvantages include the requirement of an inhaled vital capacity (Vc) in excess of 1 to 1.5 liters and a breath hold of approximately ten seconds. Although DL_{SB} is well standardized and generally easy to perform in resting conditions, it is very difficult to perform during exercise. Hence, only in well-trained, relatively normal subjects can exercise DL_{SB} measurements be obtained. In the single-breath test, DL is determined from measurements of alveolar volume (V_A), initial and final alveolar CO concentration, and breath-holding time. The details of DL measurement are reviewed in *Pulmonary Function Testing: Guidelines and Controversies.*[2]

Steady-state CO methods are recognized as being more physiologic than the DL_{SB} method and offer the advantages of measurement of DL under exercise in subjects who cannot breath hold or take large inspiratory VCs. Unfortunately, these methods suffer from the disadvantage that mean alveolar CO tension is difficult to measure under steady-state conditions. Two of these methods determine alveolar CO tension from estimation of dead space (VD); one method uses an assumed VD, the other uses physiologic VD derived from measured arterial PCO_2. At rest, small errors in estimation of deadspace volume (V_D) can grossly affect the ratio of VD to tidal volumes (V_D/V_t) and lead to gross errors in computing value for DL. If V_D is overestimated, computed DL will be falsely high; if V_D is underestimated, the computed DL will be underestimated but not to a comparable degree.[4] With exercise, the ratio of V_D/V_t falls (V_t increases considerably and V_D minimally) and calculated DL becomes relatively insensitive to changes in V_D.[4]

In general, the different methods of estimating steady-state DL give similar results. The steady-state methods give values of DL that are less than DL_{SB}. The apparent causes of this difference are the greater lung volume at which DL_{SB} is made and the cyclic nature of normal respiration. In the presence of uneven distribution of gas in the lung, the difference between DL_{SB} and steady-state DL becomes even larger, suggesting that at least one factor is important: the inspired gas is distributed better throughout the lung in DL_{SB}, in part, at least, because of the time allowed for mechanical equilibrium.

PATHOPHYSIOLOGIC RATIONALE

Factors altering the DL_{CO} are those due to changes in alveolar-capillary membrane, pulmonary circulation, distribution of ventilation and perfusion with respect to capillary diffusing surface throughout the lung, hemoglobin concentration, and miscellaneous technical factors, e.g., CO back pressure.[5]

Total membrane surface area is dependent upon the size of the patient's lungs relative to capillary blood volume. DL is affected by the simultaneously measured alveolar volume (V_A); changes in V_A result in similar but not directly proportional changes in DL. Testing normal subjects by DL_{SB}, Miller and Johnson[6] found DL to be reduced 0–12% when determined at half of total lung capacity (TLC), i.e., V_A. Other investigators have reported a decrease in DL of 10–25% when V_A was reduced by 50%. Patients with small lung volumes as a result of neuromuscular disease, chest wall disease, or poor effort will also demonstrate a reduced DL although the reduction is usually much less than the reduction in V_A. In contrast, a patient with a pneumonectomy will have a much greater reduction in DL, compared to predicted, even if the remaining lung is entirely normal, because lung resection results in an almost equal reduction of the capillary bed and V_A.[7] Thus, if one is interested in evaluating the mechanism of a reduced DL as a reflection of parenchymal disease, it is useful to relate the measured DL both with the simultaneously determined lung volume (V_A) and the measured DL relative to that predicted for a given patient's age, sex and height.[8,9]

The loss of DL can occur by loss of membrane surface independent of any primary change in lung volume. This loss of membrane surface independent of lung volume is characteristic of emphysema (the loss of the alveolar-capillary bed occurs as alveoli rupture and form larger, dilated alveolar spaces resulting in reduced diffusing capacity and reduced pulmonary capillary blood volume).

In pulmonary fibrosis, reduction in DL often parallels reduction in V_A and reflects a loss or destruction of the capillary bed through scarring and capillary obliteration, resulting in fewer functional alveolar-capillary units and a diminished alveolar-capillary bed. Alterations in the thickness of the alveolar-capillary membrane as a cause of the reduced DL in interstitial fibrosis have probably been overestimated, because in these diseases, ventilation-to-perfusion inequalities and reduction in alveolar and capillary units appear to play a greater role in the reduction of DL.[10] In pulmonary alveolar proteinosis, CO diffusion is reduced by a barrier of proteinaceous material which fills the alveoli and respiratory bronchioles. In chronic renal failure, fibrin deposition within the alveoli and interstitium have been demonstrated and may contribute to the frequent finding of impaired diffusion.[11,12]

The pulmonary circulation plays the major role in determining DL. The rate of the passage of blood through the capillaries has little influence on the uptake of DL unless alterations in pulmonary arterial pressure associated with changes in cardiac output lead to increased or decreased recruitment of capillary bed. Hence, increased capillary bed causes more blood cells to come into contact with ventilated alveoli resulting in increased uptake of CO. Classic examples of increased DL caused by recruitment of pulmonary vasculature are in exercise, changing from a sitting to a lying position (15–20% increase in DL),[13] and a left-to-right shunt.

Hb concentration has an effect on DL by altering the number of binding sites for CO.[2] This effect is very significant and changes in DL of 7% per gram Hb have been reported by Dinakara et al.[14] The current popular Hb corrections cited are those of Cotes et al.[15] and Dinakara et al.[14]

The distribution of diffusion surface relative to ventilation and perfusion probably plays a role in explaining reduced DL in those patients whose airways disease is associated with maldistribution of ventilation. This is more common when diffusion is determined by the steady-state rather than the single-breath technique.

In heavy cigarette smokers, carboxyhemoglobin saturation may approach 10–15%, create back pressure for CO in pulmonary capillary blood, and thereby reduce DL_{CO}. If back pressure has not been taken into account in this situation, a decrease in driving pressure and a slight reduction in DL may be observed.[16]

INDICATIONS

Reduced DL is a frequent and occasionally isolated pulmonary physiologic abnormality in patients with unexplained dyspnea due to early insterstitial fibrosis, vasculitis, and chronic pulmonary vascular occlusive disease. It is also extremely useful in differentiating early emphysema from asthma and bronchitis because the latter two diseases are associated with normal DL. Reduced DL may not be useful in determining the cause of hypoxemia under resting conditions but may play a role in the progressive reduction in arterial oxygen tension that commonly occurs during increasing exercise workloads in patients with interstitial fibrosis, vasculitis, alveolar proteinosis, and chronic pulmonary vascular occlusive disease.

Reduced DL has been useful in differentiating early emphysema from asthma and bronchitis. Gelb et al.[17] found that reduced DL correlated with severity of emphysema found in lobectomy specimens taken from patients with airways obstruction. In many of these patients emphysema was clinically unsuspected because lung volumes and airway resistance were relatively normal. Thurlbeck et al.[18] demonstrated close correlation between reduced DL in life and the finding of extensive morphologic emphysema at autopsy. In their study, normal DL was occasionally found in patients later demonstrated to have mild or moderate emphysema.

Reduced DL is found with high frequency in idiopathic pulmonary fibrosis[19] and is frequently abnormal before chest roentgenogram changes. Because reduced DL is common in most diffuse interstitial processes such as sarcoidosis, histiocytosis X, penumoconiosis, radiation fibrosis, lymphangitic spread of carcinoma, and oxygen toxicity, the test, in this setting, is not useful in differential diagnosis.

Reduced DL has been reported in acute and chronic pulmonary vascular occlusive disease.[20,21] It may not be as useful in acute pulmonary embolism because, in this condition, DL may be significantly reduced by ventilation maldistribution and reduced V_A caused by pleuritic pain, splinting, and increased regional airway narrowing. Reduction of DL is more marked and consistent in patients with recurrent multiple pulmonary emboli. In this condition, reduced DL is often the sole pulmonary function abnormality demonstrated.

In summary, DL should be determined in the work-up of unexplained dyspnea, obstructive airways disease, interstitial fibrosis, vasculitis, and chronic pulmonary vascular occlusive disease. In addition, DL provides a good estimate of the reduction of the pulmonary vascular bed and is, therefore, worth including as a test of normality in screening procedures.

INTERPRETATION

Examples of Abnormalities

Pulmonary disease as a cause of reduced DL is usually on the basis of the loss of pulmonary parenchyma with reduced, normal, or increased lung volume (i.e., emphysema, loss of alveolar-capillary units due to interstitial fibrosis, and pulmonary vascular occlusive disease); the resultant ventilation-to-perfusion inequalities attending these changes are important in DL_{SS}.

In emphysema, DL is frequently severely reduced and contrasts with the near-normal or normal DL observed in bronchitis and asthma, respectively. Thus, this test is a valuable method for differentiating patients with primary airways disease from those with the associated parenchymal abnormalities found in emphysema. In emphysema, the reduction of DL is due initially to the loss of alveolar surface area and, later, to the loss of capillary blood volume. Ventilation maldistribution plays a less significant role in reduction of DL when measured by the single-breath technique.

The loss of alveolar-capillary units due to fibrosis is the primary mechanism for the reduction of DL in diffuse interstitial lung disease. Frequently, the reduction in DL is more marked than the reduction in V_A and can be on the basis of alveolitis, granuloma formation in the interstitium and fibrosis. Reduction in DL is common to most diffuse interstitial lung diseases and cannot be used as a differential diagnostic point. Interestingly, although most investigators agree that DL seems to be a fairly good predictor of overall pathologic change in sarcoidosis, this is not the case in idiopathic pulmonary fibrosis.[19] Although DL is probably the measurement most widely used to follow these patients, it does not correlate directly with the amount of alveolitis and/or fibrosis present.[22]

A third and major category of reduced DL is pulmonary vascular occlusive disease. The reduction in DL is more marked with recurrent pulmonary emboli than with acute emboli.[20,21] The measurement of DL and Vc is reported by Sharma et al.[23] to improve significantly in patients with massive or submassive emboli treated with thrombolytic therapy. These observations are consistent with improved capillary perfusion and diffusion due to more complete resolution of thromboemboli with thrombolytic agents. The loss of the pulmonary capillary bed, as occurs following chronic multiple pulmonary emboli or vasculitis, is commonly associated with normal ventilation, flow rates, and lung volume (although the latter may be reduced in vasculitis).

The DL may be elevated in cardiovascular diseases associated with elevations of Vc such as left-to-right intracardiac shunts. In asthma, DL is often elevated on the basis of a more even distribution of ventilation and perfusion as a result of increased pulmonary arterial pressure.[24,25] DL is of differential diagnostic value in cases of obstructive pulmonary disease; a reduction indicates emphysema and normal values indicate chronic bronchitis and/or asthma.[26]

NORMAL VALUES FOR DL_{SB}

There are many normal predicted equations in the literature for DL_{SB}. The following list is the prediction equation for DL_{SB} developed by Crapo and Morris.[27] This equation has been normalized to a standard hemoglobin, using the accompanying Cotes' modification[15] of the relationship described by Roughton and Foster in 1957.[3]

Males: DL corrected = DL measured $1(Hb + 10.22) \div 1.7\,Hb)$.
Females: DL corrected = DL measured $1(bH + 10.22) \div 1.8\,Hb)$.

Males: DL = 0.391H − 0.196A − 25.04; 95% confidence interval = 8.5.
Females: DL = 0.267H − 0.148A − 10.34; 95% confidence interval = 5.74.

Males: Hemoglobin corrected DL/V_A = 6.93 − 0.033 A; 95% confidence interval = 1.34.

Females: Hemoglobin corrected DL/V_A = 6.94 − 0.028 A; 95% confidence interval = 1.34.

    Where H = height in cm.

    A = age in years.

    DL/V_A = diffusion per unit of alveolar volume with DL expressed as standard conditions STPD and V_A expressed as liters BTPS.

The 95% confidence interval when subtracted from the predicted value yields the lower limit of normal. Additional predicted formulae are included in *Pulmonary Function Testing: Guidelines and Controversies.*[2]

LIMITATIONS

The major limitations of DL include its lack of correlation with hypoxemia in interstitial lung disease,[19] lack of sensitivity in various disease states, and wide range of normal values, especially in older persons. In addition, the lack of uniform technique, the lack of uniform standard values of DL, and the use of different types of equipment have made it difficult to compare values obtained in different laboratories. A review of normal values from Crapo and Morris,[27] the Intermountain Thoracic Society,[28] and Teculescu[29] reveals differences of 10–20% for men 175 cm in height and 30–65 years old. Because of this amount of variability, the American Thoracic Society recommends that each laboratory check the DL equation it uses by testing at least 20 normal subjects and determining by the paired *t* test whether there is a significant difference between the observed and the predicted values. If there is, the laboratory could either develop its prediction equation or find another that would better fit its needs. Whichever equation is used, it is recommended that the laboratory establish a lower limit of normal for the equation by defining the value for DL that 95% percent of the normal population meets or exceeds. This is defined as the predicted value − 1.65 SEE. A result below this value, classified as abnormal, will more reliably identify persons with pulmonary disease whereas serial measurements may be of value in revealing trends toward worsening or improvement, as might be found in specific pulmonary disease states.

    The evaluation of a reduced D_L should take into account the simultaneously measured V_A and perhaps the ratio of DL/V_A. Conditions associated with low DL and normal or increased V_A (reduced DL/V_A) are anemia, emphysema, multiple pulmonary emboli, and pulmonary vasculitis. Reduced DL with reduced V_A can be found in lung resection (usually DL/V_A is near normal), pulmonary alveolar proteinosis, and diffuse interstitial fibrosis (Tables 10-1 and 10-2).

QUANTIFICATION OF IMPAIRMENT

Normal values for DL are commonly based on age, sex, height, hemoglobin concentration and occasionally on simultaneously measured V_A whereas DL/V_A have been based on age, gender, height, and body surface area. The normal values developed by Crapo and Morris[27] are presently being recommended by the American Thoracic Society Ad Hoc Committee on Evaluation of Impairment/Disability Secondary to Respiratory Disease.[30]

Normal DL is often cited as predicted $\pm$ 20%. Use of this cutoff may lead to unnecessary overdiagnosis. A more reasonable approach to determining the cutoff between normal and abnormal would be the use of 95% confidence limits as suggested by Crapo and Morris. In their development of normal values for DL_{SB} they found small variations in confidence limits over a large range of heights and ages, making it reasonable to substitute a single value to be subtracted from predicted to establish the lower 95% confidence limits.[27]

The reduced DL as a percent of predicted may be arbitrarily assessed as mild (60–79%), moderate (40–59%), severe (20–39%), and very severe (< 20%). This grading system is arbitrary and its correlation with pulmonary limitation often depends on the pulmonary pathophysiologic condition. For example, DL_{SB} is extremely useful in differentiating emphysema from asthma or bronchitis but not in determining the severity of limitation in chronic obstructive airways disease; dyspnea in chronic obstructive airways disease correlates best with flow impairment (FEV_1/FVC, FEV_1, and MVV). In diffuse interstitial processes, DL_{SB} of 40% or less of predicted has been found by Epler, Saber, and Gaensler to correlate best, after standard exercise testing, with severe pulmonary impairment.[31] In more than half of their patients with severe impairment due to interstitial pneumonia, the DL_{SB} was the only test that yielded results low enough for classification of severe impairment. In their criteria for severe impairment, FVC of 50% or less or DL_{SB} of 40% or less were the best correlates. This criteria when qualified for normality of DL (normal is considered a DL greater than the predicted minus the 95% confidence interval) is currently being recommended by the American Thoracic Society.[30]

Unfortunately, standard exercise testing including measurement of arterial blood gases, minute ventilation, and oxygen consumption is difficult to perform on large groups of people requiring evaluation, can be unpleasant, requires the use of sophisticated equipment, and may on occasion precipitate pulmonary and cardiac complications. In contrast, DL_{SB} is rapid, noninvasive, and suitable for screening.

Table 10-1 Alterations in D_L/V_A

Causes of low D_L with normal or increased V_A (low D_L/V_A):
Anemia
Emphysema
Pulmonary thrombosis and embolization
Pulmonary vasculitis

Causes of low D_L with low V_A (low, normal, or high D_L/V_A):
Lung resection (usually D_L/V_A is near normal).
Pulmonary alveolar proteinosis (occasionally the reduction in D_L is greater than the reduction in V_A).
Pulmonary interstitial disease, e.g., sarcoidosis, scleroderma, systemic lupus erythematosus, asbestosis, histiocytosis-X, interstitial fibrosis, and chronic hypersensitivity alveolitis.

Table 10-2 Evaluation of DL_{CO}

Abnormality	Pathophysiology	Examples
Increased DL_{CO}	1. Increase in pulmonary blood volume.	Left heart failure, left-to-right shunts (atrial septal defect, anomalous pulmonary venous return), exercise, altitude, supine position.
	2. Increase in red blood cells.	Early in polycythemia.
Decreased DL_{CO}	1. Deficiency in red blood cells.	Anemia.
	2. Loss of pulmonary capillary bed with relatively normal lung volume.	Multiple pulmonary emboli, early collagen-vascular disease, early in sarcoidosis.
	3. Loss of functioning alveolar-capillary bed with increased lung volume.	Emphysema.
	4. Loss of functioning alveolar-capillary bed with decreased lung volume.	Pulmonary resection, idiopathic interstitial fibrosis, asbestosis, scleroderma lung disease, histiocytosis-X, sarcoidosis, pneumonia.
	5. Failure of inspired air to reach alveoli (i.e., poor distribution of ventilation), with low, normal, or increased lung volume.	Severe bronchospasm, frequently with emphysema.

145

ARTIFACTS/PITFALLS

Please refer to Chapter 16 in *Pulmonary Function Testing: Guidelines and Controversies*. [24]

EXAMPLES

Case 1

LD is a 45-year-old laborer (70″, 201 lbs) who complains of progressive shortness of breath for 6 months. He had a 20-pack year history of cigarette smoking and a 20-year exposure to dusts and fumes including silica, asbestos, and paints. Study results are shown in Table 10-3.

The pulmonary function studies revealed mild airflow obstruction ($FEF_{25-75\%}$) with normal lung volumes, DL_{SB} and VC. An exercise test (data not included) revealed a heart rate of 165/min at a workload of 150 watts and an O_2 consumption of 2 liters. These studies are compatible with small airways obstruction without evidence of significant emphysema.

Case 2

EH is a 49-year-old female (62″, 123 lbs) with progressive dyspnea on exertion over 2 years. There was a 16-pack year history of cigarette smoking.

Table 10.3   Case 1

| | Measured | | |
	Before	After	Predicted
VC (liter)	4.82	4.99	4.79
FEV_1 (liter)	3.23	3.56	3.73
$FEF_{25-75\%}$ (liter/sec)	1.85	2.44	4.3
Peak Expiratory Flow (liter/min)	398.0	474.0	513.0
MVV (liter/min)	118.0	117.0	159.0
FRC (liter)	3.47	—	3.49
RV (liter)	2.13	—	2.32
TLC (liter)	7.02	—	7.04
RV/TLC%	30.0	—	33.0
DL_{SB} (ml/min/mm Hg)	33.6	—	30.9
V_A (liter) BTPS	6.9	—	7.03
D_L/V_A	4.9	—	4.5
PaO_2 (mm Hg)	78.0	—	80.0
$PaCO_2$ (mm Hg)	36.0	—	35.45
pH	7.45	—	7.35–7.45

The physical exam revealed clubbing, cyanosis, and diffuse crepitant end-inspiratory rales. A chest x-ray revealed bilateral scattered alveolar infiltrates. The study results are as shown in Table 10-4. Initial studies reveal mild restriction with severe reduction of DL and severe hypoxemia. These data are compatible with parenchymal disease and suggest either interstitial fibrosis or alveolar filling. The lung biopsy revealed PAS positive material within the alveoli and confirmed the diagnosis of pulmonary alveolar proteinosis. Repeat pulmonary studies following bilateral lung lavage revealed normalization of VC, DL_{SB}, and PaO_2.

Case 3

RW is a 45-year-old, nonsmoking black female (66″, 138 lbs) with progressive shortness of breath on exertion and a nonproductive cough of 8-months duration. A current chest x-ray revealed bilateral hilar enlargement and skin tests for tuberculosis and histoplasmosis were negative after 48 and 72 hours. Transbronchial and endobronchial biopsies revealed noncaseating granulomas; AFB and fungal stains of this material were negative. Results are shown in Table 10-5.

Pulmonary studies reveal small airways obstruction, moderate hypoxemia, and marked reduction of DL_{SB}. These abnormalities are compatible with reduction in the perfused pulmonary capillary bed and narrowing of the small airways due to sarcoid granulomas.

Case 4

MV is a 33-year-old construction worker with a 3-year history of progressive shortness of breath on exertion and sputum production. He has a 21-pack

Table 10.4 Case 2

	Measured	Postlavage	Predicted
FVC (liter)	2.15	3.23	2.88
FEV_1 (liter)	1.70	2.13	2.35
$FEF_{25-75\%}$ (liter/sec)	1.92	2.1	3.4
MVV (liter/min)	61.0	95.0	104.0
FRC (liter)	2.05	2.91	2.43
RV (liter)	1.52	1.97	1.36
TLC (liter)	3.64	5.20	4.24
DL_{SB} (ml/min/mm Hg)	7.2	19.5	19.2
V_A (liter) BTPS	3.2	4.9	4.24
D_L/V_A	2.2	3.9	4.5
PaO_2 (mm Hg)	38.0	94.0	80.0
$PaCO_2$ (mm Hg)	38.0	27.0	35–45
pH	7.47	7.50	7.35–7.45
Hematocrit (vol%)	39.0	37.0	40.0

Table 10-5   Case 3

	Measured	Predicted
FVC (liter)	3.47	3.37
FEV_1 (liter)	2.40	2.69
$FEF_{25-75\%}$ (liter/sec)	1.69	3.49
MVV (liter/min)	108.0	119.0
FRC (liter)	3.23	2.9
RV (liter)	1.4	1.7
TLC (liter)	4.87	5.07
DL_{SB} (ml/min/mm Hg)	9.3	28.2
V_A (liter) BTPS	4.5	5.1
D_L/V_A	2.1	5.5
Hematocrit (vol%)	38	40
PaO_2 (mm Hg)	54	80
$PaCO_2$ (mm Hg)	32	35–45
pH	7.45	7.35–7.45

year history of cigarette smoking. Current chest x-rays reveal hyperinflation. Test results are shown in Table 10-6.

Moderately severe airflow obstruction, hyperinflation, and reduced DL_{SB} suggest the presence of emphysema. An alpha-1 antitrypsin level was found reduced at 36 mg/dl (normal 210–400 mg/dl).

CONTROVERSIES

WHAT IS NORMAL?

Because of the differences between prediction equations for DL, each laboratory probably should check the prediction equation it is using by testing at least 20 subjects and determining whether there is a significant difference between the observed and predicted values. If a significant difference is found, the laboratory could develop its own prediction equation or find another in the literature that would fit its needs.

IS THERE A CORRELATION BETWEEN REDUCED DL AND HYPOXEMIA?

In the past, clinical investigators have tried to correlate DL with hypoxemia. Staub[1] theoretically predicted that no measurable $P(A-a)O_2$ would occur at rest until the red blood cells mean capillary transit time was less than 0.3 seconds

Table 10-6   Case 4

	Measured	Predicted
FVC (liter)	3.55	6.33
FEV$_1$ (liter)	1.1	5.0
FEV$_{25-75\%}$ (liter/sec)	0.5	4.65
MVV (liter/min)	48.0	198.0
FRC (liter)	8.51	4.22
RV (liter)	7.72	2.09
TLC (liter)	10.82	8.45
DL$_{SB}$ (ml/min/mm Hg)	16.5	29.6
V$_A$ (liter) BTPS	7.9	8.4
D$_L$/V$_A$	2.1	3.6
Hematocrit	48.0	45.0
PaO$_2$ (mm Hg)	65.0	80.0
PaCO$_2$ (mm Hg)	44.0	35–45
pH	7.36	7.35–7.45

(normal transit time = 0.75 sec), and at this shortened time the P(A-a)O$_2$ would be less than 2 mm Hg. In contrast with a severely reduced pulmonary capillary bed, regional variations in capillary transit time and thickening and reduction of alveolar membrane, significant widening of P(A-a)O$_2$ occurs. Clinical studies reveal correlation between DL and hypoxemia in patients with obstructive lung disease (OLD) as well as pulmonary fibrosis studied during exercise but not during rest.[32] This relationship is of borderline significance in OLD but is important in pulmonary fibrosis.[31] Impaired ventilation-to-perfusion ratios are at least partly responsible for the exercise-induced hypoxemia in fibrosis and are most likely responsible in obstructive disease.

How Important is Dead Space to Measurement of DL?

DL is falsely reduced when the expired gas sample is contaminated with anatomic VD gas. When DL is measured continuously during expiration of the previously inhaled VC (expired CO and helium or other inert gas related to expired volume), one observes that a rapid rise of DL occurs until anatomic VD is cleared, a plateau or a minimal rise in DL occurs until 80% of VC has been exhaled, and then a fall in DL corresponding to closing volume follows. A rise in CO concentration coming from upper lung zones implies that DL per unit volume in the upper zone is less than in the lower zones.[33] Thus, failure to clear VD will result in an underestimation of DL; this occurrence may be occasionally responsible for unusually low DL, especially in severe restrictive and obstructive disease associated with reduced VC (< 1–1.5 liters).

REFERENCES

1. Staub NC: Alveolar-arterial oxygen tension gradient due to diffusion. J Appl Physiol 18:673–680, 1963.

2. Van Kessel AL: Transfer factor for carbon monoxide (DLCO), in Clausen J (ed): *Pulmonary Function Testing: Guidelines and Controversies.* New York, Academic Press, 1982.

3. Roughton FJ, Forster RE: Relative importance of diffusion and chemical reaction rates in determining rate of exchange of gases in the human lung, with special reference to diffusing capacity of pulmonary membrane and volume of blood in the lung capillaries. J Appl Physiol 11:290–302, 1957.

4. Bates DV, Macklem PT, Christie RV: Respiratory Function in Disease (ed 2). Philadelphia, PA, WB Saunders Co, 1971, pp. 75–85.

5. Ogilvie CM, Forster RE, Blackemore WS, et al.: A standardized breath holding technique for the clinical measurement of the diffusing capacity of the lung for carbon monoxide. J Clin Invest 36:1–17, 1957.

6. Miller JM, Johnson RL Jr: Effect of lung inflation on pulmonary diffusing capacity at rest and exercise. J Clin Invest 45:493–500, 1966.

7. McIlroy MB, Bates DV: Respiratory function after pneumonectomy. Thorax 14:483, 1959.

8. Gaensler EA, Smith AA: Attachment for automated single breath diffusing capacity measurement. Chest 63:136–145, 1973.

9. Ayers LN, Ginsberg ML, Fein J, et al.: Diffusing capacity, specific diffusing capacity and interpretation of diffusion defects. West J Med 123:255–264, 1975.

10. Divertie MB, Cassan SM, O'Brien PC, et al.: Fine structural morphometry of diffuse lung disease with abnormal blood-air gas transfer. Mayo Clin Proc 51:42–47, 1976.

11. Lee H, Strelton T, Barnes A: The lungs in renal failure. Thorax 30:46, 1975.

12. Forman JW, Ayers LN, Miller WC: Pulmonary diffusing capacity in chronic renal failure. Br J Dis Chest 75:81–87, 1981.

13. Forster RE: Diffusion of gases, in Fenn WO, Rahn H (eds): *Handbook of Physiology: Respiration (vol. 1).* Washington, DC, American Physiological Society, 1965, pp. 863.

14. Dinakara P, Blumenthal WS, Johnston RF, et al.: The effect of anemia on pulmonary diffusion capacity with derivation of a correction equation. Am Rev Respir Dis 102:965–969, 1970.

15. Cotes JE, Dabbs JM, Elwood PC, et al: Iron deficiency anemia: its effect on transfer factor for the lung and ventilation and cardiac frequency during submaximal exercise. Clin Sci 42:325, 1972.

16. Frans A, Stanescu DC, Veriter C, et al.: Smoking and pulmonary diffusing capacity. Scand J Respir Dis 56:165–183, 1975.

17. Gelb A, Gold W, Wright R, et al.: Physiologic diagnosis of subclinical emphysema. Am Rev Respir Dis 107:50, 1973.

18. Thurlbeck W, Henderson J, Fraser R, et al.: Chronic obstructive lung disease. A comparison between clinical, roentgenologic, functional and morphologic criteria in chronic bronchitis, emphysema, asthma and bronchiectasis. Medicine 49:81, 1970.

19. Crystal RG, Fulmer JD, Roberts WC, et al.: Idiopathic pulmonary fibrosis: clinical, histologic, radiographic, physiologic, scintigraphic, cytologic and biochemical aspects. Ann Intern Med 85:769–788, 1976.

20. Jones N, Goodwin J: Respiratory function in thromboembolic disorders. Br Med J 1:1089–1093, 1965.

21. Nadel J, Gold W, Burgess J: Early diagnosis of chronic pulmonary vascular obstruction: value of pulmonary function tests. Am J Med 44:16–25, 1968.

22. Fulmer JD, Roberts WC, VonGal ER, et al.: Morphologic-physiologic correlates of the severity of fibrosis and degree of cellarity in idiopathic pulmonary fibrosis. J Clin Invest 63:665–676, 1979.

23. Sharma GV, Burleson VA, Sasahara AA: Effect of thrombolytic therapy on pulmonary capillary blood volume in patients with pulmonary embolism. N Engl J Med 303:842–845, 1980.

24. Ohman JL, Schmidt NW, Lawrence M, et al.: The diffusing capacity in asthma. Effect of air-flow obstruction. Am Rev Respir Dis 107:932, 1973.

25. Weitzman RH, Wilson AF: Diffusing capacity and over-all ventilation perfusion pressure in asthma. Am J Med 114:123, 1976.

26. Gonzalez E, Weil H, Ziskind M, et al.: The value of the single breath diffusing capacity in separating chronic bronchitis from pulmonary emphysema. Dis Chest 53:229, 1968.

27. Crapo R, Morris A: Standardized single breath normal values for carbon monoxide diffusing capacity. Am Rev Respir Dis 123:185–189, 1981.

28. Kanner R, Morris A (eds): Clinical pulmonary function testing: a manual of uniform laboratory procedures for the intermountain area. Salt Lake City, UT, Intermountain Thoracic Society, 1975, IV-1-13.

29. Teculescu D, Stanescu D: Lung diffusing capacity. Normal values in male smokers and nonsmokers using the breath-holding technique. Scand J Respir Dis 51:137–49, 1970.

30. Kass I, Bell C, Eper G, et al.: Evaluation of impairment/disability secondary to respiratory disease. ATS News 7:20–28, 1981.

31. Epler GR, Saber FA, Gaensler EA: Determination of severe impairment (disability) in interstitial lung disease. Am Rev Respir Dis 121:647–658, 1980.

32. Vandenberg E, Billiet L, van de Woestline K, et al.: Relationship between single-breath diffusing capacity and arterial blood gases in chronic obstructive lung disease. Scand J Respir Dis 49:92–101, 1968.

33. Wagner PD, Mazzone RW, West JB: Diffusing capacity and anatomic dead space for carbon monoxide ($C^{18}O$). J Appl Physiol 31:847–852, 1971.

CHAPTER 11

The Basics for Clinical Blood Gas Evaluation

JOHN G. MOHLER

HISTORIC BACKGROUND

The laboratory measurements and accompanying concepts that are used to describe and understand blood gases, i.e., oxygen content and pressure, carbon dioxide content and pressure, pH and titratable acidity, were developed in the early part of this century by a number of investigators including Peters, Van Slyke, Henderson, Hasselbalch, Hastings, Singer, and Barcroft.[1-3] In the succeeding several decades, advances in laboratory instrumentation by Sanz, Clark, and Severinghaus and others [4,5] have lead to the development of blood gas equipment that is reliable and easy to use. As a result, blood gas analysis is now routinely available in virtually every hospital.

INDICATIONS, SITE OF SAMPLING, AND MEASUREMENTS

Because arterial blood gases reflects gas exchange in the lung and no clinical sign [6] allows accurate estimation of pH, PO_2, or PCO_2, arterial sampling is necessary whenever clinical suspicion of respiratory dysfunction occurs. Arterial blood analysis should be obtained not only in patients with obvious respiratory insufficiency but also in patients with unexplained dyspnea or coma. Although any easily accessible peripheral artery may be used for sampling, because of convenience (and safety), most samples are obtained anaerobically from the brachial or radial arteries.

Usually, pH, PCO_2, and PO_2 are analyzed directly and oxygen saturation (SO_2) and some measure of metabolic acid/base status are calculated (bicarbon-

PULMONARY FUNCTION TESTING
INDICATIONS AND INTERPRETATIONS

ate, base excess, standard bicarbonate, etc.). Calculation of SO_2 depends upon the assumption that the curve describing the relationship between PO_2 and SO_2 is not shifted either to the right or the left (normal P_{50}, see following). Calculation of bicarbonate (HCO_3^-) depends upon the assumption that the dissociation constant (pK') of the HCO_3^-–H_2CO_3 relationship is stable. The calculation of base excess (BE) requires knowledge of the hemoglobin concentration. These calculated parameters may also be measured directly: SO_2 by spectrophotometry and total CO_2 content by gasometric or other techniques HCO_3 may be calculated from total CO_2 content by subtracting the small amount of physically dissolved CO_2.[1-3] Another measurement that often is of importance is oxygen content. O_2 content may be determined directly by gasometric techniques or calculated from the measured (or calculated) SO_2, hemoglobin, and PO_2.[7]

Concentrations of gases in arterial blood may be approximated by analysis of capillary blood from areas in which the arterial blood has been arterialized by heating.[8] Such measurements suffer primarily from exposure of the sample to room air. Mixed venous blood ($\bar{v}$) PCO_2 and pH are similar to arterial (a) blood. In general, $P\bar{v}CO_2$ is 6 mm Hg higher than $PaCO_2$ and $pH_{\bar{v}}$ is .02 lower than pHa. However, mixed venous PO_2 is usually considerably less than PaO_2. This is discussed below. Mixed venous blood is usually analyzed to obtain information about the adequacy of oxygen delivery and tissue oxygenation.

CARBON DIOXIDE

CO_2 is produced by both aerobic and anaerobic metabolism within cells. CO_2 reaches systemic capillary blood by diffusion. Although CO_2 is a gas, it is carried in blood primarily in the form of bicarbonate (70%); however, small, but significant quantities, are also transported as molecular CO_2 combined directly with hemoglobin (carbamino hemoglobin—20%) or in a hydrated but undissociated form (carbonic acid—10%).[9] Because each bicarbonate ion formed is associated with formation of a hydrogen ion, buffering of this newly formed hydrogen ion is required. Most bicarbonate is produced within erythrocytes because of the presence there of the enzyme carbonic anhydrase, which catalyzes the production of bicarbonate from CO_2 and water (carbonic acid).[10] Blockade of the activity of this enzyme does not cause marked changes in most patients but the CO_2 transport system is altered; a larger portion of CO_2 is transported in the dissolved state hence requiring higher PCO_2 values. Buffering of the hydrogen ions formed by dissociation of carbonic acid is accomplished primarily by hemoglobin, but smaller quantities of hydrogen ion are buffered by plasma proteins. Because hydrogen ions and O_2 compete with each other for binding to hemoglobin, deoxygenation of hemoglobin in tissue increases the availability of buffering sites in venous blood, thereby facilitating buffering and minimizing pH changes. Some CO_2 is reconstituted into its gaseous phase in the pulmonary capillaries by the reverse of the reaction that took place in the systemic capillaries. Gaseous CO_2 diffuses into alveoli and is removed by ventilation. Hence, the level of CO_2 in the blood represents the balance between CO_2 production by metabolism ($\dot{V}CO_2$) and alveolar ventilation ($\dot{V}_A$). Because, normally, virtually no gradient for CO_2 exists across the alveolar-capillary membrane, the partial pressure of CO_2 in arterial blood ($PaCO_2$) is approximately equal to that in alveolae ($PACO_2$). These latter relationships may be stated by the following equation:

$$PaCO_2 \doteq PACO_2 = \frac{\dot{V}CO_2\ 863}{\dot{V}_A} \qquad \text{(Eq. 1)}$$

where $PaCO_2$ and $PACO_2$ are expressed in mm Hg, $\dot{V}CO_2$ in liter/min STPD, and $\dot{V}_A$ in liter/min BTPS.

Further understanding of the physiologic interrelationships is obtained when $\dot{V}_A$ is replaced by its equivalent, total minute ventilation ($\dot{V}_E$), corrected for the fraction that is wasted, i.e., deadspace (V_D/V_T), as in the following equation:

$$PaCO_2 = \frac{\dot{V}CO_2\ 863}{\dot{V}_E\ (1 - V_D/V_T)} \qquad \text{(Eq. 2)}$$

Hence, $PaCO_2$ is elevated only when total effective (i.e., alveolar) ventilation is depressed relative to CO_2 production. This is a relationship of utmost clinical importance.

Because CO_2 is carried in the blood primarily as bicarbonate, measurement of plasma bicarbonate will also give an indication of the ratio of CO_2 production to alveolar ventilation. However, only measurement of $PaCO_2$ allows precise evaluation of the physiologic relationships stated in the preceding equations. Additionally, because ventilatory control is so sensitive and effective (see Chapter 13 this volume), $PaCO_2$ is controlled within narrow limits (40 ± 3 mm Hg). The normal limits of plasma bicarbonate and total CO_2 are much larger, in part because of technical factors relating to sample preparation and analytic techniques and, in part, because of differences in buffering between individuals.

When the metabolism/ventilation ratio is more than normal, $PaCO_2$ increases; this is termed *Respiratory Acidosis,* because, at least initially, arterial pH decreases. If the metabolism/ventilation ratio is less than normal, $PaCO_2$ declines; this is termed *Respiratory Alkalosis* because, at least initially, arterial pH increases.

Like O_2, CO_2 is transported in both the dissolved and chemically combined states. In the case of O_2, the amount dissolved is very small, but in the case of CO_2 the amount that is dissolved is an appreciable portion of the total. A CO_2 dissociation curve can be developed similar to the O_2 dissociation curve by exposing blood to a series of gases at increasing PCO_2 levels.[12] Because of the effect of O_2 on the CO_2 dissociation curve (the Christiansen-Douglas-Haldane effect, or more commonly, the Haldane effect), the CO_2 dissociation curve for saturated blood is different than that of desaturated (venous) blood. The Haldane effect plays a major role both in the transport of CO_2 and of those hydrogen ions that come from the hydration of CO_2.[9,11,13]

Hydrogen ions from CO_2 produced by tissue are, of course, present in large amounts in capillary blood; most of these immediately combine with the imidazole groups of hemoglobin that have been freed by the loss of O_2. Because the loss of 100 molecules of oxygen frees 70 buffer sites, deoxygenated hemoglobin can combine with hydrogen ions with minimal change in pH. Because in the normal resting state only about 80 molecules of CO_2 are given off from the tissue for each 100 molecules of oxygen utilized and some of the CO_2 forms carbamino groups, the transport of CO_2 is accomplished with very little change in pH. The usual resting mixed venous pH [9,11] is only about 0.02 units lower than the pH of arterial blood. Normally, at rest, central venous blood has a PO_2 of about 37 torr and a PCO_2 of about 47 torr.

METABOLIC ACID/BASE STATUS

Metabolism and diet produce a number of end products that cannot be excreted by the lung (as CO_2 is) and, hence, require renal and/or gastrointestinal elimination. Because these latter routes of excretion are not as rapid as CO_2 elimination by the lungs, even brief changes in diet or metabolism may lead to temporary accumulation of these metabolic end products. Similarly, major changes in renal or gastrointestinal function may effect end product elimination and, thereby, may lead to increase of the concentration of certain chemicals in the blood. Increased blood concentration of acid end products is termed *metabolic* (or *nonrespiratory*) acidosis whereas accumulation of alkaline end products is termed *metabolic* (or *nonrespiratory*) alkalosis.

The presence of Metabolic Acidosis or alkalosis may be inferred when $PaCO_2$ is normal (40 ± 3 mm Hg) and pH is abnormal (greater or less than 7.40 ± .02); however, this situation is relatively uncommon. More commonly, it is necessary to evaluate the type and magnitude of metabolic acid/base abnormalities in the presence of either increased or decreased $PaCO_2$. Under these more usual circumstances, it is convenient to use such parameters as BE or T_{40} bicarbonate to describe the metabolic acid/base abnormality.[12] Normal BE is O ± 2 mEq/liter and normal T_{40} bicarbonate is 24 ±2 mEq/liter. Metabolic Alkalosis is characterized by an increase of these parameters (BE greater than +2 mEq/liter or T_{40} bicarbonate greater than 26 mEq/liter). Metabolic acidosis is defined as a decrease of BE below − 2 mEq/liter or T_{40} bicarbonate less than 22 mEq/liter. The magnitude of the acid base abnormality may be inferred from by the size of the deviation from normal.

It is also possible to establish the presence of a metabolic acid/base abnormality from analysis of the magnitude of the value of pH, $PaCO_2$ and bicarbonate. Because elevation or depression of $PaCO_2$ has proportional effects upon bicarbonate, such an analysis requires reference to a nomogram. One of the principal benefits of the use of BE (extracellular fluid) is that metabolic acid/base abnormalities may be recognized from the magnitude of these parameters without reference to a nomogram.

Because, in most circumstances, the body attempts to normalize extracellular pH, primary respiratory and metabolic acid/base abnormalities are at least partially compensated by physiologic mechanisms. The major compensatory mechanisms for acidosis are renal excretion of acid by the kidney in Respiratory Acidosis [14] and hyperventilation in Metabolic Acidosis. [15] Compensation for alkalosis is less complete or may be absent; in Respiratory Alkalosis there is some renal excretion of base and, at least temporarily, increased production of acid metabolites by tissue may occur; [16] very little hypoventilation occurs in association with Metabolic Alkalosis, presumably because respiratory center control of $PaCO_2$ and/or peripheral control of $PaCO_2$ prevents hypoventilation. [17]

BODY BUFFER SYSTEM

Buffer value is the amount of an acid or base that must be added to a liter of fluid to change the pH of that fluid one unit. Buffer value has the dimensions of mEq/liter/pH unit or Slykes. The most important body buffers are proteins. [18] Most protein is intracellular, including hemoglobin in erythrocytes. The erythrocyte is particularly important because it rapidly exchanges with the plasma and, eventually, with the somatic cells. Extracellular protein is contained primarily in the plasma and is not a particularly large proportion of the total buffering power of the body. Another important buffer system is the bicarbonate–carbonic acid system. This is particularly important because CO_2 is volatile and can be quickly removed from the system by ventilation. Although phosphate and other buffer systems do exist in the body, they are quantitatively far less important than those previously mentioned. Each of the buffer systems is in equilibrium with each other within the same compartment of the body as long as hydrogen ion concentration is uniform within that compartment. If the pH is uniform through the extracellular fluid, then all of the extracellular fluid buffers must be in equilibrium with the others. Acid/base status may be evaluated by analyzing only one buffer system; usually the CO_2-bicarbonate buffer system is used for this purpose. [9,18]

CO_2-BICARBONATE SYSTEM

Because PCO_2 is routinely measured to evaluate ventilatory status, only one other measurement, usually pH, is necessary to evaluate the acid/base status of the CO_2-bicarbonate system. From the mass action interrelationships between CO_2 and bicarbonate, the Henderson equation may be written

$$K = \frac{[H][HCO_3]}{[H_2CO_3]} \qquad \text{(Eq. 4)}$$

This equation is more useful when H_2CO_3 is replaced by its equivalent PCO_2, and the bunsen coefficient (α) is incorporated into the constant K'.

$$K' = 24 = \frac{[H][HCO_3]}{PCO_2} \qquad \text{(Eq. 5)}$$

Furthermore, if the approximate relationships between hydrogen ion concentration and pH are appreciated (Table 11-1), it is possible to quickly calculate any third value, if two are known, without the direct use of logarithms. Note that for each twofold change in hydrogen ion concentration, there is a 0.3 change in pH. The equally familar Henderson–Hasselbalch equation states the same relationships in logarithmic form:

$$pH = pK + \log \frac{[HCO_3]}{PCO_2} \qquad \text{(Eq. 6)}$$

This representation is more convenient for graphic illustration (Fig 11-1).

TITRATION OF BLOOD WITH CO_2

Because CO_2 forms carbonic acid, changes in PCO_2 are equivalent to titration of the blood with carbonic acid. The nonbicarbonate buffers modify the

Table 11-1   Hydrogen Ion Concentration and pH

pH	[H+] (nmol/L)
7.0	100
7.1	80
7.2	64
7.3	50
7.4	40
7.5	32
7.6	25
7.7	20
7.8	16
7.9	12.5
8.0	10

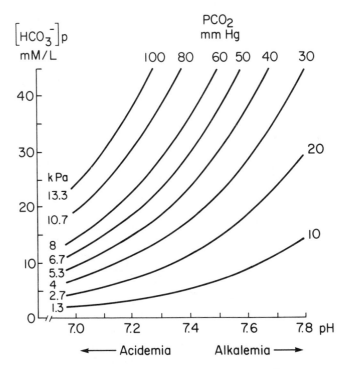

Figure 11-1. The Davenport type of diagram of acid/base interrelationships in blood. Note that the scales of the ordinate and abscissa for HCO_3 and pH are linear while the PCO_2 isobars are curvilinear.

effects of the CO_2 that is added. If the changes are plotted on the standard Davenport diagram of bicarbonate versus pH with PCO_2 values shown as isobars, then the buffer line represents a straight line across the diagram (Fig 11-2).[9] The slope of the line is the strength of the buffer in Slykes. Bicarbonate will increase stoichiometrically with the increase of CO_2 and the hydrogen ions produced will be partially buffered by nonbicarbonate buffers. Hence, the increase in bicarbonate is a measure of the actual hydrogen ions added by the increase of PCO_2. The buffer value of normal whole blood titrated with CO_2 in vitro in this way is 30 Slykes.

TITRATION OF WHOLE BODY WITH CO_2

If hypercarbia is produced by breathing elevated CO_2 mixtures, it is possible to titrate not just the blood but the entire extracellular fluid (ECF) in just a few minutes.[16,19,20] There are relatively few nonbicarbonate buffers in the interstitual fluid (ISF) compartment of the ECF. Hence, the fact that plasma rapidly equilibrates with ISF effectively reduces the buffer value of the ECF to about one

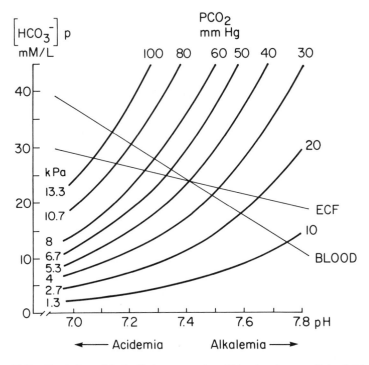

Figure 11-2.   Depiction of the buffering properties of blood and extracellular fluid (ECF, i.e., blood plus interstitial fluid) on a Davenport diagram.

third of the blood buffer value.[20] Hence, consideration of the total ECF buffer value is of much greater clinical importance than considering only the blood buffer value alone. The measured ECF buffer value is about 11.6 Slykes. The normal buffer line for ECF is also shown in the Davenport diagram (Fig 11-2).

   If noncarbonic acid or base is added to the body in vivo, the effect will be reflected qualitatively in changes of the plasma bicarbonate. Because both bicarbonate and nonbicarbonate buffer systems are involved in the reaction, there is not a direct quantitative relationship between acid or base with the bicarbonate change alone. If PCO_2 remains constant, noncarbonic acid or base change will cause the pH to move up or down on the CO_2 isobar of the diagram.

SECONDARY RESPONSES TO ACID/BASE DISTURBANCES

   There are several secondary pathways of acid/base disturbances that are much slower than the initial changes seen with acute primary events, such as ventilatory failure or diabetic ketoacidosis. For example, after a few hours, some intracellular buffering will be manifest. In about one day intracellular buffering is more or less complete following a major primary acid/base event.[18] With complete intracellular buffering, the apparent buffer value rises to about 40 Slykes, i.e., somewhat above the buffer value of blood. Further secondary changes are produced by increased renal excretion of acid or base; these changes may take up to five days for completion.[15,18] Secondary compensation for primary acid/base abnormalities tends to move arterial pH toward 7.40 but not beyond. Complete compensation to a normal pH probably never does occur except for in very mild hypercapnia. However, additional acid/base change may be caused by diuretics and other drugs as well as gastric suction; under these conditions arterial pH may exceed 7.40.

The secondary response to a Metabolic Acidosis (base deficit) is increase in ventilation. This response will be quite rapid and probably will be complete in about one day.[15] The 95% confidence bands shown on the diagram along the buffer slope for extracellular fluid represent the expected value of acute changes.[19]

The secondary responses to hypocapnia and Metabolic Alkalosis have been studied but not as greatly as hypercapnia.[16,17] In hypocapnia, there is increased renal excretion of bicarbonate, but the time course and its ultimate effectiveness has not been worked out. In Metabolic Alkalosis, there is a general decrease in hydrogen ions caused by depression of ventilation, but the data available in the literature represent a highly variable response.[16] The work of Arbus using anesthetized humans is shown in Fig 11-3.[17] The 95% confidence band is parallel to the ECF buffer line.

OXYGEN

In the normal lung, partial pressure of O_2 in arterial blood (PaO_2) is determined, in a manner similar to that for $PaCO_2$, by the ratio of O_2 consumption in the tissue to V_A. Because $PaCO_2$ is regulated within relatively narrow limits by the respiratory control centers (see Chapter 13 this volume), it might be expected that PaO_2 would also be quite constant. However, because of both normal factors (closing volume commonly exceeding functional residual capacity from the age of 45 years and upward) and pathologic factors (ventilation/perfusion mismatching, right-to-left shunting and, possibly, insufficient time or too great a distance for diffusion to complete equilibration within pulmonary capillaries), PaO_2 is frequently lower than would be expected from the level of ventilation; i.e., hypoxemia is common in diseased lungs despite hyperventilation. Hence, though P_ACO_2 is approximately equal to $PaCO_2$, PAO_2 is rarely equal to PaO_2. In the presence of disease, a large difference between PAO_2 and PaO_2 may occur. This $P(A-a)O_2$ difference may be evaluated by measuring PaO_2 and calculating PAO_2 from the alveolar gas equation.[21]

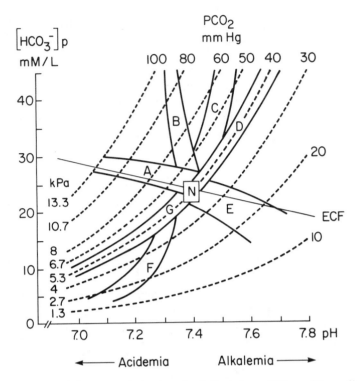

Figure 11-3. Labeled zones unless otherwise indicated are 95% confidence limits of selected studies of well-defined conditions. All areas above the ECF buffer liner represent BE; all areas below represent base deficit. **N** Normal; **A** Acute hypercapnia, acute or uncompensated respiratory acidosis; **B** Chronic hypercapnia, chronic or compensated respiratory acidosis; **C** Chronic BE, chronic or compensated metabolic alkalosis; **D** Acute BE, acute or uncompensated metabolic alkalosis. Is a theoretical area; **E** Acute hypocapnia, acute or uncompensated respiratory alkalosis. Chronic hypocapnia is not shown but is directly below the normal zone; **F** Chronic base deficit, chronic or compensated metabolic acidosis; **G** Acute base deficit, acute or uncompensated metabolic acidosis. Is a theoretical area.

$$PAO_2 = FIO_2\,(PB-47) - \frac{PACO_2}{R} + FIO_2\,(1-R)\,\frac{PACO_2}{R} \quad \text{(Eq. 7)}$$

PAO_2 may be approximated, when room air is breathed at sea level (PB = 760 mm Hg) and the respiratory exchange ratio, R, is assumed to be 0.8, by:

$$PAO_2 \doteq 147 - PaCO_2/0.8 \quad \text{(Eq. 8)}$$

Arterial pressure of O_2 and, hence, of $P(A-a)O_2$ is dependent upon several normal variables—age, position, and altitude—as well as on the disease. For instance, in one study, in subjects seated at 75 °, PaO_2 was equal to 104.2 − 0.27 years;[22] in another study, in supine subjects, PaO_2 was 109 − .43 years;[22] in mile-high Denver, mean PaO_2 is about 70 mm Hg.[11] Normal $P(A-a)O_2$ is less than 20 mm Hg in young individuals.[22,23] The difference increases with age as detailed above.

Increasing FIO_2 increases PaO_2 proportionally, except in the presence of an anatomic right-to-left shunt—congenital heart disease, pulmonary hypertension with patent foreamen ovale, pulmonary arteriovenous malformation, consolidation of lung, and so forth. Arterial PO_2 increases appropriately with O_2 administration in pathologic conditions in which pulmonary capillary blood is in contact with ventilated alveoli, such as ventilation/perfusion mismatching (bronchitis, asthma, interstitial processes, etc.), diffuse interstitial fibrotic diseases, and hypoventilation.[11,24]

TRANSPORT OF OXYGEN

THE O_2 DISSOCIATION CURVE

Knowledge of the characteristics of the O_2 dissociation curve is important for understanding O_2 transport by the blood. The O_2 dissociation curve may be obtained by exposing blood to known values of O_2 tension and analyzing the content of O_2 for a range of 0 to about 150 mm Hg. The characteristic S-shaped curve is due to progressive interactions between O_2 and hemoglobin molecules causing allosteric changes in the resulting O_2 hemoglobin complex.[25] The standard curve is commonly shown for a pH of 7.40 and temperature of 37 °C. The effect of CO_2 is qualitatively the same as that of hydrogen ions. Shift of the curve to the right is caused by either increased temperature, or increased hydrogen ion (decreased pH) or increased CO_2 tension.[24] A shift of the dissociation curve to the left is caused by the opposite changes. The process by which CO_2 shifts the curve to the right is known as the *Bohr effect*. Because of the Bohr effect, the increase in PCO_2 in systemic capillary blood augments the release of O_2 to tissue.

RELEASE OF O_2 TO TISSUE

As noted previously, the addition of CO_2 to systemic capillary blood causes the release of O_2 from hemoglobin (the Bohr effect). Additionally, shift of the oxygen dissociation curve to the right by an increase of CO_2, hydrogen ion, or 2,3 diphosphoglycerate facilitates the release of O_2 at values of PO_2 typical of venous blood (30–40 mm Hg). That is, although arterial blood contains slightly less oxygen than normal at any PO_2 value in right-shifted curves, venous blood contains considerably less oxygen than normal in right-shifted curves. Hence, for usual changes of PO_2 between arterial and venous blood (40–50 mm Hg), more oxygen will be released to tissue from blood that is right-shifted than from normal blood. Stated another way, compared to normal blood, venous PO_2 values in right-shifted blood will be higher after the release of similar amounts of O_2.

CO BINDING BY BLOOD

Blood has an affinity for CO about 250 times that for O_2.[26] The normal O_2 dissociation curve is altered in special ways by CO. CO successfully competes with O_2 for the initial binding sties. This causes the O_2 dissociation curve to function as if it has lost the lower portion up to the amount of CO saturation. Additionally, the remainder of the curve is shifted to the left starting from that point. Hence, now CO not only displaces O_2 from hemoglobin but causes the remaining O_2 to be bound more tenaciously in the presence of CO due to this functional leftward shift.[26] Because of these combined effects, coma ensues at about 60% COHb.[27]

P_{50} IN VIVO AND IN VITRO

Another way of expressing the rightward or leftward position of the O_2 dissociation curve is by means of the partial pressure of oxygen at 50% of saturation (P_{50}). The normal P_{50} for an adult is about 27 torr.[28] P_{50} is higher than 27 mm Hg in right-shifted curves and lower in left-shifted curves. P_{50} in vivo may be of critical importance in patients with severe difficulty of O_2 transport. A rule of thumb is that a 4-torr change of in vivo P_{50} requires a 25% change in the cardiac output in order to maintain the same O_2 delivery and venous PO_2. Thus, it may be readily seen that seemingly small changes in the P_{50} may have large effects on the oxygen transport system.

2,3 DIPHOSPHOGLYCERATE

Normal erythrocytes in adults contains about 15 ml/g of hemoglobin of an organic phosphate called 2,3-diphosphoglycerate (DPG).[28] This substance competes with oxygen for binding sites in the heme group. DPG is not present in fetal blood but is rapidly formed after birth, shifting the curve to the right. The initial leftward shift of fetal blood would seem to have some teleological significance because uptake of O_2 from the placenta is possibly a limiting feature of O_2 transport to the fetal tissue. DPG levels have been observed to be increased during residence at altitude and in patients with anemia.[29] Blood that has been stored in blood banks decreases its supply of DPG, causing the O_2 dissociation curve to shift markedly leftward. The administration of large amounts of bank blood may be detrimental to O_2 transport in some individuals.

MIXED VENOUS OXYGEN

Mixed venous oxygen represents an admixture of blood draining from all portions of the body. Tissues with high blood flow/metabolism ratios, e.g., kidneys, characteristically have high venous PO_2 values, while those with lower blood flow/metabolism, e.g., myocardium, have lower values. Because venous blood is approximately equal to end capillary PO_2, venous blood PO_2 may be regarded as representing a value close to the driving pressure for supply of O_2 to cells in the vicinity of the venous end of capillaries.[30] As such, venous PO_2 allows evaluation of the possibility of critical tissue hypoxia. It has been suggested that a mixed venous value of 20 mm Hg represents the minimal level before tissue hypoxia occurs, particularly in organs such as the heart and brain.[31] With modern fiberoptic techniques, mixed venous SO_2 may be monitored continuously. It may be shown that

$$S\bar{v}O_2 = SaO_2 - \frac{\dot{V}O_2}{13.7 \, (Hb) \, \dot{Q}} \qquad \text{(Eq. 9)}$$

where 13.7 is the value of O_2 in ml O_2/g hb/100 ml blood, and $\dot{Q}$ is cardiac output. Hence, the causes of low $S\bar{v}O_2$ are changes in SaO_2, O_2 consumption, hemoglobin concentration, and/or cardiac output without balancing compensatory changes, e.g., patients with anemia avoid significant decrease of $P\bar{v}O_2$ and, hence, tissue hypoxia by increasing cardiac output. Patients with lung disease and arterial saturation may increase hemoglobin and cardiac output or reduce O_2 consumption or have some combination of these physiologic functions to prevent tissue hypoxia in the face of low arterial O_2 saturation.

ARTIFACTS AND PITFALLS

A good clinical history is important in the study of acid/base problems. A patient who has developed hypercapnia may have any number of defined acid/base states depending on the time course involved and the extent of intracellular buffering or kidney compensation. When the effect of placing the patient on a ventilator and rapidly lowering PCO_2 is considered, it is clear that understanding is possible only when historic information is available.

The CO_2 tension of the arterial blood can be used without qualification as a measure of the respiratory component of acid/base status. Respiratory status may reflect primary changes or may represent secondary effects due to metabolic changes in the patient. Primary changes are often very large whereas purely secondary effects are not as large. Because purely primary changes of CO_2 tension also change bicarbonate, quantification of the metabolic component cannot be accomplished solely by consideration of bicarbonate. It is technically much easier to measure PCO_2 and pH and to compute or derive any other acid/base parameter that may be suitable for evaluation of the metabolic component.

This has led to use of derived values such as the standard bicarbonate and the T_{40} bicarbonate, which describe bicarbonate values under conditions of a constant PCO_2 of 40 torr.[12] The standard bicarbonate represents blood in vitro that has been returned to a PCO_2 of 40-torr value, and the T_{40} bicarbonate represents the bicarbonate of blood in vivo when the patient ventilatory status is such that the PCO_2 is 40 torr. It has been demonstrated that the standard bicarbonate is the least reliable clinical indicator of the metabolic state of the patient. Change of bicarbonate and T_{40} bicarbonate are better clinical guides, but the most reliable indicator of the metabolic state of the patient is the base excess (BE) of the extracellular fluid. The derivation of this value has previously been reported.[20] BE is represented on the diagram as the vertical distance on the bicarbonate axis above the buffer slope. Base deficit is the value of the vertical

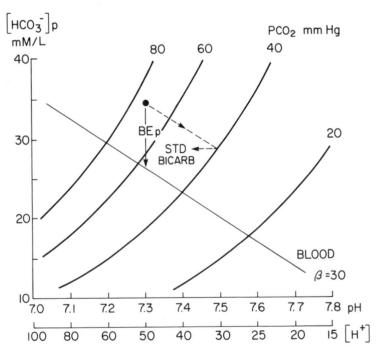

Figure 11-4.   Depiction of the derivation and calculation of the BE of the plasma (BE_p) and standard bicarbonate (Std bicarb). For details see text.

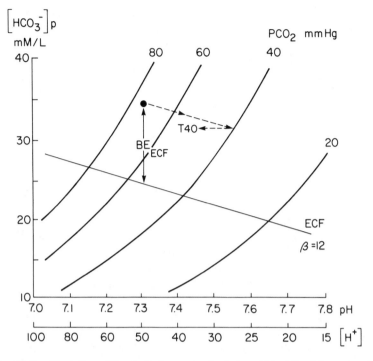

Figure 11-5. Depiction of the derivation and calculation of the BE of the extracellular fluid (BE_{ECF}) and T_{40}. For details see text.

distance below the buffer slope. The diagram also represents calculation of standard bicarbonate and T_{40} bicarbonate. These values are calculated by returning to PCO_2 40 torr on a line parallel to the buffer slope; the value of bicarbonate is then read at that point.

EXAMPLE

CASE 1

A 70-year-old woman was admitted on 8/16 at 9 PM, with a chief complaint of shortness of breath for a 3-week duration. She was known to have had chronic obstructive airways disease for many years. She had several previous admissions for pneumonia and congestive heart failure; the last admission was 4 months earlier. The patient presented with progressive shortness of breath, orthopnea, ankle swelling, and cough productions of yellow sputum. On physical examination the blood pressure was $^{110}/70$, pulse 140, respiration 25, temperature 99.6°F.

The patient was acutely dyspenic. There were moist, loud crackling rales throughout the chest both anteriorly and posteriorly. There was 2–3+ pitting edema to the midcalf. The laboratory examination revealed hemoglobin of 11.4, white blood cell count of 16,500 (83% segmented), potassium 3.9, sodium 136, BUN 34, and sugar 140. There was an apical infiltrate on the chest X ray. The patient was intubated on admission and treated with ventilatory support and O_2 therapy. She was also given bronchodilators, antibiotics, diuretics, and potassium chloride was added with the antibiotics. There were wide changes in the arterial blood gases noted secondary to changes in ventilatory settings. The arterial blood-gas summary is shown in Table 11-2.

The first blood gas was drawn after the patient received nasal O_2. Slight acidemia due to partially compensated respiratory acidosis was evident. There was also hypoxemia ($P(A-a)O_2 = 179$ mm Hg). Subsequently, following the questionable administration of 100% oxygen the next morning ($FIO_2 = 1.0$), there was increased respiratory acidosis and increased oxygenation; the failure of PaO_2 to rise to 550 mm Hg or more during 100% O_2 indicates the presence of an anatomic right-to-left shunt, e.g., pneumonia. Because of clinical deterioration, the patient was intubated and artificially ventilated. The next gas demonstrated normal pH because of lower $PaCO_2$ and low BE (mild metabolic acidosis had occurred during the period of clinical deterioration); additionally, the PaO_2 was low (44 mm Hg). Unfortunately, both the inspired O_2 and ventilator minute ventilation were increased resulting in more than adequate oxygenation and combined metabolic and respiratory alkalosis. Both inspired O_2 and ventilator minute ventilation were adjusted downward resulting in more normal pH and PaO_2 values; however, note that for this degree of metabolic alkalosis, the elevated $PaCO_2$ value of 52 mm Hg still resulted in an alkaline pH. Subsequently, PCO_2 was lowered in a more gradual manner with a consequent reduction in the BE (ECF) and better control of arterial pH.

Table 11-2   Case 1

Date	Time	pH	PCO_2 mm Hg	HCO_3 mEq/liter	BE mEq/liter	SAT %	PO_2 mm Hg	Remarks
8/16	2115	7.35	85	45	17	92	68	Nasal O_2 (40%)
8/17	0900	7.29	95	42	16	99	156	100% O_2
8/17	2400	7.39	66	39	12	77	44	Ventilator 40% O_2
8/18	0030	7.63	32	35	12	99	118	Increased ventilator, increased O_2.
8/18	0945	7.48	52	38	13	97	82	Decreased ventilator, decreased O_2.
8/21	0700	7.40	45	27	3	91	68	Decreased ventilator, decreased O_2.

QUALITY CONTROL

Quality control is usually considered the responsibility of the laboratory providing the results to the physician. However, it is also important that the physician taking care of the patient be involved in quality control of blood gases and should report inconsistent, unphysiologic, or clinically unlikely values to the laboratory. For example, as is evident from equations 6 and 7, the sum of the PaO_2 and $PaCO_2$ should not exceed 145–150 mm Hg in patients breathing air. Further, a low sum of the PO_2 and PCO_2 may suggest venous blood if the values are inconsistent with the clinical state of the patient and previous values. Rapid large changes in the BE must be explained. A sudden decrease in the BE suggests either lactic acidemia or an error in the analysis. If lactic acidemia is inconsistent with the patient's clinical state, then the analysis must be rejected as erroneous in some fashion. For this reason, it is suggested that a blood sample should not be discarded immediately upon analysis so that the clinician may have an opportunity to evaluate the results and request reanalysis should the values to be inconsistent with the clinical state in the time course of the illness. A graphic representation of acid/base relationships, such as the Davenport or a similar diagram, may be of great assistance in plotting the time course and the expected changes.

CONTROVERSIES

With the increased use of and availability of computerized interpretations of blood-gas data, standardization is needed. However, though the use of modifiers such as mild, moderate, and severe has cut-off points implicit in their meanings, there is no standard to which to refer. The following is the system utilized for a number of years at Los Angeles County General/University of Southern California Hospital. The major justification for the algorithm used is many years of experience.

Initially, PCO_2 is interpreted using the simple phrase "alveolar ventilation." If the PCO_2 is less than 36 torr, the phrase is modified to "increased." If the PCO_2 is greater than 44, "decreased" is used. These are, in turn, modified by an index term, $IND = (PCO_2 - 40) (1/2 \div 2$ integer value only). If $IND = 1$, no modifier is added; if it equals 2, "slightly" is used; if it is 3, "moderately" is used, and for 4 or more "markedly" is used. Hydrogen ion concentration ($[H+]$) is used to analyze acid/base states. $[H+]$ less than 37 is alkalemia, and greater than 43 is acidemia. These terms are further modified using the index algorithm above, substituting ($[H+] - 40$), for ($PCO_2 - 40$). The adverbs are converted to adjectives by dropping "ly."

Bicarbonate is described as "bicarbonate deficit" or "retention" if it is less than 22 or above 26 mmol/liter, respectively. The index algorithm is used but modified by substituting ($[HCO_3]-24$) for ($PCO_2 - 40$), and the integers 2, 3, and 4 derived are used to obtain the adjectives "slight," "moderate," and "marked," as above.

For the oxygen system, the concept of "oxygenation" is based upon the oxygen content. If it is a venous sample, the phrase "hypoxia" is used, which is modified as "no," "mild," "moderate," "marked," and "severe." The cut-off points for each is an O_2 content of greater than 14.5 ml/dl for "no," from 11.5 to 14.4, from 7.4 to 11.4, from 3.5 to 7.4 and less than 3.5 for each increasing in severity. If arterial blood is used, the basic phrase is "hypoxemia" and modified as above at 16.5 for "no," 13.5 to 16.4, 9.5 to 13.4, 5.5 to 9.4, and less than 5.5 for each modifier from "no" to "severe." The alveolar-arterial oxygen (A-a) O_2 difference is used to modify the phrase "ventilation/perfusion relationship" using the index above and substituting $[P(A-a)O_2 -$ predicted $P(A-a)O_2]$ for $(PCO_2 - 40)$ to modify "mismatch."

DERIVED VALUES

There is considerable disagreement on the reliability and the proper application of derived values in acid/base measurement. The difference between the CO_2 and the clinical laboratory and the bicarbonate measure from the blood-gas machine has been previously described. It is worth repeating that the further the pH is from 7.40 when the blood sample is drawn and the greater the temperature change the greater the difference between the values of the CO_2 and the clinical laboratory will be from the bicarbonate calculated from pH and PCO_2 measurements.

The use of standard bicarbonate was introduced by Van Slyke, Singer, and Hastings,[1,3] many decades ago, to describe an in vitro situation. As a result of the long tradition of this measurement, there are many who continue to use it. Subsequently, attempts to correct misuse of in vitro for in vivo states lead to the development of the T_{40} bicarbonate and subsequently the BE of the extracellular fluid.[12] Some machines report a BE of the extracellular fluid as part of their printed output. For clinical purposes many feel that the delta bicarbonate ($HCO_3 -24$) is sufficient to answer all needs. However, a delta bicarbonate of O can be calculated when there is considerable disruption in the acid/base status, both respiratory and metabolic.

ACIDOSIS AND ALKALOSIS

Acidosis and alkalosis are clinical terms that refer to the gain or loss of an acid or alkali. By definition, the suffix "osis" means excess of but is commonly used to mean "process." It is confusing to use these terms when modified as nouns such as Respiratory Acidosis or Metabolic Acidosis. Respiratory or Metabolic acidosis may or may not be accompanied by an acidemia because each may be altered by the other. Therefore, when used alone, alkalosis refers to a change in pH; but when referred to as the noun Metabolic Alkalosis, the pH state is not specified. Rigorously defined, Respiratory Acidosis represents only an increased PCO_2; a Respiratory Alkalosis conversely is synonymous with hypocapnia.

Metabolic Acidosis refers to a gain in noncarbonic or fixed acid and is represented by the term "base deficit." Conversely, Metabolic Alkalosis refers to an increase of BE. When discussing Respiratory and Metabolic Acidosis, pH must be stated. It is proper to state "the patient has Respiratory Acidosis and an Acidosis" but this is confusing as it sounds redundant. It is correct to say "respiratory acidosis" and "acidemia," but far more informative to say the PCO_2 is 80, the pH is 7.10, and the BE (ECF) is − 40.

P_{50}

The clinical usefulness of the P_{50} has not yet achieved a high degree of acceptance. This is partially due to the difficulty in the determination of the P_{50} by standard techniques. The single-point P_{50} of Collier obviates the difficulty in obtaining in vivo and in vitro P_{50} measurements, making them clinically available. Most patients are readily handled without reference to the P_{50} but clinical states involving severe cardiovascular and oxygenation problems require attention to P_{50} because apparently minor changes of P_{50} frequently require substantial changes in cardiovascular dynamics to maintain O_2 delivery. The accuracy of the single-point measurement is best when calculated from values close to 50% saturation.[32] Therefore, venous blood is a very desirable sample for the P_{50} measurement. Severely deoxygenated patients can have arterial samples comparable to the normal venous PO_2 and, therefore, provide very reliable measurements of the single-point P_{50}. However, the further the actual saturation differs from the 50% saturation, the greater the increase in the error. Therefore, there are limits to a single-point measurement. A PO_2 value for a reliable single-point P_{50} must lie between 20 and 60 torr. Furthermore, the single-point P_{50} requires evaluation of carbon monoxide.[32] Thus, it would seem that the acquisition of a relatively infrequent used value such as the P_{50} would require substantial financial outlay for equipment. However, measurement of carboxyhemoglobin is frequently of value in evaluation of the oxygen system and not just in the calculation of P_{50}.

DIAGRAMS

The use of the Davenport diagram[9] in this article may be considered a controversial issue as there are a large number of many similar diagrams available. At one count, there were as many as 33 representations of the acid/base diagram that could be used for this purpose. The Davenport diagram is selectively used here because the buffer slopes are straight lines across the face of the diagram. Furthermore, the 95% confidence limits are also straight lines across the face of the diagram as opposed to many other popular diagrams which show substantial curvilinearity to the 95% confidence bands of the acute changes. With the linearity described in the Davenport diagram it is easy to understand

and see the magnitude of the BE when the individual values are plotted. This magnitude becomes less obvious in other representations. However, many students and practitioners have found that other representatives are useful; it is certainly an individual matter which that diagram one uses.

Partial pressures of O_2 and CO_2 are thermodynamic measurements requiring that the temperature be stated. Particular problems arise with pH and deep hypothermia. Recently, Hansen [33] has drawn attention to the fact that acid/base parameters should be measured and reported at 37 °C, not body temperature, if different. Thus, PCO_2, when related to an acid/base evaluation, should be corrected to 37 °C for calculation of bicarbonate and related values. When used to calculate ventilatory values such as $\dot{V}_A$, $\dot{V}_D$, P_AO_2, and so forth, the value used should be body temperature. Because $PaCO_2$ is usually measured at 37 °C, the correct method should be to correct partial pressures related to ventilation and not correct those related to acid base; however, this approach is confusing and cumbersome. This double standard remains an unresolved problem.

REFERENCES

1. Peters JP, Van Slyke DD: Quantitative Clinical Chemistry (Vol 2) Baltimore, Williams and Wilkins Co, 1932.
2. Henderson LJ: Blood, a Study in General Physiology. New Haven, Yale Univ Press, 1928.
3. Singer RB, Hastings AB: An improved clinical method for the estimation of disturbances of the acid-base balance of human blood. Medicine 28:223, 1948.
4. Sanz MC: Ultramicro methods and standardization of equipment. Clin Chem 3:406, 1957.
5. Severinghaus JW, Bradley AF: Electrodes for blood PO_2 and PCO_2 determination. J Appl Physiol 131:515, 1958.
6. Comore JH, Jr., Botelhos: The unreliability of cyanosis in the recognition of arterial hypoxemia. Am J Med Sci 214:1, 1947.
7. Payne J, Hill D: Oxygen measurements in blood and tissue and their significance. New York, Little Brown and Co, 1966.
8. Sharp J: Measurement of pH and blood gases in arterialized capillary blood. Med Clin N Am 53:137, 1969.
9. Davenport H: The ABC of acid-base chemistry (ed 5) Chicago, Univ Chicago Press, 1969.
10. Keilin D, Mann T: Activity of carbonic anhydrase within red blood corpuscles. Nature 148:493, 1941.
11. Filey GF: Acid-base and blood gas regulation (ed 2) Philadelphia, Lea and Febiger, 1971.

12. Siggaard-Anderson O: Acid-base status of the blood (ed 2). Baltimore, Williams and Wilkins, 1964.

13. Mithoefer JC, Thibeault DW, Bossman OE: Acid-base balance and the effect of oxyhemoglobin reduction on CO_2 transport. Resp Physiol 6:292, 1969.

14. Van Ypserle de Strihou C, Brasseur L, De Coninck J: "Carbon dioxide response curve" for chronic hypercapnea. N Engl J Med 275:117, 1966.

15. Asch M, Dell R, Williams G, Cohen M, et al.: Time course for development of respiratory compensation in metabolic acidosis. J Lab Clin Med 73:610, 1969.

16. Arbus GS, Herbert LA, Levesque PR et al.: Application of "significance band" for acute respiratory alkaoosis. N Engl J Med 280:117, 1969.

17. Goldring R, Cannon P, Heinemann H, et al.: Respiratory adjustment to chronic metabolic alkalosis in man. J Clin Invest 47:188, 1968.

18. Pitts R: Physiology of the Kidney and Body Fluids (ed 2) Chicago, Year Book Med Publ, 1968.

19. Brackett N, Jr, Cohen J, Schwartz W: Carbon dioxide titration curve of normal man: Effect of increasing degrees of acute hypercapnea on acid-base equilibrium. N Engl J Med 272:6, 1965.

20. Armstrong BW, Mohler JC, Jung RC, et al.: The in vivo carbon dioxide titration curve. Lancet 1:759, 1966.

21. Rahn H: The concept of mean alveolar air and the ventilation-blood flow relationships during pulmonary gas exchange. Am J Physiol 158:21, 1949.

22. Melemgaard K: The alveolar-arterial oxygen difference. Its size and components in normal man. Acta Physiol Scand 67:10, 1966.

23. Sorbini CA, Grassi V, Solinas, et al.: Arterial oxygen tension in relation to age in healthy subjects. Respiration 25:3, 1968.

24. Shapiro B, Harrison RA, Walton JR: Clinical Application of Blood Gases (ed 3). Chicago, Year Book, 1982.

25. Perutz M: Sterochemistry of cooperative effects in hemoglobin. Nature 228:726, 1970.

26. Roughton FJW, Darling RC: The effect of carbon monoxide on the oxyhemoglobin dissociation curve. Am J Physiol 144:17, 1944.

27. Stewart RD, et al.: Experimental human exposure to carbon monoxide. Arch Environ Health 21:154, 1970.

28. Oski F, Delizonia-Papadopoulas M: The red cell, 2,3-diphosphoglycerate, and tissue oxygen release. J Pediatrics 77:941, 1970.

29. Finch C, Lenfant C: Oxygen transport in man. N Engl J Med 286:407, 1972.

30. Tenney SM: A theoretical analysis of the relationship between venous blood and mean tissue oxygen pressures. Resp Physiol 20:283, 1974.

31. Bendixen HH, Laver MB: Hypoxia in anaesthesia: A review. Clin Pharmacol Ther 6:510, 1965.

32. Collier CR: Oxygen affinity of human blood in the presence of carbon monoxide. J Appl Physiol 40:487, 1976.

33. Hansen J: Letter to the editor. N Engl J Med 303:341, 1981.

CHAPTER 12

Exercise Testing

JAMES E. HANSEN

HISTORY AND REVIEW OF METHODS

Exercise testing has traditionally been used to evaluate athletes, students, soldiers, and those with disturbed nutrition or exposure to extremes of heat or physical exertion. Today, surgeons and physicians specializing in cardiovascular and pulmonary medicine use exercise testing to detect abnormalities that are not apparent when the patient is measured at rest. A diversity of equipment, techniques, and strategies have evolved for clinical exercise testing in the respiratory and cardiovascular laboratories.[1-6]

Exercise requires not only lung function but also heart function and two circulations for gas transport. There is no single correct way to equip an exercise laboratory. Often, simple cardiovascular and respiratory measurements during exercise suffice. The minimum measures required for diagnostic evaluation are inspired or expired minute ventilation, ventilatory frequency, work rates, a single-lead electrocardiogram, and the recording of symptoms. Some clinicians would also include multiple-lead electrocardiography. For selection of O_2 therapy in patients with obvious respiratory impairment, measurement of arterial blood O_2 saturation or pressure at rest may not be sufficient and measurement during exercise may be required. The understanding of pathophysiology and the thoughtful application of a few measures may lead the discerning clinician to the correct decision, whereas a large number of measures, especially when of questionable accuracy, may obscure the truth.

The examples presented in this chapter use incremental cycle exercise, but the same principles can be used to interpret steady-state or incremental exercise on either the treadmill or cycle.

PULMONARY FUNCTION TESTING
INDICATIONS AND INTERPRETATIONS

PHYSIOLOGY OF EXERCISE

To perform external work, energy must be derived from the metabolism of foodstuffs which depends on the transfer of O_2 from the inspired air through the lungs, pulmonary circulation, heart, and peripheral circulation to the muscle. Concurrently, CO_2 is transferred from the muscle to the expired gas.[7,9] Only a trivial quantity of CO_2 is excreted by the kidney as bicarbonate. The respiratory quotient (RQ) of the tissues is the ratio of the moles of CO_2 produced to the moles of O_2 consumed. The aerobic metabolism of carbohydrate yields an RQ of 1, whereas that of fatty acids is approximately 0.71. The ratio of CO_2 output to O_2 uptake at the lung is the respiratory exchange ratio, or R. In the steady state the R is similar to the RQ of the fuel metabolized; but it can be increased temporarily with hyperventilation or metabolic acidosis. The oxygen stores of the body are limited to the few liters: the gas phase in the lung and that combined chemically with hemoglobin and myoglobin. The CO_2 stores are much greater and include carbonates and bicarbonates. The fuel utilized by the muscle during exercise depends not only on the substrate but also on the supply of O_2. With sufficient oxygen, carbohydrate is metabolized aerobically to yield approximately 38 moles of adenosine triphosphate (ATP) per mole of glucose. With insufficient oxygen, some of the pyruvate is not metabolized via the citric acid cycle but is converted to lactic acid. This lactic acid is buffered in the blood and tissue with the production of CO_2 in excess of that which comes from aerobic metabolism.[10] This excess CO_2 causes a temporary rise in R during exercise and early recovery. The R declines in later recovery as O_2 stores are replenished and the metabolic acidosis subsides.

During incremental exercise performed in the upright position, the cardiac stroke volume rises initially but then plateaus. The heart rate (HR), expired ventilation ($\dot{V}_E$), oxygen uptake ($\dot{V}_{O_2}$), and carbon dioxide output ($\dot{V}_{CO_2}$) continue to rise progressively. In a healthy person, $\dot{V}_{O_2}$ increases approximately tenfold from the resting level while cardiac output and arterial-mixed venous (a-$\bar{v}$) oxygen difference each increase threefold to fourfold.[11] Both the increase in HR and cardiac output are linearly related to $\dot{V}_{O_2}$ and work rate.[2,12]. The maximum HR gradually declines with age.[2] The oxygen pulse, which is the ml of O_2 uptake per heart beat, is a useful index of both gas exchange and cardiovascular response. With valvular heart disease or physical deconditioning, the HR may be higher and the effective stroke volume and O_2 pulse lower than predicted for a given work rate or $\dot{V}_{O_2}$.

Physiologically, one may think of the tidal volume (V_T) as consisting of an alveolar volume (VA) which contributed to CO_2 elimination and a physiological dead space volume (V_D) which did not participate in gas exchange. The ratio of physiologic dead space to tidal volume (V_D/V_T) is approximately one third at rest, and is lower in those with higher V_T. Normally during exercise, the V_D/V_T

declines to 0.15–0.30 or less.[2,8,18] When there is uneven ventilation and perfusion of lung units causing some ventilation/perfusion relationship($\dot{V}/\dot{Q}$) ratios to be increased relative to others, the V_D and V_D/V_T are increased.

Minute ventilation ($\dot{V}_E$) is more closely related to $\dot{V}_{CO_2}$ than to $\dot{V}_{O_2}$. The ratios of $\dot{V}_E$ to $\dot{V}_{CO_2}$ and $\dot{V}_{O_2}$ are defined as the ventilatory equivalents for CO_2 and O_2, respectively. These ratios decrease normally with moderate exercise to approximately 23 for O_2 and 27 for CO_2.[3] With anaerobic metabolism, there is an additional increase in CO_2 due to the buffering of lactic acid. The increased $PaCO_2$ stimulates ventilation and $\dot{V}_E$ rises faster than $\dot{V}_{O_2}$. The point just before the appearance of lactic acid or its consequence, excess CO_2 production, is called the anaerobic threshold (*AT*).[10] Exercise cannot be continued indefinitely above the *AT* due to increasing metabolic acidosis. The *AT* can usually be accurately identified noninvasively by serial measurements of gas exchange (a rise in partial pressure of end-tidal O_2 ($P_{ET}\,O_2$), ventilatory equivalent of O_2 ($\dot{V}_E/(\dot{V}_{O_2})$, and *R* with a stable $P_{ET}CO_2$ and $\dot{V}_E/\dot{V}_{CO_2}$).

In the normal person, incremental exercise usually stops well before maximum $\dot{V}_E$ at $\dot{V}_{O_2}$ max ($\dot{V}_E$ max) reaches maximum voluntary ventilation (MVV), although $\dot{V}_E$ max approach MVV in well-motivated individuals and exceed it in patients with severe ventilatory impairment.

Exercise capacity can be assessed by measuring *AT* and maximum oxygen uptake ($\dot{V}_{O_2}$ max). In normals, $\dot{V}_{O_2}$ max is usually characterized by a brief plateau of $\dot{V}_{O_2}$ while the work rate increases. In patients, such a plateau may not be seen and $\dot{V}_{O_2}$ max is considered to be the highest $\dot{V}_{O_2}$ reached. By itself, $\dot{V}_{O_2}$ max does not indicate whether the physiologic limitation is the skeletal muscles, peripheral circulation, heart, pulmonary circulation, lungs, or chest wall.

PATHOPHYSIOLOGY OF EXERCISE

As partially described elsewhere,[9,13] the following diseases or pathologic conditions, listed numerically, may be associated with the following anatomic and physiologic defects, and findings.

1. Obstructive lung disease:
   (a) increased airway resistance causes a decrease in flow rates;

   (b) $\dot{V}/\dot{Q}$ mismatch causes an increase in V_D, V_D/V_T, $\dot{V}_E/\dot{V}_{CO_2}$, $\dot{V}_E/\dot{V}_{O_2}$, P(A-a)O_2, and positive arterial end-tidal CO_2 difference in mm Hg (P(a-ET)CO_2);

   (c) Hypoxemia causes an increase in ventilatory equivalents; and

   (d) the combination causes a decrease in maximum working capacity and an increase in $\dot{V}_E$max/MVV and may result in inability to exercise above *AT.*

2. Restrictive disease:
   (a) decreased lung compliance causes a decrease in V_T and an increase in frequency;
   (b) the reduced pulmonary capillary bed and the $\dot{V}/\dot{Q}$ mismatch cause an increase in V_D/V_T and $P(A\text{-}a)O_2$;
   (c) hypoxemia causes an increase in $\dot{V}_E/\dot{V}_{O_2}$ and $\dot{V}_E/\dot{V}_{CO_2}$; and
   (d) the combination causes an increase in $\dot{V}_E max/MVV$ and a reduced work capacity.

3. Exercise induced bronchospasm:
   (a) increased airway resistance caused by cooling of the airways associated with high ventilation and acidemia result in a decrease in expiratory flow rates at the end of or following heavy exercise.

4. Pulmonary vascular disease:
   (a) reduction of recruitable pulmonary capillary bed, and
   (b) accompanying $\dot{V}/\dot{Q}$ mismatch causes an increase in $\dot{V}_E/\dot{V}_{CO_2}$, $\dot{V}_E/\dot{V}_{O_2}$, V_D, V_D/V_T, and pulmonary artery pressure, a reduced maximum work capacity and O_2 pulse, and a normal or decreased heart rate at $\dot{V}_{O_2}max$ (HRmax).

5. Chest wall disease:
   (a) limitation to ventilation causes a reduced MVV with a resulting increase in $\dot{V}_E max/MVV$, and a decrease in maximum work capacity.

6. Valvular or hypertensive cardiovascular disease:
   (a) reduction in stroke volume may cause a decrease in work capacity, $\dot{V}_{O_2}max$, O_2 pulse max, and $\dot{V}_E max/MVV$.

7. Coronary artery disease:
   (a) myocardial ischemia and reduced contractility may cause a worsening rhythm disturbance, decrease in systolic blood pressure, pulse pressure, and stroke volume despite increasing demands; and
   (b) decreased myocardial perfusion may cause arrhythmia, ST segment changes, angina, or dyspnea with a resulting decrease in *AT*, maximum work capacity, and associated values.

8. Peripheral vascular disease:
   (a) inability to increase blood flow to the exercising muscle may cause muscle pain, an increase in lactic acid production, and metabolic acidosis; and

(b) limited ability to work causes a decrease in $\dot{V}_{O_2}$max, O_2 pulse max, and HRmax.

9. Deconditioning:
   (a) low stroke volume and poor distribution of blood flow is likely to cause a decrease in $\dot{V}_{O_2}$max, *AT,* and O_2 pulse max.

10. A disinclination to work or psychogenic disease:
    (a) cortical or autonomic influences may cause hyperventilation, regular rapid or irregular breathing, and/or tachycardia at rest which tend to normalize with increasing exercise;
    (b) if exercise is prematurely terminated, the lack of significant anaerobic metabolism yields no evidence of cardiovascular or ventilatory limitation, i.e., there is a low HRmax, low$\dot{V}_E$max/MVV, slight decline in arterial bicarbonate, and a small rise in *R* during recovery; and
    (c) if exercise is continued, a normal *AT.*

11. Obesity:
    (a) the increased metabolic requirement to move the legs and body causes an increase in $\dot{V}_{O_2}$ at unloaded pedalling or walking with normal work efficiency thereafter;
    (b) basilar atelectasis causes hypoxemia at rest with improvement during exercise as V_T increases.

12. Anemia or carboxyhemoglobinemia:
    (a) the reduced O_2 content of the blood causes a decrease in $\dot{V}_{O_2}$max, O_2 pulse max, and *AT.*

INDICATIONS

Exercise testing is useful to the pulmonary physician or cardiologist and beneficial to the patient for diagnosis, quantification of impairment, evaluation of therapies, and understanding physiology and pathophysiology. Exercise is particularly useful in evaluating patients with dyspnea, whether or not accompanied by chest pain or fatigue. Exercise is also useful in assessing chronic obstructive lung disease (OLD) including exercise-induced bronchospasm, interstitial lung disease, neuromuscular diseases, obesity, anxiety-induced hyperventilation, pulmonary vascular disease, unfitness, coronary artery disease, or other circulatory diseases. In each case, the patterns of data may be distinctive. In patients with multiple disorders, evaluation may allow identification of the dominant disorder.

It is frequently necessary to quantify impairment, as when evaluating patients for disability or when deciding on the necessity for O_2 therapy. Examples of problems that may be helped by serial evaluation include the response of interstitial lung disease to corticosteroids, the response of OLD disease to O_2 therapy or physical conditioning programs, or the response of alveolar proteinosis to lung lavage.

INTERPRETATIONS

PATTERNS OF ABNORMAL RESPONSE TO EXERCISE

Abnormal Gas Exchange

Increasing Hypoxemia and Widening of P(A-a)O₂. This pattern is particularly striking in interstitial lung disease, where the PaO_2 may decline to 40 mm Hg or lower and occurs to a variable degree in obstructive airway disease. In such patients, however, exercise appears to be terminated because of ventilatory limitation rather than hypoxemia per se. P(A-a)O₂ and PaO_2 are age dependent. Only rarely, except in the elderly or highly motivated does PaO_2 decline in normals to below 80 mm Hg.[18]

Decreasing Hypoxemia and Narrowing of P(A-a)O₂ With Exercise. Obese patients often have abnormal P(A-a)O₂ while they are at rest sitting in a chair. P(A-a)O₂ usually improves without change in $PaCO_2$ or R when they move to the cycle ergometer, presumably because the belly falls forward and the diaphragm drops, with resultant opening of the basal airways. In such patients, P(A-a)O₂ rises to normal during exercise, indicating the primary cause of the hypoxemia and $\dot{V}/\dot{Q}$ disturbance is extrapulmonary.

Positive P(a-ET)CO₂ and Abnormally Elevated $\dot{V}_E/\dot{V}_{CO_2}$ and V_D/V_T. The V_D/V_T normally declines with exercise as V_T increases twofold to fourfold and physiologic V_D increases minimally. In patients with pulmonary vascular disease, whether due to embolism or secondary to diseases such as emphysema or scleroderma, V_D/V_T may decline only minimally with increasing exercise as ventilation increases more to poorly rather than well-perfused airspaces. In such patients, $\dot{V}_E/\dot{V}_{CO_2}$ does not decline below 30 and the $PaCO_2$ may be higher than PETCO₂. In patients with anxiety-induced tachypnea without lung disease, V_D/V_T and $\dot{V}_E/\dot{V}_{CO_2}$ may also remain high. Usually with encouragement, familiarization with equipment, and re-exercise after a few minutes of recovery, the tachypnea of anxiety will be reduced and the patient will develop a more normal breathing pattern.

Ventilatory Limitation

Usually it is the cardiovascular system or strength of the working muscles that limit the ability to sustain a progressive workload. In normals, the maximum sustained ventilation, measured for four minutes, is approximately 70% of the MVV, calculated from 15 seconds of voluntary hyperventilation.[15] Ventilatory limitation to exercise may occur at high altitude, in extremely fit and well-motivated athletes, or perhaps in healthy older people. When $\dot{V}_E$max approaches or exceeds MVV, a ventilatory limitation to exercise is implied. In patients with variable obstructive disease, MVV should be remeasured on the day of exercise testing. Upper airway or neuromuscular disease or lack of motivation should be suspected if MVV is much less than FEV_1 multiplied by 40. The ventilatory rate at maximal exercise often reaches 70 to 90 per minute in the patient with restrictive lung disease, but rarely exceeds 50 in patients with OLD. If exercise-induced bronchospasm is suspected, forced expiratory maneuvers should be obtained approximately 2, 5, 10, and 15 minutes after 6 to 10 minutes of exercise to exhaustion. With exercise-induced bronchospasm, the peak flow, or FEV_1, falls to 80% or less of pre-exercise levels at one of these times with later recovery. There may or may not be simultaneous abnormal auscultory findings.

Circulatory Limitation

The Fick equation ($\dot{V}_{O_2}$ equals cardiac output times $C(a-\bar{v})O_2$) indicates that $\dot{V}_{O_2}$max is dependent on maximal values of HR, stroke volume, and arterial oxygen content and minimal values of mixed venous O_2 content. Similarly, maximal O_2 pulse ($\dot{V}_{O_2}$/HR) is dependent on maximal values of stroke volume and arterial O_2 content and minimal values of mixed venous O_2 content. Although hematocrit and therefore O_2 capacity may rise approximately 10% with heavy exercise, the maximal arterial oxygen capacity and content is necessarily decreased with anemia and with carboxyhemoglobinemia. The HRmax may be far below the predicted normal value because of cardiovascular, neuromuscular, skeletal, or respiratory disease. In fact, the most common cause of a reduced HRmax in patients studied in our laboratory is reduced exercise capacity of ventilatory-limited patients with pulmonary disease. Maximum HR may also be decreased by beta blockade, but such blockade appears to be accompanied by an increase in stroke volume, so that the maximum O_2 pulse rises above control values.[16] Coronary artery disease may also cause a reduction in HRmax because the physician stops the test, or because of angina, arrhythmias, or other reasons that are not identified.[17] The stroke volume may be less than predicted with pulmonary vascular disease, peripheral vascular disease, high peripheral resistance, hypertensive cardiovascular disease, metabolic disorders, valvular or coronary artery disease, neurocirculatory asthenia, or unfitness.

The *AT* may be reduced in any of the above disorders. Even in the presence of other limiting factors, a circulatory disorder can be diagnosed if there is a low

AT. A small increase in *AT*, resulting from a training program, may result in a major improvement in the patients ability to walk or work. Thus, treatment of secondary circulatory disorders such as anemia, carboxyhemoglobinemia, or unfitness may be of major clinical benefit.

High Metabolic Requirement for External Work

The prime example of increased metabolic requirement occurs with obesity, when the work of moving the legs without accomplishing measurable external work may take more than one third or one half of the total O_2 uptake. High output states, hypertensive cardiovascular disease, and OLD may also cause a small increase in requirement for $\dot{V}_{O_2}$ and $\dot{V}_{CO_2}$.

Improvement in Symptoms or Work Capacity with Supplemental Oxygen

In many respiratory laboratories, the primary purpose of exercise testing may be to ascertain the effect of O_2 supplementation on blood gases, saturation, ventilation, dyspnea, or endurance in patients with severe lung disease.

Supplemental O_2 increases PIO_2, PAO_2, PaO_2, SaO_2, and CaO_2. Even though the increase in CaO_2 may be minimal, the increase in PaO_2 may cause a significant decrease in exercise ventilation due to carotid body inhibition. The decrease in exercise ventilation with supplemental O_2 is correlated with the severity of hypoxemia, at least in OLD.[18] With such a response, the patient will be less hypoxemic and dyspneic for the same level of exercise and should be able to increase activity and degree of fitness.

NORMAL VALUES AND QUANTIFICATION OF IMPAIRMENT

Work Capacity

The capacity to work to exhaustion in a few minutes correlates well with the $\dot{V}_{O_2}$max, whereas the capacity to work for hours correlates with the *AT*. In our clinical laboratory we base the predicted $\dot{V}_{O_2}$max on Bruce's study of an adult American population.[19] In obese patients the cycle $\dot{V}_{O_2}$max in ml STPD/min = $(0.79H - 60.7)(50.7 - 0.372Y)$ for men and $(0.79H - 68.2)(40.0 - 0.372Y)$ for women, where H = height in cm and Y = age in years. In nonobese or underweight patients the cycle $\dot{V}_{O_2}$max in ml STPD/min = $K(50.7 - 0.372Y)$ for men and $K(40.0 - 0.372Y)$ for women, where K = weight in kg. The predicted treadmill values are 111% of the predicted cycle values. In our clinical population the values derived from these data[19] seem reasonable for men but low for women. The SD of this study[19] approximates 12%; therefore a reduction of over 20% should occur in only 1 of 20 normal adults. Although such a division is arbitrary, we suggest that a reduction to 80–89% of predicted normal is borderline, to 65–79% is mild, to 50–64% is moderate, and 49% or below is severe.

In the untrained normal, the mean *AT* is 56% of the predicted $\dot{V}_{O_2}$max.[18] A reduction of the *AT* below 40% of the predicted $\dot{V}_{O_2}$max is abnormal, whether due to disease or unfitness.

Cardiovascular

The HR max of our normal population better fits the equation 220 - Y (20) than 210 - 0.65 Y (2), where Y = age in years. Because HR rises approximately threefold with maximum exercise, and $\dot{V}_{O_2}$ approximately tenfold, the HRmax will decline less than the $\dot{V}_{O_2}$max for the same severity of disease. Arbitrarily, we suggest the following quantifications for reduction in the HRmax: 90–94% of predicted is borderline, 85–89% is mild, 75–84% is moderate, and 74% or less is severe. Digitalis and the beta-blocking drugs reduce the expected HRmax.

Ventilation

In normal individuals, with valid measures of MVV, the $\dot{V}$Emax is usually less than 70-80% of the MVV (directly measured for 15 seconds at rest) and the breathing reserve (MVV-$\dot{V}_E$max) exceeds 15 liter/min.[18] In patients with ventilatory impairment, the ratio of $\dot{V}_E$max/MVV may approach or exceed 1.0, and the breathing reserve becomes zero or negative. In the absence of neuromuscular disease or upper airway obstruction the validity of the MVV maneuvers should be questioned if the MVV does not equal or exceed the FEV_1 times 40. Occasionally the $\dot{V}_E$max rises in an athlete or very well-motivated person above the MVV.

Gas Exchange

In 77 shipyard workers age 34–74 years without evidence of cardiovascular or parenchymal lung disease, it was unusual to find a PaO_2 less than 80 mm Hg, $P(A-a)O_2$ greater than 38 mm Hg, $P(a-ET)CO_2$ greater than 1 mm Hg, or a V_D/V_T greater than 0.28 at maximal exercise.[18] Using the following arbitrary numbers, gas exchange may be considered severe if: PaO_2 declines below 50 mm Hg at sea level, V_D/V_T remains above 0.40, or $V_E/\dot{V}_{O_2}$ does not decline to 40 with exercise.

ARTIFACTS, PITFALLS, AND QUALITY CONTROL

Poor exercise tests can result from improperly used or inaccurate equipment; improperly calibrated cycles or gas analyzers; slipping treadmill belts; alinear volume, flow, or fractional gas-measuring devices; leaking valves, tubes, or bags; improper timing or matching of volumes and fractional gas concentrations; improper blood collection; or inaccurate blood gas analyzers. Lack of knowledge of the exact water vapor pressure of the expired gas at the time of

Table 12-1   Exercise Test in Patient with Interstitial Lung Disease

Time min	Work wt	BP mmHg	HR min-1	RR	$\dot{V}_E$ BTPS L/min	$\dot{V}_{CO_2}$ STPD L/min	$\dot{V}_{O_2}$ STPD L/min	O_2 pulse ml/bt	R	PET O_2 (mmHg)	PA O_2	Pa O_2	Aa O_2	PET CO_2 (mmHg)	Pa CO_2	aET CO_2	pH	HCO$_3$ meq L	$\dfrac{\dot{V}_E}{\dot{V}_{CO_2}}$	$\dfrac{\dot{V}_E}{\dot{V}_{O_2}}$	$\dfrac{VD}{VT}$
0.5			77	15	9.4	0.20	0.26	3	0.77	106		74		35	35		7.47	25	43	33	
1.0			74	19	9.0	0.16	0.20	3	0.80	112				33					50	40	
1.5			79	21	8.0	0.12	0.16	2	0.75	112				33					58	43	
2.0			74	22	9.5	0.14	0.18	2	0.78	112				33					60	47	
2.5			72	24	8.9	0.14	0.18	3	0.78	110				34					55	43	
3.0		119/68	76	19	8.3	0.14	0.17	2	0.82	112	108	65	43	33	36	3	7.45	25	52	43	0.40
3.5	0		78	20	10.3	0.22	0.30	4	0.73	104				36					42	31	
4.0	0		79	25	12.9	0.26	0.36	5	0.72	103				37					45	32	
4.5	0		78	34	12.9	0.18	0.24	3	0.75	105				36					62	47	
5.0	0		78	23	11.3	0.23	0.29	4	0.79	107				35					44	35	
5.5	0		82	29	12.9	0.24	0.31	4	0.77	110				33					48	37	
6.0	0	125/68	77	24	12.6	0.25	0.32	4	0.78	109	107	70	37	34	35	1	7.44	24	45	36	0.35
6.5	15		73	20	8.7	0.18	0.25	3	0.72	102				38					43	31	
7.0	15		82	32	12.0	0.22	0.31	4	0.71	101				38					48	34	

7.5	30		91	22	15.4	0.37	0.49	5	0.76	105				36					39	29	
8.0	30	131/ 68	95	23	17.1	0.42	0.56	6	0.75	104	103	68	35	37	37	0	7.44	25	38	28	0.31
8.5	45		98	26	19.1	0.46	0.59	6	0.78	106				36					39	30	
9.0	45		102	23	17.6	0.46	0.58	6	0.79	103				38					36	28	
9.5	60		107	28	23.8	0.62	0.73	7	0.85	109				36					36	31	
10.0	60	146/ 75	113	29	25.9	0.69	0.80	7	0.86	108	106	68	38	37	39	2	7.43	25	35	31	0.31
10.5	75		114	31	29.8	0.79	0.86	8	0.92	111				36					36	33	
11.0	75		117	30	29.9	0.82	0.91	8	0.90	110				37					35	31	
11.5	90		123	37	36.2	0.96	1.01	8	0.95	112				36					36	34	
12.0	90		127	37	37.8	1.03	1.05	8	0.98	112				36					35	34	
12.5	105		132	42	43.8	1.15	1.13	9	1.02	115				35					36	37	
13.0	105	190/ 78	134	50	47.0	1.18	1.13	8	1.04	110	115	64	51	40	36	−4	7.42	23	38	39	0.31
13.5	120		143	51	54.9	1.39	1.29	9	1.08	118				33					38	41	
14.0	120	190/ 81	149	53	58.4	1.47	1.35	9	1.09	119	116	61	55	33	36	3	7.41	23	38	41	0.32
14.5			128	45	46.6	1.22	1.16	9	1.05	115				36					36	38	
15.0			104	41	37.6	0.95	0.83	8	1.14	117				36					38	43	
15.5			93	41	30.7	0.68	0.58	6	1.17	119				34					42	49	
16.0		162/ 65	83	34	23.1	0.51	0.48	6	1.06	116	115	80	35	35	37	2	7.36	21	42	45	0.36

wt = watts, BP = blood pressure, HR = heart rate, RR = respiratory rate, AaO$_2$ = P(A−a)O$_2$, aETCO$_2$ = P(a−ET)CO$_2$.

measurement and improper calculations are major causes of errors. Because of noise and movement associated with cycle or treadmill exercise, measurement of arterial blood pressure with a cuff, sphygmomanometer, and stethoscope is difficult.

Poor tests can also result from patient anxiety, especially when there has been insufficient practice and orientation on the cycle or treadmill, or selection of an improper work rate. Rarely is poor patient motivation alone a factor. If the work increment is too small, the patient may terminate exercise because of boredom, general fatigue, or discomfort, rather than a cardiovascular or pulmonary limitation. If the work rate increment is too large, the patient may terminate exercise because of local muscle weakness and not for cardiovascular or pulmonary reasons. Therefore, work increments causing exhaustion in 6 to 12 minutes seem optimal, regardless of the age, gender, strength, or infirmity of the patient. For normals, we base the increment on treadmill[10] or cycle[7] data; for patients, we use subjective judgements.

EXAMPLES

The following examples will be presented and discussed with the complete exercise data in the format available in our clinical laboratory.[2] Each patient will then be discussed as if he or she were exercised incrementally with only the following measures available: HR with single-lead EKG recording, expired ventilation rate and volume, work rate, and ear oximetry.

Interstitial Lung Disease

Table 12-1 and Figure 12-1 show an exercise study in a 37-year-old woman with interstitial lung disease before treatment with corticosteroids. A brachial artery catheter was inserted. The pulse rate, expired flow, and fractional gas concentrations were measured repeatedly at rest, during unloaded pedalling on a cycle ergometer, during incremental exercise to exhaustion, and during early recovery. At intervals the blood gases and arterial pressure were measured. In the first study, the patient developed increasing hypoxemia and widening of the $P(A-a)O_2$ during exercise, typical findings in interstitial disease. This pattern has also been reported even in patients with normal chest X rays.[3] Abnormal values derived from noninvasive measurements are high $\dot{V}_E/\dot{V}_{CO_2}$ (1d, f), which should decline to less than 30, the low HRmax (1b, e), high $\dot{V}_E$max/MVV (1 g), and low $\dot{V}_{O_2}$max (1c, e), all of which are typical of patients limited by lung disease. The rise of respiratory frequency above 50 (1 g) is typical of restrictive lung disease. The anaerobic threshold is estimated as the $\dot{V}_{O_2}$ at the point before $\dot{V}_E/\dot{V}_{O_2}$ rises while $\dot{V}_E/\dot{V}_{CO_2}$ remains stable (1c, f). The timing of the anaerobic threshold is confirmed to be at 45 watts of exercise in the graphs of R and $P_{ET}O_2$ (arrows in 1h, i). The abnormally high V_D/V_T and the positive $P(a-ET)CO_2$

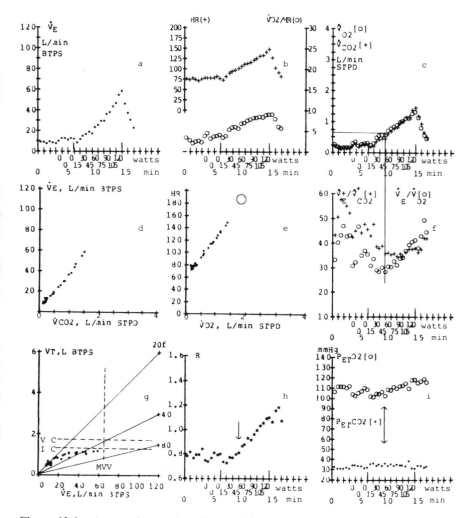

Figure 12-1. An exercise test in a 37-year-old woman with interstitial lung disease. From left to right, upper panels are (a) minute ventilation versus time and work rate; (b) HR and O₂ pulse in ml/beat versus time and work rate; and (c) O₂ uptake and CO₂ output versus time and work rate. Middle panels are (d) minute ventilation versus CO₂ output; (e) HR versus O₂ uptake; and (f) ventilatory equivalents for O₂ and CO₂ versus time and work rate. Lower panels are (g) V$_T$ versus minute ventilation; (h) respiratory exchange ratio versus time and work rate; and (i) end-tidal O₂ and CO₂ pressures versus time and work rate. In panel e the circle indicates the predicted maximum HR and O₂ uptake based on gender, age, and size; in panel g the dashed horizontal lines indicate VC and inspiratory capacity, the dashed vertical line indicates the 15-second MVV, and the solid diagonal lines indicate ventilatory frequencies of 20, 40, and 80 per minute. In panels c, f, h and i the solid vertical lines and arrows indicate the *AT*, which is then marked with a solid horizontal line in panel c.

(Table 12-1) are typical of $\dot{V}/\dot{Q}$ mismatch that may occur with obstructive, restrictive, or vascular lung disease.

After corticosteroid therapy, (Fig. 12-2), the improvement in the noninvasive measures ($\dot{V}_E/\dot{V}_{CO_2}$, $\dot{V}_E$max, HRmax, $\dot{V}_{O_2}$max, V_T, AT) was striking, indicating improvement in lung function and improved cardiovascular fitness. The invasive measures, P(A-a)O_2, P(a-ET)CO_2, and V_D/V_T, although not presented, also showed striking improvement and became normal.

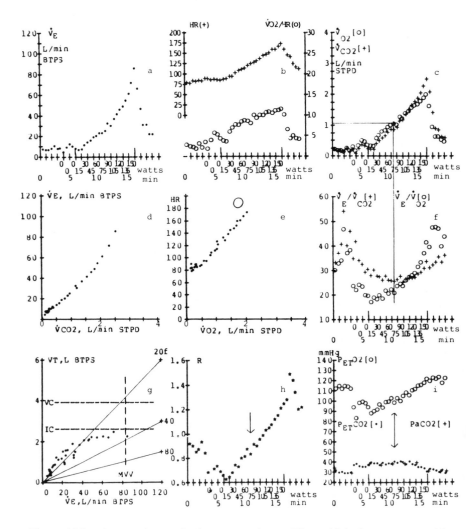

Figure 12-2. An exercise test in the same patient as Figure 12-1 after treatment with prednisolone. Symbols are as in Figure 12-1. Arterial CO_2 pressure has been added to panel i.

Using only the simple measures, one could discern arterial desaturation with increasing exercise, a high respiratory rate and $\dot{V}_E$max/MVV, and a low HRmax and work capacity on the first test. It would also be evident that the patient was initially ventilatory limited and hypoxemic and that she improved strikingly with treatment. The improvement in cardiovascular function as measured by the O_2 pulse and *AT* would not be evident.

OLD and Obesity

The patient depicted in Figure 12-3 and Table 12-2 is a 50-year-old man with a 50-pack year smoking history, industrial asbestos exposure, and obesity.

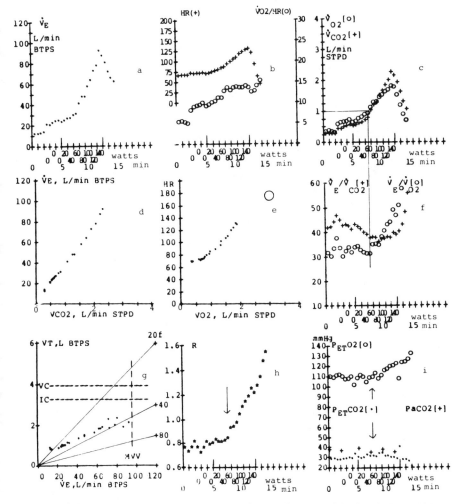

Figure 12-3. An exercise test in an obese 50-year-old man with chronic bronchitis. Symbols are as in Figures 12-1 and 12-2.

Table 12-2   Exercise Test in Obese Man with Chronic Bronchitis*

Time min	Work wt	BP mmHg	HR min-1	RR	V̇E BTPS L/min	V̇CO2 STPD L/min	V̇O2 STPD L/min	O2 pulse ml/bt	R	PET O2	PA O2 mmHg	Pa O2	Aa O2	PET CO2	Pa CO2 mmHg	aET CO2	pH	HCO3 meq L	V̇E/V̇CO2	V̇E/V̇O2	VD/VT
0.5		131/ 88	68	14	12.4	0.28	0.37	5	0.76	110		71		30	37		7.41	23	42	32	
1.0			69	16	12.6	0.28	0.39	6	0.72	109				31					42	30	
1.5			69	17	13.3	0.28	0.37	5	0.76	111				30					44	34	
2.0		138/ 88	69	18	14.0	0.28	0.35	5	0.80	112	107	73	34	29	36	7	7.38	21	47	38	0.41
2.5	0		73	25	21.5	0.45	0.60	8	0.75	110				30					45	34	
3.0	0		71	25	20.9	0.46	0.65	9	0.71	107				31					43	30	
3.5	0		73	25	23.3	0.51	0.68	9	0.75	107				31					43	32	
4.0	0		73	24	24.6	0.55	0.69	9	0.80	110				31					42	34	
4.5	0		74	26	25.2	0.58	0.75	10	0.77	101				35					41	32	
5.0	0	150/ 88	72	26	23.7	0.52	0.66	9	0.79	108	104	74	30	32	38	6	7.39	22	43	34	0.41
5.5	20		73	26	25.4	0.57	0.70	10	0.81	111				31					42	34	
6.0	20		76	27	27.0	0.62	0.78	10	0.79	109				32					41	33	

6.5	40		79	28	27.9	0.66	0.83	11	0.80	104	109	74	35	34	34				40	32	0.30
7.0	40	156/ 88	81	27	30.2	0.74	0.92	11	0.80	109				32		2	7.42	21	39	31	
7.5	60		85	29	31.6	0.80	0.96	11	0.83	109				33					38	31	
8.0	60		88	30	41.5	1.05	1.14	13	0.92	113				32					38	35	
8.5	80		95	32	47.8	1.22	1.31	14	0.93	107				36					38	35	0.32
9.0	80	169/ 94	101	31	47.8	1.28	1.33	13	0.96	111	112	91	21	36	37	1	7.36	20	36	35	
9.5	100		106	35	58.1	1.52	1.47	14	1.03	116				32					37	38	
10.0	100		110	35	64.4	1.68	1.54	14	1.09	117				33					37	41	
10.5	120		119	39	73.3	1.87	1.65	14	1.13	120				32					38	43	
11.0	120	200/100	124	39	78.3	2.02	1.72	14	1.17	120	120	97	23	32	34	3	7.35	19	38	44	0.30
11.5	140	206/106	129	43	92.6	2.28	1.84	14	1.24	123				30					40	49	
12.0	140		131	45	87.3	2.18	1.81	14	1.20	108				42					39	47	
12.5		131/ 72	122	34	80.9	1.96	1.55	13	1.26	124				29					40	51	
13.0		113/ 63	94	31	71.9	1.63	1.22	13	1.34	124				29					43	58	
13.5		88/ 44	64	34	66.1	1.33	0.91	14	1.46	127				28					48	71	
14.0		75/ 31	46	34	62.7	1.09	0.71	15	1.54	133				22					56	86	

*See Table 12-1 for abbreviations.

His resting values include height of 174 cm, weight of 113 kg, VC of 3.95 liter, FEV_1 of 2.53 liter, MVV of 96 liter/min, and PaO_2, $PaCO_2$, and pH at sitting rest of 70 mm Hg, 37 mm Hg, and 7.41. For his age and height, his ideal weight was 77 kg, his predicted $\dot{V}_{O_2}$max was 2.47 liter/min, and predicted HRmax was 178.

The patient exercised on a cycle ergometer with a 20-watt increment every minute until he stopped at 140 watts because of dyspnea and fatigue. His $\dot{V}_E$max was 93 liter/min, HRmax was 129, and $\dot{V}_{O_2}$max was 1.84 liter/min; $\dot{V}_E/\dot{V}_{O_2}$ and $\dot{V}_E/\dot{V}_{CO_2}$ were elevated. The high $\dot{V}_E$max/MVV ratio with a low pulse rate indicates ventilatory limitation at the end of exercise; $\dot{V}/\dot{Q}$ mismatching is indicated by the high V_D/V_T and positive $P(a\text{-}ET)CO_2$. The wide $P(A\text{-}a)O_2$ at rest (34 mm Hg) decreases during exercise, suggesting that much of the $\dot{V}/\dot{Q}$ mismatch is due to the basilar atelectasis of obesity which improves as V_T increases.

In this man, simple measures would reveal a high $\dot{V}_E$max/MVV, arterial desaturation improving with exercise, and a low HRmax, all evidence for ventilatory limitation, hypoxemia due to obesity, and an absence of cardiovascular limitation. The subtle evidence of $\dot{V}/\dot{Q}$ mismatching (high V_D/V_T and positive $P(a\text{-}ET)CO_2$) would not be available.

Differential Diagnosis of Dyspnea

The patient is a 47-year-old male executive referred for evaluation because of dyspnea. Three years previously, in 1978, he had been resuscitated following an acute anteroseptal myocardial infarction associated with ventricular fibrillation. He had a coronary artery bypass operation; his postoperative course was complicated by recurrent left lower lobe atelectasis and hypoxemia. After he recovered from the operation he began a rehabilitation program but stopped participating because of dyspnea. The dyspnea occurred during but not after exercise. He was a heavy smoker and had asthma in childhood, but not as an adult. He denied angina or other chest pain, edema, and wheezing. He was receiving diuretics and digoxin but no beta blockers. A recent radionuclide study showed a left ventricular ejection fraction of 55%. His height was 170 cm, and weight 86 kg, with an ideal weight of 73 kg. He had a normal VC, FEV_1, FEV_3, FEV_1/VC, $FEF_{25-75\%}$, MVV (141 liter/min), DL_{CO}, and TLC, but the FEV_3/VC was slightly reduced. He was apprehensive at the time of exercise testing. There were inspiratory rales and rhonchi in the left lower lobe area which did not clear with cough. The resting EKG showed poor precordial R wave progression and occasional premature ventricular contractions. His predicted exercise values were HRmax of 179, $\dot{V}_{O_2}$max of 2.45 liter/min, O_2 pulse max of 14 ml/beat, and *AI* over 1.0 liter/min.

He exercised on a cycle ergometer with 10-watt increments every minute plus blood-gas measurements and a 12-lead EKG every other minute (Table 12-3 and Fig. 12-4). During exercise, the blood pressure rose appropriately and the EKG remained unchanged except for an increase in rate. He stopped exercising because of calf fatigue and dyspnea. The $\dot{V}_E$max was 72 liter/min (well below his MVV). The HRmax of 158, V_{O_2}max of 1.82, and O_2 pulse max of 12 ml/beat were all low; his *AT* approximated 1.0 liter/min. These values suggest a cardiovascular rather than a ventilatory limitation to exercise and cause of dyspnea. This cardiovascular limitation could be on the basis of intrinsic cardiac disease or physical deconditioning. His anxiety and mild obesity aggravate his condition.

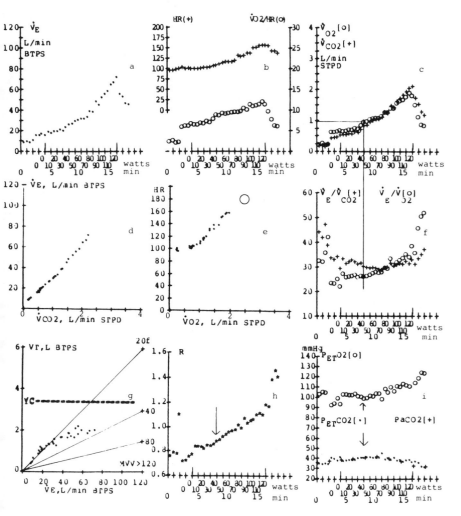

Figure 12-4. An exercise test in a 47-year-old man with heart and lung disease. Symbols are as in Figures 12-1 and 12-2.

Table 12-3 Exercise Test in Patient with Heart and Lung Disease*

Time min	Work wt	BP mmHg	HR min-1	RR	$\dot{V}_E$ BTPS L/min	$\dot{V}_{CO_2}$ STPD L/min	$\dot{V}_{O_2}$ STPD L/min	O_2 pulse ml/bt	R	PET O_2 mmHg	PA O_2	Pa O_2	Aa O_2	PET CO_2	Pa CO_2	aET CO_2	pH	HCO$_3$ meq L	$\dfrac{\dot{V}_E}{\dot{V}_{CO_2}}$	$\dfrac{\dot{V}_E}{\dot{V}_{O_2}}$	$\dfrac{VD}{VT}$
0.5		131/ 75	97	26	8.8	0.17	0.23	2	0.74	103		93		37	34		7.47	25	44	33	
1.0			96	23	9.5	0.20	0.26	3	0.77	105				36					42	32	
1.5			99	27	8.9	0.16	0.21	2	0.76	104				36					47	36	
2.0		125/ 75	100	18	10.6	0.25	0.23	2	1.09		116	90	26	36	36	0	7.44	24	39	42	0.29
2.5	0		104	20	15.8	0.44	0.63	6	0.70	91				42					34	24	
3.0	0		101	20	15.9	0.45	0.64	6	0.70	93				41					33	23	
3.5	0		102	20	17.4	0.48	0.65	6	0.74	98				39					34	25	
4.0	0	150/ 81	100	17	16.1	0.52	0.69	7	0.75	93	103	86	17	43	37	-6	7.42	24	29	22	0.16
4.5	10		101	19	18.9	0.54	0.66	7	0.82	102				39					33	27	
5.0	10		101	16	18.1	0.55	0.67	7	0.82	102				39					31	26	
5.5	20		102	18	19.5	0.58	0.71	7	0.82	101				40					32	26	
6.0	20	144/ 75	103	20	19.7	0.57	0.71	7	0.80	101	105	86	19	40	38	-2	7.41	24	33	26	0.26
6.5	30		104	21	21.6	0.64	0.77	7	0.83	102				40					32	27	
7.0	30		105	21	20.3	0.62	0.75	7	0.83	100				41					31	26	
7.5	40		107	20	23.7	0.72	0.86	8	0.84	100				42					32	26	

8.0	40	156/ 75	109	20	26.3	0.84	0.9/	9	0.87	98	106	84	22	42	39	−3	7.40	24	30	26	0.23
8.5	50		112	21	27.0	0.87	0.99	9	0.88	99				43					30	26	
9.0	50		114	21	29.8	0.97	1.07	9	0.91	101				43					30	27	
9.5	60		117	23	30.9	1.00	1.08	9	0.93	100				42					30	28	
10.0	60	169/ 81	118	20	32.0	1.05	1.11	9	0.95	103	108	86	22	42	40	−2	7.39	24	30	28	0.24
10.5	70		117	20	31.7	1.06	1.11	9	0.95	103				42					29	28	
11.0	70		120	27	33.8	1.12	1.16	10	0.97	97				46					29	28	
11.5	80		132	23	39.2	1.28	1.28	10	1.00	108				40					30	30	
12.0	80	175/ 81	130	23	38.5	1.25	1.28	10	0.98	104	111	86	25	42	38	−4	7.39	22	30	29	0.21
12.5	90		132	28	48.6	1.49	1.41	11	1.06	109				39					32	33	
13.0	90		138	27	45.1	1.44	1.41	10	1.02	105				42					30	31	
13.5	100		138	31	52.4	1.64	1.58	11	1.04	110				39					31	32	
14.0	100	188/ 81	150	30	55.6	1.73	1.65	11	1.05	110	116	93	23	40	35	−5	7.39	21	31	33	0.19
14.5	110		152	29	58.9	1.84	1.70	11	1.08	112				38					31	34	
15.0	110		156	34	64.7	1.95	1.78	11	1.10	111				39					32	35	
15.5	120		158	33	66.7	2.07	1.91	12	1.08	110				40					31	34	
16.0	120	194/ 81	158	35	71.9	2.12	1.82	12	1.16		122	98	24	37	31	−6	7.37	18	33	39	0.14
16.5			156	25	55.7	1.75	1.52	10	1.15	114				38					31	36	
17.0			144	25	53.0	1.55	1.13	8	1.37	118				37					33	46	
17.5			144	25	46.8	1.30	0.90	6	1.44	124				33					35	51	
18.0		144/ 75	138	24	45.9	1.20	0.86	6	1.40	123	127	111	16	33	30	−3	7.35	16	37	52	0.20

*See Table 12-1 for abbreviations.

There was no gas exchange abnormality as evidenced by the normal blood gases, ventilatory equivalents, and V_D/V_T.

In this patient, simple measures would reveal a normal SaO_2, a low $\dot{V}_E$max/ MVV, and a low HRmax. The evidence for normal gas exchange (normal V_D/V_T, $\dot{V}_E/\dot{V}_{CO_2}$, $P(A-a)O_2$, and $P(a-ET)CO_2$) would not be available. The high R and 9 milliequivalent/liter fall in bicarbonate during recovery (lactate ions replace bicarbonate ions), indicating that the patient exercised maximally, would not be available. The low O_2 pulse would not be measured. Thus, simple measures would not identify that he had maximally exercised and was cardiovascularly limited.

Oxygen Supplementation in OLD

The patient is a 63-year-old man with chronic cough and dyspnea. He is 178 cm tall, weights 70 kg, and on repeated testing has a VC of 2.91 to 3.63 liter, a FEV_1 of 1.03 to 1.32 liter, a MVV of 54 liter/min, a TLC of 8.65 liter, and a single-breath DL_{CO} of 15.6 ml/min/mm Hg (57% of predicted). His exercise data are shown in part in Table 12-4. At every work rate there is a lesser V_E, V_{CO_2} and higher Pa_{CO_2} as the FIO_2 is increased, presumably due to suppression of the carotid body. With O_2 supplementation there was a lower effective alveolar ventilation and less dyspnea, but also a greater respiratory acidosis, especially with 100% O_2. With O_2 supplementation more work can be performed. The V_E/ V_{CO_2} and V_D/V_T are elevated in all tests. Note the similar $V_E$max on 21% and 33% O_2. The V_{O_2} cannot be measured on 100% O_2 but the O_2 pulses were similar on the 21 and 33% O_2 tests. This study illustrates that O_2 supplementation may allow a significant improvement in oxygenation and maximal work capacity with concurrent reduction in CO_2 output and ventilatory requirement.

CONTROVERSIES

EQUIPPING A LABORATORY

There is no single "best" way to equip an exercise laboratory. Several approaches, simple to complex, have been presented elsewhere.[1-6] The difference between cycle and treadmill ergometry, and steady-state and incremental tests were previously discussed.[3] Exercise stresses both the cardiovascular and respiratory systems. Whether the exercise is performed in the respiratory or cardiac laboratory, the minimal diagnostic measures are heart, respiratory, and work rates, and inspired or expired ventilatory volumes. Twelve lead EKGs and ear oximetry add considerable information. The addition of end-tidal and mixed expiratory gases and arterial blood gases yields more information. The clinician should become familiar with the biologic and technical variability of each measure. Therefore, the thoughtful application of a few accurate and simple mea-

Table 12-4 Three Incremental Exercise Tests in a Man with Chronic Bronchitis and Emphysema Breathing 21%, 33%, and 100% Oxygen.

Watts	% O$_2$	HR min^{-1}	RR min^{-1}	$\dot{V}_E$ L,BTPS	$\dot{V}_{CO_2}$ L,STPD	Pa$_{CO_2}$ mm Hg	Pa$_{O_2}$ mm Hg
0	21	99	23	27	.63	44	57
0	33	99	19	19	.44	43	90
0	100	88	18	16	.36	57	482
20	21	103	26	29	.64	42	57
20	33	104	19	22	.53	44	91
20	100	90	21	20	.47	58	520
40	21	115	28	36	.88	44	51
40	33	114	21	28	.72	45	89
40	100	100	23	24	.63	58	489
60	21	116	35	43	1.09	46	52
60	33	129	25	38	1.05	48	94
60	100	122	27	29	.85	56	496
80	21	unable					
80	33	133	32	43	1.24	50	96
80	100	138	34	36	1.18	61	487

sures is more likely to lead to a correct assessment than the use of a plethora of unreliable parameters.

STAFFING FOR EXERCISE TESTS

It is necessary to have an adequate number and quality of personnel during exercise testing to insure patient safety and measurement accuracy. In our teaching hospital setting, a physician interviews and examines the patient, inserts and removes the arterial catheter, obtains arterial blood specimens, and monitors the patient and output devices during the exercise period. A trained technician calibrates equipment and assists before, during, and after the procedure. Other personnel are available in the next room should an emergency arise. I believe the training, teamwork, and experience of the operator and assistants in the exercise laboratory are more important than their official titles or certifications. In other settings, after the physician evaluates the patient, it might be appropriate for some, or all, of the procedures to be performed by nonphysicians.

PREDICTION OF Vo_2MAX

Traditionally, Vo_2max has been measured in populations and the resulting normal values have been based on age, gender, and weight. Sometimes smoking history or an estimate of physical activity have been added. It seems logical to base predicted values on these parameters.

On the other hand, the patients seen in the respiratory or cardiovascular laboratory often are older, more obese, and less physically fit than the normal population from which the formulae were derived. Predictive equations for lung volumes and flow rates are based almost exclusively on age, gender, and height, with weight seldom reducing the variance significantly.

A normal man initially weighing 60 kg and gaining 20 kg of excess weight should not have a 33% improvement in his Vo_2max or O_2 pulse max because there would be no appreciable increase in his maximum stroke volume, $(a-\bar{v})$ O_2 difference, or lean body mass. Thus, we prefer basing his predicted $V_{O2}max$ on his height and predicted normal weight rather than his actual weight.[18]

If this same individual were 5 to 10 kg under his predicted weight, one might base his predicted Vo_2max on either his predicted or actual weight, although we use the latter.

REFERENCES

1. Consolazio CF, Johnson RE, Pecora LJ: Physiological Measurements of Metabolic Functions in Man. New York, McGraw-Hill, 1963.
2. Jones NL, Campbell EJM: Clinical Exercise Testing (ed 2). Philadelphia, WB Saunders, 1982.

3. Hansen JE: Exercise Testing. in Clausen JL (ed),: Pulmonary Function Testing: Guidelines and Controversies. New York, Academic Press, 259-279, 1982.

4. Wilson PK, Bell CW, Norton AC: Rehabilitation of the Heart and Lungs. Fullerton, Beckman Instruments, 1980.

5. Ellestad MH: Stress Testing: Principles and Practice. Philadelphia, F.A. Davis, 1975.

6. Exercise Testing and Training of Individuals with Heart Disease or at High Risk for its Development: A Handbook for Physicians. American Heart Association, Dallas, 1972.

7. Wasserman K, Whipp BJ: Exercise physiology in health and disease. Am Rev Respir Dis 112:219-249, 1975.

8. Wasserman K, Van Kessel Al, Burton CG: Interaction of physiological mechanisms during exercise. J Appl Physiol 22:71-85, 1967.

9. Wasserman K: Use of Exercise in Cardiopulmonary Assessment of Exertional Dyspnea, in Baum GL (ed): Textbook of Pulmonary Diseases (ed 3). Boston, Little Brown, 1982.

10. Wasserman K, Whipp BJ, Koyal SN, et al.: Anaerobic threshold and respiratory gas exchange during exercise. J Appl Physiol 35:236-243, 1973.

11. Astrand P, Cuddy TE, Saltin B, et al.: Cardiac output during submaximal and maximal work. J Appl Physiol 19:268-274, 1964.

12. Durand J: Circulatory Response to Exercise, in Moret PR, Weber J, Haissley J-Cl, et al. (ed): Lactate Physiologic, Methodologic and Pathologic Approach. Berlin, Springer-Verlag, 25-34, 1980.

13. Hansen JE, Wasserman K: Exercise Testing, in Chusid EL, (ed): Selective and Comprehensive Testing of Adult Pulmonary Function. New York, Futura, 1983.

14. Holmgren A, McIlroy MB: Effect of temperature on arterial blood gas tensions and pH during exercise. J Appl Physiol 19:243-246, 1964.

15. Freedman S: Sustained maximum voluntary ventilation. Respir Physiol 8:230-244, 1970.

16. Sue DY, Van Meter LR, Hansen JE, et al.: Effect of beta-adrenergic blockade on gas exchange during exercise. J Appl Physiol 55:529-533, 1983.

17. Powles ACP, Sutton JR, Wicks JR, et al.: Reduced heart rate response to exercise in ischemic heart disease: the fallacy of the target heart rate in exercise testing. Med Sci Sports 11:227-233, 1979.

18. Hansen JE, Sue DY, Wasserman K: Predicted values for clinical exercise testing. Am Rev Respir Dis 129:S49-S55, 1984.

19. Bruce RA, Kusumi F, Hosmer D: Maximal oxygen intake and nomographic assessment of functional aerobic impairment in cardiovascular disease. Am Heart J 85:546-562, 1973.

20. Astrand PO, Christiansen EH: Aerobic work capacity, in Dickens F, Neil E, Widdas WF (ed): Oxygen in the Animal Organism. New York, Pergamon Press, 295, 1964.

21. Giovani B, Goldman RF: Predicting metabolic energy cost. J Appl Physiol 30:429-433, 1971.

22. Sue DY, Hansen JE, Blais M, et al.: On-line measurement and analysis of gas exchange during exercise using a programmable desk-top calculator. J Appl Physiol 49:456-461, 1980.

23. Epler GR, McLoud TC, Gaensler EA, et al.: Normal chest roentgenograms in chronic diffuse infiltrative lung disease. N Engl J Med 298:934-939, 1978.

CHAPTER 13

Control of Ventilation

BRIAN J. WHIPP
SUSAN A. WARD

The control of ventilation is the primary means whereby the fluid milieux of the various tissues of the body are maintained within the relatively narrow pH range and at a PO_2 compatible with their function. The ventilatory control system is, however, enormously complex and tests to discern the site(s) of impaired function should, wherever possible, be designed to challenge a particular component—or components—of the control loop. These include the transmission of primary humoral stimuli from their sites of generation to the sensing elements (the peripheral and central chemoreceptors); the integration of chemoreceptor afferent activity within the brainstem "respiratory centers"; the generation of motor discharge patterns which, depending upon current ventilatory demands, may involve not only the diaphragm but also the intercostal and abdominal muscles and accessory muscles of respiration; neuromuscular transmission at the respiratory muscles; and, finally, the generation of appropriate pressure gradients within the respiratory system to provide adequate airflow and ventilation.

In order to discern the extent to which a particular response is abnormal, it needs to be considered within the frame of reference of the distribution of normal values. We provide typical or representative values for the normal ventilatory responses to the stressors, when they are available from the literature. These unfortunately are, at present, typically not available in the sense that the normal range for indices of forced expired airflow or lung volumes may be referred to in pulmonary function testing.

PULMONARY FUNCTION TESTING
INDICATIONS AND INTERPRETATIONS

INHALED GAS CHALLENGES

Inhalation of hypercapnic and hypoxic gas mixtures is widely utilized to estimate the normalcy of ventilatory "chemoreflex" sensitivity. And while abnormal ventilatory responsiveness to CO_2 and hypoxia may be readily documented, the ability to locate precisely the specific site of dysfunction is limited by the inaccessibility of the majority of the control elements. Furthermore, interpretation of the pattern of ventilatory response to CO_2 or hypoxia must incorporate consideration of the intervening portions of the control system and should be viewed as an overall "input–output" relationship whose characteristics are determined by the interaction of the constitutent elements.

ESTIMATION OF VENTILATORY RESPONSE TO INHALED CO_2

The most common technique used to estimate overall ventilatory CO_2 responsiveness is to establish the relationship between ventilation ($\dot{V}_E$) and arterial or alveolar PCO_2.[1] Characteristically, this relationship is linear in healthy individuals (Fig. 13-1), with a slope which averages some 1.5 liter/min/m²/mm Hg.[2] This slope is often taken to reflect the CO_2 responsiveness of participating chemoreceptors. These include the central "chemoreceptors" on the ventral medullary surfaces and, if the level of arterial PO_2 is not excessive, the peripheral chemoreceptors (predominantly, if not exclusively, the carotid bodies in humans). However, as the CO_2 responsiveness of the carotid bodies increases

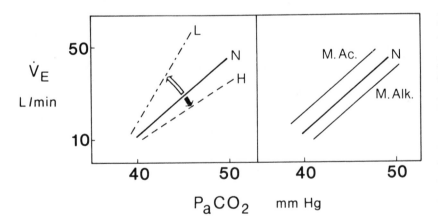

Figure 13-1. Characterization of the steady-state ventilatory response to inhaled CO_2. N represents the slope with normal euoxia, L with simultaneous low PO_2, H with high PO_2, M.Ac. with chronic metabolic acidosis, and M.Alk. with chronic metabolic alkalosis. The different levels of oxygenation affect the slope of the response curve, whereas the metabolic acid/base changes induce locational shifts without significant change of slope.

with reductions of arterial PO_2 below normal values, it is crucial to the interpretation of the $\dot{V}_E$-$PaCO_2$ relationship that PaO_2 be maintained constant throughout the CO_2 inhalation.

Implicit in the methods of CO_2 inhalation currently in use is the existence of a reasonably (although not precisely known) relationship between arterial PCO_2 and the PCO_2 at each set of chemoreceptors, and thence the local $[H^+]$, i.e., apparently the modality actually sensed by the chemoreceptors.[3] The time required to establish equilibrium at the chemoreceptors following an alteration in $PaCO_2$ depends upon factors such as the local perfusion, CO_2 production, CO_2 capacitance, $[H^+]$ buffering capacity, and metabolic acid/base status. And although the interaction of these factors is poorly understood, it is generally assumed that the equilibrium process at the carotid body chemoreceptors is rapid, but is considerably delayed at the central chemoreceptors.

The time required for equilibration of $[H^+]$ at the chemoreceptors will therefore dictate the duration of a particular CO_2 inhalation procedure. With the classical steady-state approach, it is generally agreed that some 15–20 minutes are needed for the full ventilatory response to develop. And, as characterization of the $\dot{V}_E$-$PaCO_2$ relationship by this procedure realistically demands four or so levels of PCO_2, it constitutes a lengthy and therefore stressful undertaking for the patient. Two expedients may be utilized to shorten the duration of the steady-state test by hastening equilibration: (a) by transiently "overshooting" P_ICO_2 beyond its required level, the new steady-state level of $PaCO_2$ can be achieved with little delay and (b) $\dot{V}_E$ can more rapidly reach its steady-state by overshooting $PaCO_2$. A serious drawback to these techniques, however, is that complex instrumentation or a high degree of manipulative gas-mixing skills is required to achieve the desired profiles of PCO_2.

It therefore was of significant procedural utility that the rebreathing test described by Read[4] would give the same values of CO_2 responsiveness ($\Delta\dot{V}_E/\Delta P_ACO_2$) as the steady-state (presumably hyperoxic) test, while taking a small fraction of the time to perform. Furthermore, the locational shift of the rebreathing relationship to the right of the steady-state relationship (Fig. 13-2) is predictable, based on the transit delays between the lungs and the sites of chemoreception and on the kinetic characteristics of the system. And although the test is not steady state in the conventional sense, it is presumed to provide a constant rate of change of PCO_2 at the chemoreceptor sites and, hence, the rate of change of $\dot{V}_E$ may appropriately be compared with the rate of change of P_ACO_2.

This rebreathing test, having been validated in numerous laboratories, not surprisingly is currently in widespread use. The normal range of values for the response slope is, however, quite wide,[5] with values of 0.5–8 l/min/mm Hg having been reported in healthy adults. The cause of this intersubject variability is presently unclear, although genetic factors and variations in lung size may be involved.[5] Surprisingly, the zero-ventilation intercept, or the magnitude of the rightward locational shift in the curve, has received little attention. Unfortu-

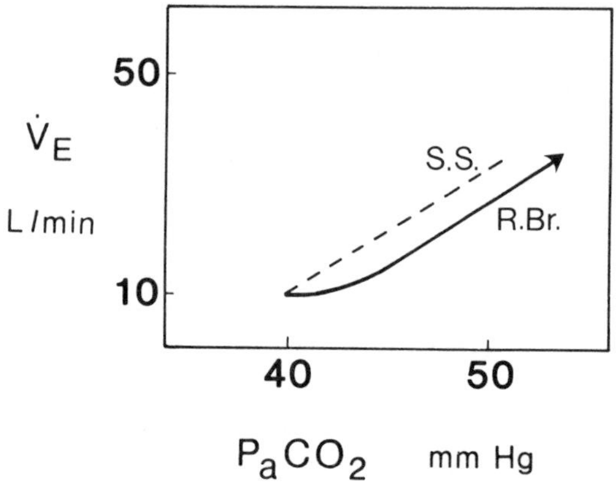

50
$\dot{V}_E$
L/min
S.S.
R.Br.
10
40
50
P_aCO_2 mm Hg

Figure 13-2. The pattern of ventilatory response resulting from a rebreathing test. Note that following a lag phase, the rebreathing (R.Br) slope becomes equal to the steady-state (S.S.) slope.

nately, estimations of CO_2 responsiveness obtained by this approach reflect only the activity of the central chemoreflex, the background hyperoxia serving to silence the peripheral component of the response. Typically, therefore, some form of hypoxic test is utilized for the latter purpose.

Estimation of ventilatory response to hypoxia

The ventilatory responsiveness to hypoxia is traditionally represented by the curvilinear $\dot{V}_E$-PaO_2 relationship (Fig. 13-3) which, if defined under isocapnic conditions, is considered solely to reflect the activity of the peripheral chemoreceptors. Both steady-state and rebreathing techniques have been successfully utilized for this purpose.

The steady-state approach is far easier to implement than was the case for CO_2, largely as a consequence of a shorter $\dot{V}_E$ response time (about half a

30
$\dot{V}_E$
L/min
10
H
N
L
45
60
75
90
P_aO_2 mm Hg

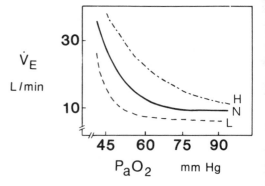

Figure 13-3. Relationship between ventilation and arterial PO_2 performed at three constant levels of $PaCO_2$: N, the normal eucapnic level; H, with high PCO_2; and L, with low PCO_2.

minute, typically). It is therefore feasible to obtain sufficient data for the adequate definition of the $\dot{V}_E$-PaO_2 relationship in a reasonably short period of time. The approach of progressive hypoxia induced by rebreathing may, however, prove to be superior because a far greater density of data can be obtained in a significantly shorter interval. The requirement for isocapnia throughout the test does demand a degree of sophistication in the design of the rebreathing circuit (specifically in the geometry of the CO_2-absorbing system).

A potential drawback to the interpretation of the $\dot{V}_E$-PaO_2 data obtained by these techniques is that hypoxemia may lead to depression of brainstem respiratory neurones. Considerable debate surrounds the critical level of PaO_2 required to elicit this effect and whether this threshold is time-dependent. It is therefore advisable to minimize the duration of the hypoxic episodes. With the steady-state approach, this can be achieved by switching the patient to air or even a mildly hyperoxic mixture between successive hypoxic steady states. In the case of the rebreathing approach, the likelihood of a significant central depressant action of hypoxia developing during the procedure is probably small, as the duration of the entire test can be reasonably short.

A hyperbolic function has been traditionally utilized to describe the isocapnic $\dot{V}_E$-PaO_2 relationship:[1,6]

$$\dot{V}_E = \dot{V}_E(o) + A/(PaO_2 - C) \qquad \text{(Eq. 1)}$$

where $\dot{V}_E$ is the ventilatory response at a particular PaO_2, $\dot{V}_E(o)$ is the response during hyperoxia (when the peripheral chemoreceptors are assumed to be silent); C is an asympototic level of PaO_2; and A is the area constant of the hyperbolic function and is regarded as the index of hypoxic responsiveness.

At least two functional interpretations have been placed on the hyperbolic parameter of hypoxic responsiveness. The one, which has been advocated by Weil and his colleagues,[7] simply ascribes the hypoxic responsiveness to parameter A. In contrast, Cunningham and Lloyd[1,6] have proposed that this parameter is defined not only by the hypoxic responsiveness but also by the value of $\dot{V}_E$ during hyperoxia, so that equation 1 becomes:

$$\dot{V}_E = \dot{V}_E(o) + \dot{V}_E(o) \cdot A/(PaO_2 - C)$$

$$\text{or} \quad \frac{\dot{V}_E}{\dot{V}_E(o)} = 1 + A/(PaO_2 - C) \qquad \text{(Eq. 2)}$$

Normal average values for Weil's A and Cunningham and Lloyd's A, derived under normocapnic conditions, are 127 ± 53 (SD) 1 liter/min/mm Hg[7] and 23 mm Hg,[1] respectively. The parameter C has been empirically determined to average 32 mm Hg,[1] and this value is indeed often assumed.

Additionally, hypoxic ventilatory responsiveness has been characterized by an exponential function[8] of the form:

$$\dot{V}_E - \dot{V}_E(o) = [\dot{V}_E(\infty) - \dot{V}_E(o)] \cdot e^{-PaO_2/K} \qquad \text{(Eq. 3)}$$

where $\dot{V}_E$ is the ventilatory response at a particular PaO_2; $\dot{V}_E(o)$ is the response during hyperoxia; $\dot{V}_E(\infty)$ is the response for an infinitely high level of hypoxia; and K, the exponent, is the index of hypoxic responsiveness. An average value of 24.5 ± 7.4 (SD) mm Hg has been reported for parameter K by Kronenberg and his colleagues.[8]

Currently, however, there are no strong physiologic grounds for distinguishing between the hyperbolic and exponential descriptions of the ventilatory response to hypoxia (although the former has been more widely employed). These conflicting issues regarding the most appropriate index for hypoxic responsiveness appear to have been resolved (at least on technical and empirical grounds) by the demonstration that the curvilinear $\dot{V}_E$-PaO_2 relationship can be transformed into a linear relationship[5] by substituting arterial O_2 saturation (SaO_2) for PaO_2:

$$\dot{V}_E = -G.SaO_2 + \dot{V}_E(o) \qquad \text{(Eq. 4)}$$

In this equation, the slope parameter G provides the index of hypoxic responsiveness. A normal average value for this parameter is 1.47 ± 0.97 (SD) 1 liter/min/ % decrease of SaO_2.[5]

Severinghaus,[9] however, has demonstrated that the exponential equation:

$$1 - SaO_2 = 1.89\,e^{-0.05PaO_2} \qquad \text{(Eq. 5)}$$

accurately describes the standard (pH = 7.4, t = 37 °C) human oxyhemoglobin saturation curve to within 1% over a saturation range from 35–100%. Consequently, both exponential and saturation displays are likely to be equally appropriate for characterizing the ventilatory response to hypoxia in this range.

However, as SaO_2 can now be monitored continuously and noninvasively by ear oximetry, this modification considerably facilitates estimations of the ventilatory responsiveness to hypoxia. It should be emphasized, however, that the expression of hypoxic drive in terms of SaO_2 rather than PaO_2 is an empirical expedient, and should not be taken to imply that the peripheral chemoreceptors are responding to saturation rather than to partial pressure.[5]

Severinghaus[9] has also suggested an ingenious conceptual approach to testing hypoxic responsiveness ($\Delta\dot{V}_{40}$), based upon the recognition (first demonstrated by Nielsen and Smith[10]) that the *potentiation* (or *steepening*: Fig. 13-1) of the CO_2 response curve by hypoxia is a specific result of increased peripheral chemoreceptor gain. The test determines hypoxic responsiveness as the increase in $\dot{V}_1$ between a hyperoxic CO_2 response curve, i.e., peripheral chemoreceptors effectively silenced, and a curve established at a PaO_2 of 40 mm Hg at a specific level of $PaCO_2$, typically approximately 40 mm Hg in normal subjects (Fig. 13-4). A normal, average value for $\Delta\dot{V}_{40}$ of 19.9 ± 13.5 (SD) liter/min/m² has been reported.[8] This test, however, is not as simple to perform as the isocapnic, progressive hypoxia test recording O_2 saturation.

A further test that depends upon hypoxic ventilatory responsiveness being isolated to the peripheral chemoreceptors is the hypoxia-withdrawal test of Dejours.[11] If a particular level of PaO_2 is established by inhalation of an hypoxic gas mixture (or if the patient is already hypoxemic, noting the spontaneous PaO_2), then the abrupt but surreptitious administration of 100% O_2 will cause $\dot{V}_E$ to fall rapidly. The maximum decrease in $\dot{V}_E$ is given as a fraction of the total hypoxic $\dot{V}_E$ to provide an index of hypoxic responsiveness.

The validity of the Dejours test depends upon: (a) the hypoxic response being exclusive to the peripheral chemoreceptors; (b) such high levels of PO_2 actually "silencing" the carotid bodies—this is probably the case in humans but not in animals such as cat and dog; and (c) the $\dot{V}_E$ decrement reaching its nadir prior to the consequently increased $PaCO_2$ (caused by the reduced $\dot{V}_E$) arriving at and influencing central sites of CO_2 responsiveness. And as the nadir of the response commonly occurs some 20–25 seconds after the hypoxic-hyperoxic transition, there is some uncertainty regarding this latter point. This test of hypoxic responsiveness is quite easy to perform and provides a useful qualitative estimate; it remains to be precisely standardized and quantified.

MECHANICAL LOADING

Techniques are available for assessing the ventilatory responses to both elastic and resistive loads. And although the pattern and magnitude of such

Figure 13-4. Scheme for computing $\Delta\dot{V}_{40}$. This is derived from the difference in $\dot{V}_1$ between a hyperoxic steady-state CO_2 response curve and one generated at a PaO_2 of 40 mm Hg for a specific level of $PaCO_2$. The arrow represents the normal (surface-area scaled) $\dot{V}_1$ from which the ventilatory increment is determined.

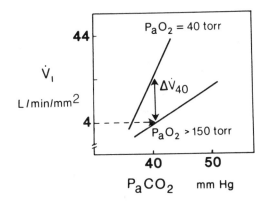

responses are reasonably well documented (in healthy individuals, at least), their functional basis is more questionable. However, airway and chest wall mechanoreceptors are commonly invoked as the primary mediators of the responses, with a secondary involvement of the ventilatory chemoreceptors if alterations in arterial blood-gas tensions result. Thus, in situations in which the primary response is of particular interest, the experimenter should ensure that $PaCO_2$ and PaO_2 are held at constant levels throughout the testing procedure, by appropriate manipulation of the inhaled gas composition. In the event of such a response appearing abnormal, its specific functional basis can be further explored.

In addition to analyzing the ventilatory responses to applied mechanical loads, a further crucial aspect concerns respiratory "sensation." It has been demonstrated that patients with COPD can evidence a significantly higher threshold to the perception of applied loads.[12] And while the precise relevance of this observation to the genesis of dyspnea is not yet clear, it is important to incorporate considerations of respiratory sensation into the analysis of ventilatory control.

ESTIMATION OF VENTILATORY RESPONSE TO ELASTIC LOADING

The simplest technique for applying an elastic load to the respiratory system is to cause a subject to breathe from a rigid, airtight container. The applied load can then be quantitated in terms of its elastance ($\Delta P/\Delta V$), which is greater the smaller the container. In healthy individuals, elastic loads of up to some 30 cm H_2O/liter are typically utilized.

There is, however, no good concensus on how best to apply elastic loads. For example, periods as short as one breath or as long as five minutes have been employed. Furthermore, the load may not be applied throughout the entire respiratory cycle, but rather specifically during either the inspiratory or expiratory phases.

For the present purpose, it is perhaps most appropriate to consider the "steady-state" ventilatory response to prolonged elastic loading, which is maintained throughout each successive breathing cycle; a period of five minutes probably sufficing for the attainment of the new steady state. Because $\dot{V}_E$ in this new steady state may well be different from the control (or unloaded) value, manipulation of the inhaled CO_2 fraction may be necessary for maintenance of a constant $PaCO_2$ throughout the procedure. Alternatively, the influence of the elastic load may be examined in terms of its influence on the ventilatory response to inhaled CO_2.[13] Typically, the form of the $\dot{V}_E$-$PaCO_2$ relationship obtained by Read's rebreathing technique[4] is investigated.

A crucial index to be established is the threshold elastic load required to elicit ventilatory compensation. This approach, however, has yet to be incorporated systematically into evaluations of the ventilatory effects of elastic loading, though considerable progress has been made recently with respect to the threshold for perceptual load detection.

Insight into the nature of the ventilatory compensation for elastic loading may usefully be gained from an analysis not only of $\dot{V}_E$ but also of the associated breathing pattern responses. There is, for example, general agreement that steady-state elastic loading is attended by an increase in breathing frequency (both inspiratory and expiratory durations being shortened) and a decrease in tidal volume.[14,15] The variability in the adequacy of the ventilatory response is unclear at present (but may be clarified when more consideration is given to the magnitude of a particular elastic load relative to the threshold level), although it has been postulated that the maintenance of an adequate level of ventilation in these conditions is primarily dependent upon the magnitude of the breathing frequency response,[15] rather than the inspiratory drive (as assessed from inspiratory occlusion pressures or electromyographic indices, see further discussion that follows).

The major problem encountered in evaluating ventilatory responses to elastic loading is the definition of an "abnormal" response. As yet, there is not a sufficient body of data to warrant such judgement except, perhaps, in cases of extreme dysfunction. For this reason, there appears to be little to recommend the use of transient bouts of elastic loading at present, although dynamic analysis of the ventilatory response to elastic loading is likely to assume considerable importance in patient evaluation in the future.

Finally, it should be recognized that the use of such simple elastic loads bears little resemblance to the elastic loads encountered in pulmonary disease states. And, therefore, the technique of chest strapping has been introduced, as it at least provides the opportunity to effect regional variations in pulmonary compliance. Again, however, the "normal" pattern and range of ventilatory response associated with this procedure is poorly documented.

ESTIMATION OF VENTILATORY RESPONSE TO RESISTIVE LOADING

The evaluation of the ventilatory compensation for added resistive loads is subject to much the same criticisms and limitations as is that for elastic loading. Thus, while the resistive load itself may be simple in concept (typically, a fine wire-mesh inserted in the external airway), its mode of application may be quite variable. Again, the simplest approach is likely to be that of steady-state resistive loading, in which the load is applied until the associated ventilatory response has stabilized. Typically, resistive loads may range up to about 15 cm H_2O/liter/sec in normal individuals.

As the characteristic response to resistive loading is hypoventilation,[14] it is impossible to reduce the inspired CO_2 fraction to maintain isocapnia unless, of course, the subject was previously made hypercapnic. Therefore, it is most usual to evaluate the effects of resistive loading with respect to the $\dot{V}_E$-$PaCO_2$ relation-ship.[14] As was suggested for elastic loading, it does seem crucial to establish the threshold for ventilatory compensation with resistive loads.

Both inspiratory occlusion pressures and electromyographic indices have been usefully employed in discerning the role of inspiratory drive in the compen-satory response to resistive loading. Less emphasis, however, has been placed on the contribution of breathing frequency and its components.

The major drawback to the evaluation of responses to resistive loading is, as described earlier for elastic loading, the lack of a suitable body of normal data for comparison.

EXERCISE

The most common stress to the ventilatory control system is provided by the variations in metabolic rate that take place with physical activity. Therefore, we shall consider for this review any activity-induced increments of metabolic rate to be "exercise." And, unlike the contrived stimuli commonly used to assess ventilatory responsiveness, hyperoxic hypercapnia, exercise imposes the most naturally occurring stimulus to the ventilatory control system.

The ventilatory response to exercise may be characterized with respect not only to metabolic rate but also to changes in $\dot{V}_D$ (most commonly expressed as the physiologic dead space fraction, V_D/V_T) and in the operating- or set-point for $PaCO_2$. These influences are best represented by the equation:

$$\dot{V}_E(BTPS) = \frac{863\ \dot{V}CO_2(STPD)}{PaCO_2\ (1-V_D/V_T)} \qquad \text{(Eq. 6)}$$

Up to the onset of sustained metabolic acidosis (the anaerobic threshold, Θ_{an}), the ventilatory response to exercise is a highly linear function of metabolic rate[16] but most precisely of CO_2 output ($\dot{V}CO_2$). This linear response, however, intercepts at a positive $\dot{V}_E$ of about 3 liter/min in normal humans.[17] As a consequence, despite the fact that the slope of the $\dot{V}_E - \dot{V}CO_2$ relationship (i.e., $d\dot{V}_E/d\dot{V}CO_2$) is constant for this moderate intensity of exercise (the slope averag-ing some 25 liter/min $\dot{V}_E$ per l/min $\dot{V}CO_2$ in normal subjects), the ventilatory equivalent for CO_2, (i.e., $\dot{V}_E/\dot{V}CO_2$) decreases progressively with increasing work rate from a resting value of 30–40 to approximately 25 at Θ_{an}). Thus, in an attempt to establish the normalcy of a ventilatory response to exercise, either the slope and the intercept of the $\dot{V}_E$-$\dot{V}CO_2$ relationship, must be defined or a value of $\dot{V}_E/\dot{V}CO_2$ normalized to a particular level of $\dot{V}CO_2$.

Incremental exercise tests (in which the work rate is incremented progres-sively for constant intervals of time up to the limit of tolerance) have proved to be most useful in characterizing the appropriateness of the ventilatory response to exercise. Thus, when the ventilatory response at each work rate is plotted as a function of $\dot{V}CO_2$, the nature of the work rate increment (i.e., rapid or slow) appears to be unimportant, allowing fairly short work increments to be used for a valid interpretation.

Clearly, factors such as hypoxia, metabolic acidosis, and anxiety which result in a decreased $PaCO_2$ will be associated with an increased ventilatory response to exercise. A large physiologic dead space, such as occurs in patients with COPD or pulmonary vascular occlusive disease, also results in an abnormally high ventilatory response to exercise,[18] as evidence by an increased slope of the $\dot{V}_E$-$\dot{V}CO_2$ relationship. In contrast, a diminished response to exercise occurs in the presence of factors such as resistive loads that elicit an increase of $PaCO_2$.[19] However, when arterial blood sampling is available, the measurement of $PaCO_2$ functionally integrates these influences and allows judgements of whether the ventilatory response is appropriate or otherwise for the current metabolic demand.

At work rates greater than Θ_{an}, ventilatory compensation for the metabolic acidosis results, largely from stimulation of the carotid bodies by the lowered arterial pH. And, therefore, any increase in $\dot{V}_E$ above that predicted from the extrapolation of the linear $\dot{V}_E$-$\dot{V}CO_2$ relationship beyond Θ_{an} may be regarded as the component that normally provides the respiratory compensation. (This assumes, of course, that alveolar ventilation also changes with this general pattern. In the case of a relatively abrupt increase in V_D/V_T, such an inference could not be made.) Therefore, an analysis of this additional increment in ventilation during heavy and severe exercise provides a reflection of the degree of carotid body responsiveness to the induced metabolic acidosis of exercise. Unfortunately, the techniques for quantifying and characterizing this response above Θ_{an} have not been standardized to date.

In addition to assessing the general ventilatory response to exercise and the pattern of breathing by which this is attained, exercise may also be used as an expedient to assess carotid body function under conditions in which the investigator may not wish to establish a prior hypoxic background as a prelude to the Dejours test (see preceding discussion). Thus, as exercise causes a greater ventilatory drive which can be attributed to the carotid bodies, the abrupt and surreptitious substitution of 100% O_2 for air as the inspirate allows the proportional contribution from the carotid bodies to be discerned.

A further and highly important application of exercise testing to the evaluation of appropriate or inappropriate ventilatory responses lies in the interpretation of the maximal exercise ventilation and its relationship to the maximum voluntary ventilation (MVV). Clearly, under conditions in which maximal exercise $\dot{V}_E$ reaches (or, in some cases, exceeds) MVV, mechanical limitation to breathing can be characterized, and often results in less than maximal metabolic or cardiovascular stress as considered by the relatively low maximal O_2 uptake, heart rate (HR), and blood lactate levels at the limit of tolerance in patients with severe

COPD. Thus, the range of normal physical activities inducing such responses may then be defined.

A more precise analysis of mechanical limitation to breathing may be brought about by measurements of the flow-volume curve especially during the expiratory phase, and comparing that spontaneously generated during exercise with the maximum (or forced) curve. These curves have been shown to coincide during exercise both in patients with limited MVVs (e.g., severe COPD[20]) and in highly fit athletes (i.e., those having a normal flow-volume curve but an excessively large ventilatory requirement[21]). In both these cases, therefore, a mechanical limitation to ventilation at high work rates may be inferred: a condition which is likely to predispose to, or exacerbate any developing, respiratory muscle fatigue.

ANALYSIS OF VENTILATORY RESPONSES

Ventilatory responses can be conveniently partitioned into inspiratory "drive" and "timing" components. This approach is conceptually attractive because it has been demonstrated that these components are controlled by functionally discrete mechanisms; being widely regarded as the efferent manifestations of particular elements in the pontobulbar respiratory centers.[22] Thus, a given ventilatory response may be described in the following manner:

$$\dot{V}_I \text{ or } \dot{V}_E = \frac{V_T}{T_I} \cdot \frac{T_I}{T_T} \qquad \text{(Eq. 7)}$$

where V_T/T_I is the mean inspiratory flow and T_I/T_T is the inspiratory duty cycle (denoting the fraction of the periodic cycle that is "energetically active"[22]).

Over a wide range of ventilatory stimulation by factors such as CO_2, hypoxia and exercise, mean inspiratory flow increases in a quantitatively similar fashion to $\dot{V}_E$. The usefulness of this variable as an index of inspiratory drive is limited, however, to situations where the flow-generating mechanisms function normally. Thus, with the development of techniques to monitor indices of inspiratory drive upstream of the flow generation, it has become possible to discriminate between an impaired response originating at the airways and one deriving from sites functionally closer to the brainstem respiratory centers.

The most widely used of these indices is the inspiratory occlusion pressure response[22] which may be presented as P_{100} (the pressure developed against an occluded airway at FRC or end-expiratory lung volume) or dP/dt_{max} (the maximum rate of change of pressure that occurs at 100ms of an occluded inspiration). These indices are regarded as providing estimates of the efferent inspiratory drive to the pressure-generating mechanisms, and therefore should be uninfluenced by altered airways resistance per se. (An increased P_{100} response typically attends resistive loading in normal subjects, but this is thought to represent a reflex ventilatory compensation for the applied load.) Thus, for example, a patient whose ventilatory impairment is confined largely to the airways themselves would be most likely to evidence an essentially normal slope for the P_{100}-$PaCO_2$ relationship but abnormally low slope for both the $\dot{V}_E$-$PaCO_2$ and $\dot{V}_E$-P_{100} relationships. On the other hand, when the ventilatory impairment is, for example, of central neural or of chemoreceptor origin with little involvement of the airways, both the P_{100}-$PaCO_2$ and $\dot{V}_E$-$PaCO_2$ relationships will evidence abnormally low slopes, while that for the $\dot{V}_E$-P_{100} relationship may be reasonably normal.

Caution is required when interpreting inspiratory occlusion pressure responses solely in terms of efferent drive from the brainstem respiratory centers. For example, it has been documented that functional residual capacity (FRC) decreases in normal subjects upon going from rest to exercise. The length-tension characteristic of skeletal muscle predicts that, as a consequence, the muscles of inspiration should contract more forcefully in response to a given neural drive from the respiratory centers. Furthermore, the lowering of FRC might possibly induce a secondary modulation of ventilation or its pattern. In contrast, hyperinflation is a typical feature of the emphysematous patient, and therefore P_{100} measurements would tend to underestimate inspiratory drive. An additional complicating feature in patients with pulmonary disease is the considerable deformation of the chest wall which is frequently encountered.

Electromyographic indices[22] of respiratory muscle activity (the diaphragm, most typically) overcome many of the problems associated with inspiratory occlusion pressure measurements, but it must be recognized that they only sample the active inspiratory musculature. The techniques are, however, necessarily invasive and suffer from the limitation of being difficult to compare responses between subjects or even from the same subject on different occasions, consequent to relocation of the recording electrode.

A further index, namely, the phrenic neurogram[22,23] has also been utilized. However, owing to technical complexities, its use has largely been restricted to experimental animals.

The contribution of breathing frequency and its components, the durations of inspiration and expiration (T_I, T_E), to a given ventilatory response can be assessed in several ways. For example, the *Hey* relationship expresses the ventilatory response in terms of tidal volume (V_T) and frequency.[22,24] Generally, with increasing ventilatory drive from factors such as CO_2, hypoxia, and exercise, $\dot{V}_E$ increases as a linear function of V_T up to a critical V_T which, in healthy individuals, is about 50% of VC. This range of response has been termed "range 1", and can be described in the following form:

$$\dot{V}_E = m.V_T - c \qquad \text{(Eq. 8)}$$

where *m* is the slope and *c* is the $\dot{V}_E$ intercept.

The contribution of breathing frequency to the ventilatory response in range 1 is variable. In some instances, the $\dot{V}_E$–V_T relationship intercepts at the origin (i.e., $c = 0$), indicating that increases in V_T alone contribute to the $\dot{V}_E$ response; the constant value of breathing frequency in this range being defined by the slope parameter m. This form of ventilatory pattern response is characteristic, for example, of individuals who entrain their breathing cadence to some unit multiple of their cycling or stride frequency during exercise. In other instances, however, both V_T and f may contribute to the ventilatory response in this range (typically for CO_2 inhalation). Thus, the $\dot{V}_E$–V_T relationship, while still linear, evidences a positive intercept on the V_T axis (Fig. 5), which implies that frequency is increasing progressively in a hyperbolic fashion as $\dot{V}_E$ rises, (i.e., as $f = \dot{V}_E/V_T$).

Beyond range 1, the characteristics of the ventilatory pattern response evidence a marked change. In this higher range of response, termed "range 2", the $\dot{V}_E$–V_T relationship becomes strikingly more steeper than in range 1 (Fig.13-5), even approaching the vertical in some individuals. Clearly, therefore, the increase in $\dot{V}_E$ in range 2 is achieved largely, if not exclusively, by a progressively greater increase in breathing frequency. Finally, if the ventilatory drive is sufficiently intense (as is encountered, for example, in exhausting exercise), a third component of the ventilatory pattern response may emerge (range 3), in which further increases of ventilation are effected by disproportionately large increases in breathing frequency. V_T may therefore actually fall in this range, with the $\dot{V}_E$–V_T relationship demonstrating a negative slope (Fig. 13-5).

The contribution of inspiratory and expiratory durations to the analysis of ventilatory responses may be assessed by means of the *Euler* relationships,[6,25] which express the V_T response in terms of T_I or T_E (Fig. 13-6). Typically, the

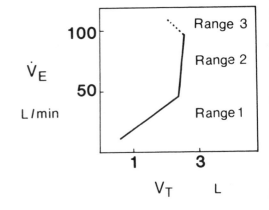

Figure 13-5. Normal relationship between $\dot{V}_E$ and V_T during induced hyperpnea. In range 1 both V_T and f contribute to the hyperpnea. In range 2 (at high V_T) the response is predominantly through breathing frequency. A range 3 is occasionally observed, especially in high-intensity exercise when the hyperpnea is so marked that V_T can actually decrease.

increase of V_T in range 1 is accompanied by a hyperbolic shortening of T_E. Besides the passive effects of increasing elastic recoil with increasing lung volume, this shortening is thought to be achieved by factors such as a progressive attenuation of postinspiratory diaphragmatic discharge, the recruitment of abdominal muscles, and decreased laryngeal resistance.[26] There is, however, some variability in the form of the range 1 T_I response. In some instances, the $V_T - T_I$ relationship resembles that for T_E, with T_I evidencing a hyperbolic shortening as V_T increases. In others, the relationship is effectively vertical, T_I remaining constant throughout range 1. The reason for this discrepant behaviour of T_I is not clear. In range 2, both the $V_T - T_I$ and $V_T - T_E$ relationships display a more striking curvilinearity than in range 1, demonstrating that the marked increase of breathing frequency in this range is achieved by a shortening of T_I and T_E. Finally, in range 3 (when present) T_I and T_E shorten further.

This analysis can be extended to a consideration of the inspiratory duty cycle (T_I/T_T) response, which allows the relative behavior of T_I and T_E to be established. Thus, as is evident from the form of the *Euler* relationships (Fig. 13-6), T_I/T_T typically increases in normal subjects as the degree of ventilatory

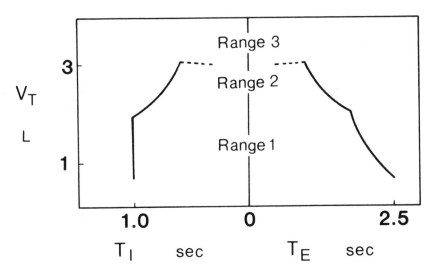

Figure 13-6. Normal relationship between V_T and inspiratory and expiratory durations during induced hyperpnea. Note that in range 1 the breathing frequency changes are largely the result of T_E shortening, whereas both T_I and T_E shorten in range 2. There is more considerable shortening of T_I and T_E at the highest ventilatory levels (often associated with a decreasing phase of V_T).

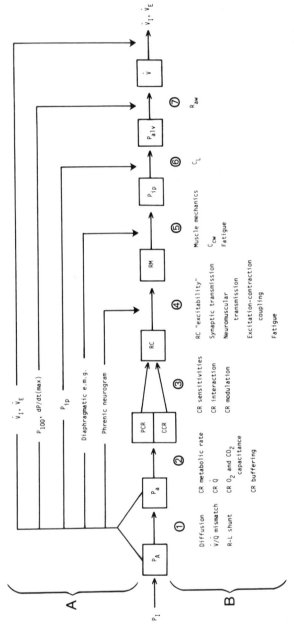

Figure 13-7. Schematic representation of physiologic mechanisms that intervene between the application of an inhaled gas stimulus at the mouth (P_I) and the ventilatory response ($\dot{V}_I$, $\dot{V}_E$). Bracket A represents examples of measurement and the system's access points that allow more precise localization of sites of impaired responsiveness. Bracket B represents factors that modify the transform between sequential elements in the control loop.

stimulation increases.[22] This reflects the greater contribution to the breathing frequency response from expiratory duration.

The precise mechanisms responsible for the strikingly different ventilatory pattern responses of range 1, range 2, and range 3 are uncertain at present. Possible factors might, however, include (a) mechanical influences relating to the disproportionately large increase in the elastic work of breathing required as ventilation becomes high; and (b) the attainment of a critical lung volume threshold for activation of vagal pulmonary and somatic chest wall mechanoreceptors whose reflex actions are exerted on breathing pattern.

However, while these ventilatory pattern responses have received considerable attention with respect to their form and their controlling mechanism, no established range of the limits of normal response are available at present.

CONCLUSION

This account has addressed approaches to the evaluation of the ventilatory control processes that are currently in use. In particular, we have attempted to characterize the portions of this system that may be functionally "isolated" for interpretation by the judicious choice of test and "access point" for measurement. Although such approaches can provide considerable information on the effects of disease-induced dysfunction, it is clear that interpretation is severely limited by our inability to "dissect" adequately the various control loops involved. Future technical and conceptual developments will likely improve our ability to undertake such analyses.

We have stressed the complexity of the ventilatory control system and that, in order to interpret a ventilatory control test in the context of a specific site of dysfunction, it is necessary to go beyond a simple determination of ventilatory response to some applied stimulus. Rather, as schematized in Figure 13-7, it is necessary to determine responses at appropriate access points in the control loop. Rapid advances are taking place in this area, utilizing techniques such as electromyography of the respiratory muscles and phrenic electroneurography. At present, however, these techniques are necessarily limited by what Eldridge[23] has termed "aliquotting" a sample of the output rather than the output itself, and also by the lack of appropriate ranges of standardized normal responses with which to compare putatively abnormal behavior. Even so, the future appears exciting in this regard.

Finally, we have deliberately refrained from addressing the dynamic control features of ventilatory responsiveness in systems-analytic terms. There is little doubt that the characteristics of elements of a control system are most strikingly displayed when the system is challenged by appropriate dynamic forcing techniques. Even so, the application of systems-analytic techniques to various aspects of the ventilatory control system is not widespread at present. In the future, however, such approaches will undoubtedly be more widely adopted.

REFERENCES

1. Lloyd BB, Cunningham DJC: Quantitative approach to the regulation of human respiration, in Cunningham DJC, Lloyd BB (eds): The Regulation of Human Respiration. Oxford, Blackwell, 1963, pp 331-344.
2. Kronenberg R, Severinghaus JW: Chemical control of ventilation, in Altman PL, Dittmer DS (eds): Biological Handbooks, Respiration and Circulation. Bethesda, Federation of American Societies for Experimental Biology 1971, p 104.
3. Mitchell RA: Cerebrospinal fluid and the regulation of respiration, in Caro CG: Advances in Respiratory Physiology. London, Arnold, 1966, pp 1-47.
4. Read DJC: A clinical method for assessing the ventilatory response to carbon dioxide. Australas Ann Med 16:20-32, 1967.
5. Rebuck AS, Slutsky AS: Measurement of ventilatory responses to hypercapnia and hypoxia, in Hornbein TF (ed): Regulation of Breathing. New York, Dekker, 1981, pp 745-772.
6. Cunningham DJC: Integrative aspects of the regulation of breathing: A personal view, in Widdicombe JG (ed): MTP International Review of Science, Ser. 1, Physiology, Vol. 2, Respiration. Baltimore, University Park Press, 1974, pp 303-369.
7. Weil JV, Byrne-Quinn E, Sodal ID, et al.: Hypoxic ventilatory drive in normal man. J Clin Invest 49:1061-1072, 1970.
8. Kronenberg R, Hamilton FN, Gabel R, et al.: Comparison of three methods for quantitating response to hypoxia in man. Respir Physiol 16:109-125, 1972.
9. Severinghaus JW: Proposed standard determination of ventilatory responses to hypoxia and hypercapnia in man. Chest 70(suppl):129-131, 1976.
10. Nielsen M, Smith H: Studies on the regulation of respiration in acute hypoxia. Acta Physiol Scand 24:293-313, 1952.
11. Dejours P: Control of respiration by arterial chemoreceptors. Ann NY Acad Sci 109:682-695, 1963.
12. Howell JBL: Effects and associations of disturbed airway resistive and ventilatory control, in Pengelly LD, Rebuck AS, Campbell EJM (eds): Loaded Breathing. Toronto, Longman, 1974, pp 3-9.
13. Cherniack NS, Altose D: Respiratory responses to ventilatory loading, in Hornbein TF (ed): Regulation of Breathing. New York, Dekker, 1981, pp 905-964.
14. Freedman S, Dalton KJ, Holland D, et al.: The effect of added elastic loads on the ventilatory response to CO_2 in man. Respir Physiol 14:237-250, 1972.
15. Lopata M, Pearle JL: Diaphragmatic EMG and occlusion pressure response to elastic loading during CO_2 rebreathing in humans. J Appl Physiol 49:669-675, 1980.
16. Wasserman K, Van Kessel AL, Burton GG: Interaction of physiological mechanisms during exercise. J Appl Physiol 22:71-85, 1967.
17. Whipp BJ, Ward SA: Ventilatory control dynamics during muscular exercise in man. Int J Sports Med 1:146-159, 1980.
18. Wasserman K, Whipp BJ: Exercise physiology in health and disease. Am Rev Respir Dis 112:219-249, 1975.
19. Zechman F, Hall FG, Hull WE: Effect of graded resistance to tracheal air flow in man. J Appl Physiol 10:356-362, 1957.

20. Potter WA, Olafson S, Hyatt RE: Ventilatory mechanics and expiratory flow limitation during exercise in patients with obstructive lung disease. J Clin Invest 50:910–919, 1971.

21. Grimby G, Saltin B, Wilhelmsen L: Pulmonary flow-volume and pressure-volume relationship during submaximal and maximal exercise in young well-trained men. Bull Physiopathol Resp 7:157–168, 1971.

22. Milic-Emili J, Whitelaw WA, Grassino AE: Measurement and testing of respiratory drive, in Hornbein TF (ed): Regulation of Breathing. New York, Dekker, 1981, pp 675–743.

23. Eldridge FL: Quantification of electrical activity in the phrenic nerve in the study of ventilatory control. Chest 70(suppl)154–157, 1976.

24. Hey EN, Lloyd BB, Cunningham DJC, et al.: Effects of various respiratory stimuli on the depth and frequency of breathing in man. Respir Physiol 1:193–205, 1966.

25. Clark FJ, Euler C von: On the regulation of depth and rate of breathing. J Physiol (Lond) 222:267–295, 1972.

26. Gautier H, Remmers JE, Bartlett D, Jr: Control of duration of expiration. Respir Physiol 18:205–221, 1973.

CHAPTER 14

Respiration and Sleep

CHRISTIAN GUILLEMINAULT

A HISTORIC OVERVIEW

The relationship between sleep and breathing, two basic, vital biologic functions, is often ignored. Breathing and its control are affected by sleep and sleep states, and sleep abnormalities affect breathing. It is only recently, however, that sleep-related respiratory studies have been performed systematically.

Rapid eye movement (REM) sleep was clearly identified in 1953, with publication of the landmark article by Aserinsky and Kleitman.[1] In 1965, Aserinsky indicated that diaphragmatic pauses could be observed in normal subjects during sleep in association with bursts of rapid eye movements.[2] The same year, Gastaut and his colleagues, studying obese patients complaining of daytime somnolence ("Pickwickians"), reported that obstructive apnea could be monitored during sleep.[3] In 1968, Kuhlo et al.[4] reported the first cases of Pickwickians who were helped by tracheostomy, and in 1972 Lugaresi and Sadoul chaired the first international meeting, held in Bologna (Italy), on "Hypersomnie et Respiration Periodique,"[5] which brought together for the first time sleep researchers and pulmonary specialists. In 1973, Duron published his studies on the effect of REM sleep on intercostal muscles, indicating the existence of REM–sleep-related inhibition.[6] Steinschneider, in the fall of 1972 (in English),[7] and we ourselves, in the spring of 1973 (in French),[8] published observations of apnea during sleep in infants and children, and questioned the relationship between abnormal breathing patterns during sleep and the sudden infant death syndrome (SIDS). In 1972, we published, in collaboration with F.E. Eldridge, the first report on the central sleep apnea syndrome and insomnia.[9] In

PULMONARY FUNCTION TESTING
INDICATIONS AND INTERPRETATIONS

1977 the Kroc Foundation sponsored an international meeting on sleep apnea syndromes.[10] Several meetings were held on the subject of the control of breathing during sleep, one in Sweden under the auspices of the Karolinska Institute,[11] and one in Sydney, Australia, in 1980.[12] Finally, the first textbook on the "Physiology in Sleep" was published in 1981.[13] During the past 15 years, first in Europe and then in North America, there has been an increase in the number of studies on central controls of various organs in relation to the different states of alertness. This has led to the progressive development of a subspecialty, somnology-sleep medicine. The official society in the United States is the Association of Sleep Disorders Centers, formed in 1975. The first examinations for the certificate of "Clinical Polysomnographer" were held in 1977.

PATHOPHYSIOLOGIC MECHANISMS OF SLEEP-RELATED BREATHING DISORDERS

When evaluating breathing problems during sleep, it is first necessary to consider the nature of sleep physiology. Sleep is a behavior controlled by central structures, including the hypothalamus and the brainstem. Certain neurotransmitters and/or neuromodulators are known to contribute to the control of sleep and the two specific sleep states: REM sleep and nonrapid eye movement (NREM) sleep. However, no model has yet been developed that accounts for all current pharmacologic or chemical control of sleep can be given.

Sleep appears to be influenced by genetic factors in mammals, including humans. Sleep, especially REM sleep, is tied to circadian rhythms; the relationship between REM sleep and the 24-hour core temperature rhythm is complex but is well understood. This is important because cardiovascular and respiratory function also are modulated by circadian rhythms; at times, the combined influences of sleep and the various rhythms may produce a serious breathing problem in the middle of the night.

The structure of sleep in humans changes from birth through old age, with the most important variations occurring during infancy and early childhood. Puberty also affects sleep and sleepiness in both sexes. REM sleep—called *active sleep* in infancy—decreases during the first 24 months of life. *Delta sleep* (stages 3–4 NREM, or slow-wave sleep) appears at about 3–4 months of age. The amount of delta sleep seen is highest in prepubertal childhood; it then decreases slowly until old age. The most regular breathing patterns can be observed during delta sleep, and chemical control of ventilation also is seen here in its purest form.

The fact that humans sleep lying down has an influence on breathing during sleep; the position affects tidal volume (V_T) and O_2 saturation and may lead to specific problems in patients with disorders such as kyphoscoliosis, abdominal obesity, and thyroid enlargement. Because the recumbent position tends to intensify breathing disorders, it is unfortunate that most human physiologic studies are performed on standing or seated subjects. Sorbini et al.[14] have demonstrated that PaO_2 decreases at a rate of 0.42 mm Hg per year after the age of 14 years in awake, supine subjects.

Physiologic changes can also be related to the different sleep states. During REM sleep, continuous antigravity muscle atonia is present, involving the accessory respiratory muscles and, as demonstrated by Duron,[6,15] the intercostal muscles. The Toronto school has studied the sudden laxity of the rib cage induced by intercostal muscle atonia during REM sleep in infants.[16] In patients who have borderline ventilation while awake, such as those with muscle disorders involving the thorax, thoracic deformities, or lung diseases, muscle atonia unquestionably plays an important role in REM–sleep-related hypoxia.[17-20]

During REM sleep, respiration is rapid and irregular, and brief episodes of hypopnea and apnea occur. Breathing irregularities during REM sleep often are associated with eye movements and myoclonic twitches. Also, during NREM sleep, the respiratory rate and minute ventilation decrease. This may be related to the loss of wakefulness stimuli, as hypothesized by Fink in 1961.[21]

A certain number of airway reflexes are altered during sleep. Laryngeal stimulation in dogs produces different responses depending on the state of alertness, with the appearance of reflex apnea during sleep.[22] In cats, upper airway resistance increases during sleep; this is probably related to the decrease in muscle tone of upper airway dilating muscles.[23] Ventilatory studies performed on sleeping humans have had controversial results. During REM sleep, a small increase in arterial PCO_2 and a shift of the CO_2 responses to higher CO_2 pressures were found; these changes were less marked in men than in women. During REM sleep, several studies have shown a depressed ventilatory response to CO_2 as compared to NREM sleep. This response may be intact during tonic REM sleep but impaired in phasic REM sleep.[24] Others have found no significant difference between REM and NREM sleep. Ventilatory responses to hypoxia are present during NREM sleep, but the extent of these responses during REM sleep also is controversial.

The arousal response is an important respiratory defense mechanism during sleep. It can be altered by many factors, such as ingestion of alcohol or other central nervous system depressant drugs, or sleep deprivation and sleep fragmentation. In such cases, this important defense may be impaired.[25,26]

This brief review of sleep-related physiologic changes[13] may explain why some patients face a risk of developing cardiorespiratory problems during sleep, and may be placed in life-threatening circumstances that are not foreseen during waking hours.

METHODS

The technologic approach to studying the effects of the different states of alertness on normal subjects and patients has been labeled *polysomnography*. This term was strongly attacked by some sleep specialists because it should more properly be either *polyhypnography* or *multisomnography*, but it had been recognized as the official terminology by different health agencies in the state of California and had already been printed in lists of official state nomenclature. The potential cost of reprinting these books led to the decision to accept the term.

Polysomnography

To evaluate the physiologic functioning of patients during sleep, a polysomnogram is performed. Polysomnography is the complex evaluation during sleep of a patient's central nervous system, respiratory, cardiac, and other functions; the comparison of these values with those obtained during wakefulness; and a quantitative evaluation of sleep/wake parameters. Several techniques are used to evaluate respiration during sleep; some are more invasive than others. When selecting a monitoring protocol, one should keep in mind that patient's sleep should be disturbed as little as possible. Several protocols, performed on successive nights, may be necessary to obtain an accurate picture of the problems of patients.

States and Stages of Sleep

Based on polygraphic criteria,[27] two different sleep states have been defined: NREM sleep (also called orthodox sleep or S state) and REM sleep (also called paradoxical sleep, D state, and desynchronized sleep). NREM sleep has been subdivided into four stages. Stage 1 is a transition phase between full wakefulness and unambiguous sleep; it is identified by a relatively low-voltage, mixed-frequence EEG with a predominance of activity in the range of 3–7 cycles per second (cps). Stage 1 is of short duration; in normal subjects it represents less than 4% of total sleep time (TST). Stage 2 sleep is marked by the appearance of *sleep spindles* (bursts of waves with a frequency of 12–14 cps) and *K complexes* (large, independent waves with an amplitude greater than 75 microvolts [μV]). Stages 3 and 4, also called slow wave sleep or delta sleep, are defined by an EEG record showing at least 20% of waves with a frequency of 0.5 to 3 cps and an amplitude of greater than 75 μV peak-to-peak during one epoch. An epoch is usually defined as 20 or 30 seconds, depending on the equipment used. REM sleep alternates with NREM sleep at approximately 100-minute intervals. The EEG pattern during REM sleep resembles that of stage 1 NREM, but with the addition of random saw-tooth waves. During this state, skeletal muscle tone is low, especially in the muscles of the neck and chin, but sudden twitches are monitored against the atonic background. Rapid eye movements appear singly or in bursts; heart and respiratory rates are irregular.

A standard polysomnographic recording generally includes all-night monitoring of the following variables: electroencephalogram (C_3/A_2-C_4/A_1 of the 10–20 international EEG placement system); electrooculogram (EOG); digastric electromyogram (EMG); electrocardiogram (ECG) (usually lead II). The criteria and procedures for recording and scoring sleep parameters are fully described in *A Manual of Standardized Terminology, Techniques and Scoring System for Sleep Stages of Human Subjects.*[27]

Various types of apparatus are used to screen for respiratory problems during sleep. The classic approach is to measure airflow with nasal and buccal thermistors and respiratory effort with mercury-filled thoracic and abdominal strain gauges. O_2 saturation is measured using an ear oximeter (the Hewlett-Packard [Palo Alto, CA] 47201A is used most commonly and is the most accurate model currently available).

Use of the respiratory inductive plethysmograph system (Respitrace [Ambulatory Monitoring, Inc. Ardsley, NY]) allows monitoring of changes in rib cage and abdominal compartments that occur with breathing. This system can be used simultaneously with devices designed to detect airflow, but by itself may give sufficient information to determine accurately the presence or absence of upper airway obstruction and the presence or absence of rib cage and abdominal movements. The advantages of respiratory inductive plethysmography are that it can be calibrated such that the monitored signal reflects V_T. The calculated accuracy of the instrument is within 10% of expected values. Calibration must be performed using a spirometer or a spirobag before sleep onset;[28] the data cannot be quantified easily using strain gauges and thermistors alone. Analysis of the rib cage and abdominal signals of the Respitrace allows assessment of the contribution and phase relationships of each of these to breathing. Obstructive apnea can be recognized on the basis of paradoxical rib cage and abdominal motions, and the absence of V_T.[28]

More elaborate protocols may be performed for evaluation of specific respiratory variables, although, as already mentioned, less sleep usually is seen when more equipment is used. The expired CO_2 may be monitored. The percent of expired CO_2 can be determined accurately for each breath if appropriate calibration has been performed using reference gases.

The following invasive techniques have a significant impact on sleep and sleep states; these observations should be kept in mind when the results are interpreted. Light sleep (stage 1) may be present for hours, and the breathing pattern seen with it may be misinterpreted because it mimics Cheyne-Stokes breathing. REM sleep may not occur at its usually scheduled time, or may be aborted very quickly, particularly during the early part of the night. Stages 3–4 NREM (slow-wave) sleep will not be present. Patients may become hyperaroused at the beginning of the night, and sleep deprived as morning approaches. (In certain patients, the ear oximeter may cause similar problems.) Nonetheless, despite these equipment-induced sleep changes, accurate assessment of certain sleep-related disorders is now possible.

The measurement of esophageal pressure may help to determine the type of apnea or hypopnea present during sleep. It may be associated with simultaneous measurement of gastric pressure and diaphragmatic EMG activity, using intraesophageal electrodes. Phenomena such as diaphragmatic fatigue can be evaluated in this manner.

Esophageal pH may be monitored if there is a suspicion of gastroesophageal reflux (GER) during sleep. This is particularly likely to occur in obese patients, whether or not they have obstructive apnea during sleep. GER may be responsible for esophagitis or secondary repetitive lung infections.

Blood-gas determinations may be made during sleep, either alone or in association with hemogynamic studies. Each individual has a distinctive movement pattern during sleep, but arms are more likely to be involved in sleep-related movements than thighs. Therefore, despite the potential risks associated with replacement of cathethers in the femoral artery or vein, if a line is needed for blood sampling during sleep, better sleep and more appropriate sleep staging will be obtained using femoral rather than upper limb placement. If cardiac output must be calculated during sleep, the most commonly used technique is that of thermodilution. But the injection of ice water can cause systematic arousals, and thus most of the data will be obtained while the subject is in stage 1 NREM sleep, or is just drowsy; so, despite the increase in the margin of error, the use of room temperature water is recommended.

We also recommend use of the 24-hour Holter ECG to screen for certain types of breathing problems during sleep (see following discussion).

INDICATIONS FOR POLYSOMNOGRAPHY

When should a polysomnogram be performed? This question is sometimes a source of strong disagreement. We do not discuss here all possible indications for polysomnography in infants, children, and adults; a large overview of such indications has been presented in two recent publications sponsored by the Association of Sleep Disorders Centers.[29,30] However, some indications for polysomnography are very clear. The first step is to have a complete interview and a thorough physical evaluation of the patient. The clinical symptoms associated with obstructive sleep apnea syndrome are well known by now.[31] They include excessive daytime somnolence, fatigue, tiredness, morning headaches, and automatic behavior during the daytime; these symptoms are usually associated with a history of repetitive heavy snoring and restless sleep. Reports by bed partners of observed abnormal breathing patterns during sleep are also very common. These symptoms clearly point to the diagnosis of obstructive sleep apnea syndrome. Other symptoms that may be found in relation to the nocturnal sleep periods are of value in making the diagnosis; these include abrupt sleep-related dyspnea or abrupt awakenings with a burning (acidic) sensation in the throat or mouth. These clinical symptoms should lead to a referral to a sleep specialist if there is any doubt about the diagnosis; as in any other field of medicine, the responsibility of deciding for or against performing a polysomnogram should be the result of this consultation. The specialty of sleep/wake medicine has increased in complexity, and there are now over 60 centers in the United States that are available for consultations.

As already mentioned, the 24-hour Holter ECG may be helpful in the evaluation of patients suspected of presenting complete or partial, continuous or intermittent airway obstruction during sleep. The Holter processing laboratory must have the capability of plotting the R-R interval over time in a readable way. These capabilities are lacking in many cases, despite the fact that the programming is easy to implement. Figure 14-1 shows a typical tracing, with progressive bradycardia during complete or partial obstruction and hypoxia, and tachycardia with relief of the abnormal event. These R-R changes are also enhanced due to the fact that the abnormal event occurs during sleep, when the autonomic nervous system balance in various organs is modified. For example, during NREM sleep and even more during REM sleep, there is an increased activity of the vagus nerve on the heart. The R-R changes also reflect the fact that a complete or partial Müller maneuver is induced during complete or partial airway obstruction with, once again, autonomic nervous system stimulation.

This technique does not give any indication of the severity of the problem, because the hypoxia of central apnea may lead to similar R-R swings, although these are usually less pronounced. But after reviewing 500 Holter ECGs of patients presenting sleep apnea syndrome, we have not found a single Holter ECG without this pattern in the absence of severe autonomic lesions (e.g., heart transplant patients, Shy-Drager syndrome, and severe autonomic neuropathy). Based on these findings, two private companies are developing microcomputerized systems that will allow outpatient, ambulatory screening with immediate interpretations using small computers. These ambulatory systems will permit economic screening for sleep apnea syndrome.

But sleep apnea syndrome is not the only indication for polysomnography. Patients who are obese may develop significant hypoxia and secondary cardiac arrhythmia during sleep. When daytime pulmonary function tests are performed,

228

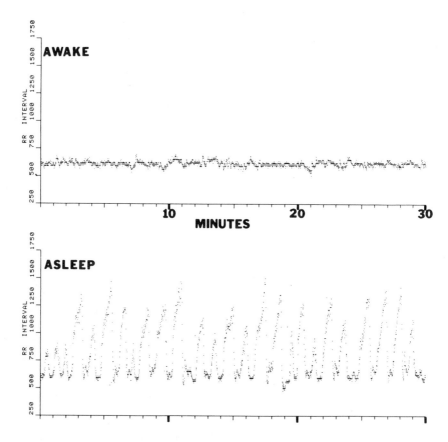

Figure 14-1. A computer print-out of a Holter ECG recording. The top of the figure represents 30 minutes of R-R intervals during quiet wakefulness; the bottom represents 30 minutes of R-R intervals during NREM sleep. As mentioned in the text, computer analysis of the R-R interval can be used as a screening technique for breathing abnormalities during sleep, if the clinician is familiar with the ECG pattern associated with the breathing irregularity, such as is seen in this plot.

In association with abnormal breathing patterns, stimulation of the autonomic nervous system occurs. In association with apnea and hypopnea, progressive bradycardia develops; when breathing resumes, with concomitant arousal, a substantial sympathetic response is observed. Plotting of the R-R interval displays a very characteristic pattern, similar to saw-tooth waves. Computer analysis is essential because some of the changes in the R-R interval occur between 500 and 1200 msec and may not be seen clearly with simple visual screening techniques. The peak-to-peak distance between each saw-tooth wave may indicate the duration of the abnormal breathing event, or even its type (e.g., apnea or hypopnea).

In this figure, the pattern associated with sleep-related obstructive apnea is clearly visible. Ambulatory monitors are now being developed to recognize such characteristic patterns; these should provide easy and inexpensive screening methods.

changes related to body habitus will be demonstrated. Probably, more pathology would be noted if these tests were performed on a supine patient who had been kept in dorsal decubitus for an hour (an evaluation that is only rarely performed).

Patients with impairment of the diaphragm or rib cage related to kyphoscoliosis or muscle weakness (muscle disorder or neurologic disorders involving a motor component impinging on thoracic motor neurons, the phrenic nerves, or on the sensory segment of the loop, such as patients with autonomic neuropathies) also need to be carefully evaluated during sleep.

The abnormal breathing process often involves the lungs. Patients with COPD, for example, have been investigated by several groups.[19,20,32,33] The association of COPD with obstructive apnea, which was originally reported by us,[34] has been confirmed by others.[35] This type of patient seems to be diagnosed more frequently in sleep clinics than in pulmonary clinics, probably because the systematic search for sleepiness is not commonly performed in lung-oriented departments. But the obstructive apnea issue is not the only one. A certain number of COPD patients present a functional depression of their respiratory neuronal network during sleep. It is commonly accepted that nocturnal administration of low-flow oxygen may allow longer survival of patients with severe COPD. This view was recently reinforced by two multicenter studies (the N.O.T.T. study[36] and the British Medical Council Study.[37]) However, in individual cases, O_2 administration may have an undesired effect, with progressive worsening of CO_2 retention and, once again, its eventual cortege of secondary cardiovascular changes.

Other lung diseases, particularly diseases of the lung in which ventilation, perfusion, and diffusion relationships are severely deranged in their internal relationship secondary to distorting diseases of the pulmonary parenchyma, such as fibrosing tuberculosis or other problems such as cystic fibrosis,[38] may be associated with important sleep-related worsening, as observed in our clinic.

A lesion of the neuronal respiratory network is an indication for systematic monitoring of the patient during sleep. Very often, patients with clear brainstem vascular lesions present with other obvious neurologic symptoms. But patients with encephalitis, including Reye's syndrome, may also develop primary or idiopathic alveolar hypoventilation syndrome secondarily, with differing degrees of respiratory impairment during NREM sleep. These adult patients have acquired lesions. The congenital central (or primary) alveolar hypoventilation syndrome can be diagnosed within weeks,[39] occasionally months, after birth by polysomnographic monitoring. There is a group of patients in whom alveolar hypoventilation is more difficult to recognize; in these patients, the presence of encephalitis or cerebrovascular lesion can not be clearly identified; nevertheless, they present with blunted responses to hypoxia and hypercapnia during NREM sleep and an inadequately driven ventilatory apparatus during this sleep state. Some patients with obesity-hypoventilation syndrome (although certainly not all of them) also present this problem, which disappears after weight loss.[40]

The effect of aging on the control of ventilation is not very well understood, but some elderly patients who complain of nocturnal sleep disturbance (insomnia) experience repetitive central respiratory pauses during sleep which greatly increase in number when central nervous system depressant drugs (including hypnotics) are administered.[41] Once again, this syndrome can only be diagnosed with sleep recording.

Finally, there are two other patient populations that may benefit from polysomnography: (a) patients with chronic mountain sickness, who appear to present repetitive severe hypoxia and apnea during sleep; and (b) patients receiving chronic doses of strong diuretics, who develop metabolic alkalosis leading to functional depression of the ventilatory system. In these patients, hypoxia and apnea are also first seen during sleep. Similarly, these patients with renal disease undergoing hemodialysis may, at times, present with respiratory abnormalities during sleep.

SUMMARY

The ventilatory apparatus can be impaired at many levels, and internists must keep in mind that very frequently the respiratory abnormality will be seen during sleep before being suspected while the patient is awake. The various categories of patients indicated above have all been seen and monitored in our clinic. Sleep-related hypoxia leads to secondary cardiovascular changes. Resetting of the sympathetic and parasympathetic systems during the two sleep states compared to wakefulness may also favor the appearance of cardiac arrhythmia when there is a ventilatory dysfunction. One must evaluate the patient's functioning while asleep as well as awake to propose a safe and adequate treatment.

CONTROVERSIES

The main controversies in the field of sleep research have been educational, financial, and technical.

EDUCATIONAL CONTROVERSIES

Sleep medicine is not yet fully recognized as a separate specialty. However, a specialty board on somnology and clinical polysomnography was established six years ago, and an educational program has been offered. Sleep medicine has been looked upon with some suspicion by other fields of medicine, mainly because most physicians are not familiar with sleep physiology. In the United States, another factor has been the initial strong dominance of psychiatrists and psychologists in the field (i.e., "What do *they* know about medicine?"). The complete absence of medical school teaching programs on sleep-related physiology and pathology seems to be an American idiosyncrasy, and is not necessarily true in other parts of the world. This explains why most of the initial work on sleep physiology came from Europe. Because sleep and sleep states imply changes of the central nervous system control of multiple internal functions and readjustments of autonomic nervous system controls, neurologists and neurophysiologists have been the most involved specialists in this field on the other side of the Atlantic. Sleep research is integrated into the departments of clinical neurophysiology, neurology, or internal medicine as a division. However, the first handbook devoted to the physiology of sleep was published in the United States in 1981,[13] and the first attempt to describe the indications and techniques of sleep medicine was also published in 1981.[30] Because a third of the life of each individual is spent in sleep, it would seem appropriate to include systematic study of sleep medicine in the curriculum of all medical schools.

FINANCIAL CONTROVERSIES

"Polysomnography is expensive!" is a frequently heard complaint. In our clinic, patients finally sent to us after a series of consultations have spent a mean of $5000 on various tests, without finding the basis of their problems. Polysomnography does not cost one tenth of this amount. It is less expensive than computerized tomography (CT) scans, which are performed on almost all excessively sleepy patients. In California, a long-term (four-hour) electroencephalogram costs about as much as an all-night sleep study. A 24-hour Holter ECG with an R-R interval plot costs two thirds as much as an all-night sleep recording, and provides much less information. Finally, most patients who need polysomnography are chronically ill and require continuous medical support and funds for treatment. If any technique can help avoid worsening of a chronic illness, can prevent serious complications leading to chronic disability, or can lead to better therapeutic adjustment, such a technique should be strongly supported. Most patients referred to our clinic for a breathing-related disorder during sleep have experienced difficulties on the job and loss of gainful employment due to their disease. A survey of the patients with sleep-related breathing disorders who were seen in our clinic during 1978 and 1979 indicates that 78% of them went back to full gainful employment after the appropriate diagnosis and treatment.

TECHNICAL CONTROVERSIES

There is no doubt that there is always room for technical improvement, and it is a healthy exercise to question the current techniques. Some of the current technical questions concern the length of the recording and its interpretation.

Length of polygraphic recording

How long should polysomnography last? Sleep studies, obviously, have to be performed while the patient is asleep, but the question remains as to whether the studies can be performed during daytime naps, following sleep deprivation, or after administration of sleep-inducing medication. Although this is clearly more convenient than night-time recordings, there are several arguments against this suggestion. Sleep is divided into two states: NREM and REM sleep; the latter state is associated with complete muscle atonia and a major increase in parasympathetic tone. It is obvious that monitoring of REM sleep is necessary for full evaluation of the impact of this sleep state on the cardiorespiratory status of the patient. However, REM sleep follows a circadian cycle, with a low between 12:00 PM and 5:00 PM and a peak between 2:00 AM and 5:00 AM. The longest uninterrupted REM sleep period is usually between 3:00 and 5:00 AM. Performing sleep monitoring during the daytime greatly reduces the chance of observing REM sleep and consequent changes; even if REM sleep does occur, it may not last long enough to allow a full evaluation of its impact on the patient's cardiorespiratory status.

A second problem with nap recording is related to the duration of sleep. A study performed on children with sleep apnea[42] has indicated that there is a relationship between the duration of uninterrupted sleep and frequency of apnea; that is, the longer the sleep time, the greater the frequency of apneic events. This means that to evaluate a patient's problem fully several hours of sleep monitoring are much more effective than just one. It seems obvious that if alveolar hypoventilation develops during sleep, hypoxia and hypercapnia may have a feedback effect on the respiratory neuronal network. This feedback may be a negative one in some patients, with more impairment of the brain structure due to the blood-gas changes. The hemodynamic consequences have also been proven to be more pronounced after several hours of sleep-related respiratory dysfunction.[43]

Sleep medicine is integrally related to circadian medicine. Many physiologic variables show cyclic variation. We know that some cancerous cells will have a 75% destruction rate if irradiation occurs at a particular point of the circadian rhythm and only a 25% destruction rate if irradiation occurs at a different time. We have integrated the notion that hormonal values can only be interpreted with relation to the 24-hour cycle. The respiratory rate and HR also have a circadian distribution, and tend to exhibit the greatest amount of pathologic depression between 2:00 AM and 5:00 AM. Once again, daytime nap monitoring would completely miss this aspect of the problem.

There are also problems with the administration of hypnotics to induce sleep for daytime monitoring. Usage of central nervous system depressant drugs should be carefully controlled because they may induce abrupt respiratory failure during sleep. Administration of a CNS-depressant drug during investigation of CNS control systems appears self-defeating, and adds another factor that is difficult to interpret. Sleep deprivation for daytime nap recordings also has its drawbacks. It has been well demonstrated that sleep deprivation has a direct impact on polysynaptic reflexes. The work of Phillipson et al.[25] with dogs and our own studies[26] of sleep apneic patients with moderate problems have clearly demonstrated the impact of sleep deprivation on hypoxic and hypercapnic responses, arousal threshold, and the amount of apnea. Once again, the results of sleep monitoring would be difficult to interpret under these conditions.

A study was performed by our clinic and the Henry Ford Hospital Sleep Disorders Clinic in Detroit analyzing the results obtained in a total of 35 unselected sleep apneic patients during all-night monitoring versus a long (90-minute) afternoon nap. The results obtained during the nap were significantly different in 23 subjects. The conclusion is that in the most severe cases, a nap recording obtained without pharmacologic induction may give some information, but in most cases the nap recording will be insufficient for appropriate diagnosis and treatment.

Evaluation of the polysomnograph recording

A polysomnographic recording is used to evaluate the type of abnormal respiratory events seen, their duration, impact on O_2 saturation, blood gases, cardiac rhythm, hemodynamic variables, and sleep. It is also used to evaluate the relationship between specific sleep states and respiratory events, and, of course, to guide therapeutic recommendations.

Apnea may be seen in normal individuals of all ages during sleep. It appears that gender, and endocrine status in women, influence the normal values for apneic and hypopneic events during sleep. In order to evaluate the severity of a sleep apnea syndrome, an apnea and hypopnea index ([A&H]I) has been developed. It is defined as the number of respiratory irregularities per sleep hour, and is calculated as follows:

$$\frac{(\text{Total number of apnea}) + (\text{Total number of hypopnea})}{\text{Total sleep time in minutes}} \times 60$$

An index of 5 is considered within normal range.

The evaluation of apneic and hypopneic events should include scoring of associated O_2 desaturations. Different scoring methods have been proposed to represent adequately the severity of respiratory disturbances during sleep. These include measurement of the total number of apneic and hypopneic events of each type, the longest apneic event seen during NREM and REM sleep, the mean duration of abnormal respiratory events during NREM and REM sleep, the total amount of time spent in a given sleep state or in total sleep time without air exchange, the lowest O_2 saturation observed during NREM and REM sleep, the number of respiratory events associated with a given range of O_2 saturation (e.g., between 90% and 80%, 80% and 70%, 70% and 60%, etc.), and the mean duration time spent with O_2 saturation within a given range (as above). Originally, these data were collected with handscoring techniques; a process both laborious and time consuming, particularly when correlations between abnormal respiratory events, types of events, O_2 saturation levels, cardiac arrhythmias, and sleep states were tabulated. In the recent past, introduction of computer programs designed for small, portable computers, and/or microprocessors has eased this task somewhat. The most commonly used program analyzes ear oximetry variations during sleep. Different software packages have been developed by different clinics; the sophistication varies among them. Some programs generate a plot (see Fig. 14-2) as well as numbers. One recently developed microprocessor [44] simultaneously analyzes signals obtained from ear oximetry and respiratory inductive plethysmography. Quantitative measurement and analysis of breath-by-breath (V_T), minute ventilation ($\dot{V}_E$), breathing frequency (f), total breath duration (Ttot), inspiratory time (T_i), and fractional inspiratory time (T_i/Ttot), can be obtained and associated with ear oximetry measurements. Similar programs currently are being studied by several groups. The most difficult computer analysis to develop remains that of sleep states. Efforts are being made, using physiologic variables such as EEG, chin EMG, actogram (which records the number and intensity of movements of the nondominant arm), and ECG, to differentiate the various sleep states with computers.

Although apnea and hypopnea during sleep originally received great attention, syndromes associated with abrupt hypoxemia during specific sleep states have been investigated more recently. Examples of polysomnographic findings are presented in Figures 14-2 through 14-5.

Other controversies regarding the technical aspects of polysomnography have concerned the number of variables to be monitored rather than the techniques to be used. Such controversies should not exist if the medical problem is well analyzed before performing the test. Wake/sleep states can be identified with three channels: an electroencephalographic (EEG) lead (C_3/A_2 or C_4/A_1), an interocular derivation (EOG), and one chin electromyogram recording. This montage will not show all EEG changes with hypoxia, and may miss some small independent eye movements, but it is generally sufficient for sleep staging and recognition of state of alertness.

Most problems arise because sleep can easily be disturbed by invasive techniques. One should remember that, at times, multiple questions may not be answered with one nocturnal recording, and several successive monitorings may be needed to evaluate complex problems.

CONCLUSION

To perform an adequate evaluation, sleep expertise and good technology, sometimes involving costly equipment, are necessary. As research in the field of sleep medicine continues, good understanding of sleep physiology and of the

235

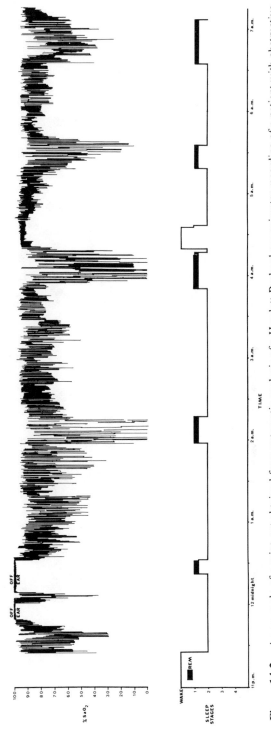

Figure 14-2. An example of a print-out obtained from automatic analysis of a Hewlett-Packard ear oximeter recording of a patient with obstructive sleep apnea syndrome. The sleep plot was obtained from a simultaneous polygraphic recording and was added to the ear oximetric plot after manual analysis. Note the marked desaturation occurring during REM.

236

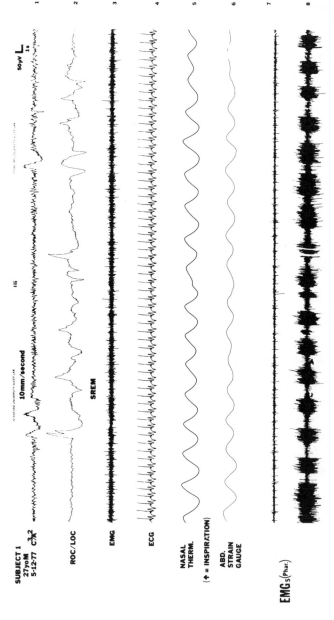

Figure 14-3. An example of a simple screening recording including, from top to bottom, the following variables: EEG, eye movements, chin EMG, ECG, airflow (indicated by nasal thermistor), abdominal strain gauge. Monitoring of the oropharyngeal muscle EMG (two bottom channels—an infrequently performed monitoring) was added to this simple recording. This is a 60-sec segment of a recording of a 24-year-old, normal volunteer, during REM sleep.

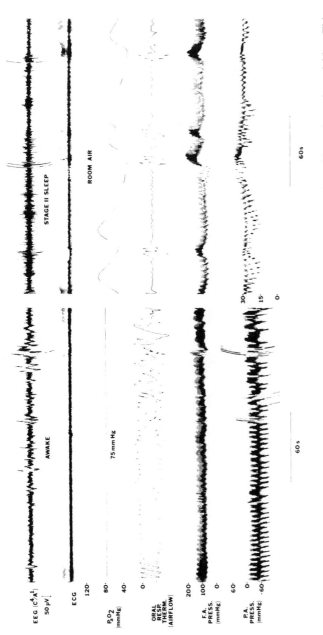

Figure 14-4. An example of a more complex montage that includes continuous monitoring of hemodynamic variables. This recording was obtained from a 48-year-old man with a history of severe obstructive sleep apnea syndrome. On the left of the figure, the patient is awake, supine. On the right, he is in stage II NREM sleep. Femoral arterial and pulmonary arterial pressures vary with changes in O_2 saturation. The interruption of airflow is associated with repetitive drops in O_2 tension; cardiac arrhythmias develop with apnea. Progressive increases in femoral arterial and pulmonary arterial pressures are related to hypoxia and to the Muller maneuver that occurs with obstruction. The impact of the Muller maneuver (inverse Valsalva) is seen clearly on the F.A. pressure channel, with the abrupt burst of pressure.

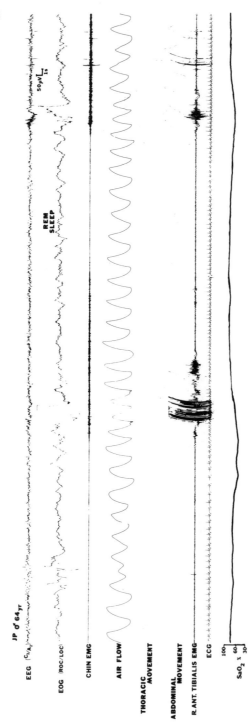

Figure 14-5. Monitoring during sleep of a 64-year-old, male patient with chronic COLD presenting abrupt hypoxia in association with REM sleep. During NREM sleep, the patient had normal O_2 saturation during sleep. Note that cardiac arrhythmias develop progressively with O_2 desaturation. An arousal, indicated by a change in the EEG and a leg movement, is triggered when O_2 reaches low values.

techniques used to monitor sleep will aid our knowledge of disorders that appear, or increase in severity, during sleep. After all, because all of us spend one-third of our lives asleep, medicine should not let this aspect of our existence remain a mystery.

REFERENCES

1. Aserinsky E, Kleitman N: Regularly occurring periods of eye motility and concomitant phenomena during sleep. Science 118:273–274, 1953.
2. Aserinsky E: Physiological activity associated with segments of the rapid eye movement periods, in Evants E, Kety S, Williams H (eds): Sleep and Altered States of Consciousness. Baltimore, Williams and Wilkins, 1967, pp. 335–350.
3. Gastaut H, Tassinari C, Duron B: Etude polygraphique des manifestations épisodiques (hypniques et respiratoires) diurnes et nocturnes du syndrome de Pickwick. Rev Neurol 112:568–579, 1965.
4. Kuhlo W, Doll E, Franck MC: Erfolgreiche dehandlung eines Pickwick syndroms durch eine dauertrachealkanule. Dtsch Med Wochenschr 94: 1286–1290, 1969.
5. Sadoul P, Lugaresi E (eds): Les hypersomnies avec respiration periodique. Bull Physiol Pathol Respir 8:967–1292, 1972.
6. Duron B: Postural and ventilatory functions of intercostal muscles. Acta Neurobiol Exp 33:355–380, 1973.
7. Steinschneider A: Prolonged apnea and the sudden infant death syndrome: clinical and laboratory observations. Pediatrics 50:646–654, 1972.
8. Guilleminault C, Dement WC, Monod N: Syndrome "mort subite du nourrisson" apnees au cours du sommeil. Nouv Presse Med 2:1355–1358, 1973.
9. Guilleminault C, Eldridge FL, Dement WC: Insomnia, narcolepsy and sleep apnea. Bull Physiopathol Respir 8:1127–1138, 1972.
10. Guilleminault C, Dement W (eds): Sleep Apnea Syndromes. New York, Alan R. Liss, Inc, 1978.
11. von Euler U, Lagercrantz H: Central Nervous Control Mechanisms in Breathing. New York, Pergamon Press, 1979.
12. Sullivan C, Henderson-Smart DJ, Read DJC (eds): The control of breathing during sleep. Sleep 3:221–465, 1980.
13. Orem J, Barnes CD (eds): Physiology of Sleep. New York, Academic Press, 1981.
14. Sorbini CA, Grassi V, Solinas E, et al.: Arterial oxygen tension in relation to age in healthy subjects. Respiration 25:3–13, 1968.
15. Duron B, Marlot D: Intercostal and diaphragmatic electrical activity during wakefulness and sleep in normal unrestrained adult patients. Sleep 3:269–281, 1980.
16. Muller N, Gulston G, Cade D, et al.: Diaphragmatic muscle fatigue in the newborn. J Appl Physiol 46:688–695, 1979.
17. Skatrud J, Iber C, McHugh W, et al: Determinants and hypoventilation during wakefulness and sleep in diaphragmatic paralysis. Am Rev Respir Dis 121:587–593, 1980.
18. Coccagna G, Mantovani M, Parchi C, et al.: Alveolar hypoventilation and hypercomnia in myotonic dystrophy. J Neurol Neurosurg Psychiatry 38:977–984, 1975.

19. Leitch AG, Clancy LJ, Legget RJE, et al.: Arterial blood gas tension, hydrogen ions, and electroencephalogram during sleep in patients with chronic ventilatory failure. Thorax 31:730–735, 1976.

20. Douglas NJ, Legget, RJE, Calverly PMA, et al.: Transient hypoxemia during sleep in chronic bronchitis and emphysema. Lancet 1:1–14, 1979.

21. Fink BR: Influence of cerebral activity in wakefulness on regulation of breathing. J Appl Physiol 16:15–20, 1961.

22. Sullivan CE, Murphy E, Kozar LF, et al.: Waking and ventilatory responses to laryngeal stimulation in sleeping dogs. J Appl Physiol 45:681–689, 1978.

23. Orem J, Lydic R: Upper airway function during sleep and wakefulness: experimental studies on normal and anesthetized cats. Sleep 1:49–68, 1968.

24. Sullivan CE, Murphy E, Kozar LF, et al.: Ventilatory responses to CO_2 and lung inflation in tonic versus phasic REM sleep. J Appl Physiol 47:1304–1310, 1979.

25. Phillipson EA, Bowes G, Sullivan CE, et al.: The influence of sleep fragmentation on arousal and ventilatory responses to respiratory stimuli. Sleep 3:281–288, 1980.

26. Guilleminault C: Sleep apnea syndromes: impact of sleep and sleep states. Sleep 3:227–246, 1980.

27. Rechtschaffen A, Kales A: A Manual of Standardized Terminology, Techniques, and Scoring System for Sleep Stages of Human Subjects. Los Angeles, Brain Information Service/Brain Research Institute, 1968.

28. Cohn MA, Rao BVA, Davis B, et al.: Measurement of tidal ventilation and forced vital capacity in normals and patients with obstructive lung disease with a respiratory inductive plethysomograph, in Stott FD, Raftery EB, Goulding L (eds): ISAM 1979: Proceedings of the Third International Symposium on Ambulatory Monitoring. London, Academic Press, pp. 355–365, 1980.

29. Roffwarg HP, Clark RW, Guilleminault C, et al.: Diagnostic classification of sleep and arousal disorders, (ed 1). Association of Sleep Disorders Centers. Sleep 2:3–137, 1979.

30. Guilleminault C (ed): Disorders of Sleep and Waking: Indications and Techniques. Menlo Park, CA, Addison Wesley, 1981.

31. Guilleminault C, Tilkian A, Eldridge FL, et al.: Sleep apnea syndrome due to upper airway obstruction: A review of 25 cases. Arch Intern Med 137:296–300, 1977.

32. Wynn JW, Block AJ, Hemenway J, et al.: Disordered breathing and oxygen desaturation during sleep in patients with chronic obstructive lung disease. Am J Med 66:573–579, 1979.

33. Cocagna G, Lugaresi E: Arterial blood gases and pulmonary and systemic arterial pressure during sleep in chronic obstructive pulmonary disease. Sleep 1:117–124, 1978.

34. Guilleminault C, Cummiskey J, Motta J: Chronic obstructive airflow disease and sleep studies. Am Rev Respir Dis 122:397–406, 1980.

35. Littner MR, McGinty DJ, Arand DL: Determinants of oxygen desaturation in the course of ventilation during sleep in chronic obstructive pulmonary disease. Am Rev Respir Dis 122:349–357, 1980.

36. Nocturnal oxygen therapy trial group. Continuous or nocturnal oxygen therapy in hypoxaemic chronic obstructive airways disease. Ann Int Med 93:391–398, 1980.

37. Report of the medical research council working party. Long term domiciliary oxygen therapy in chronic hypoxic cor pulmonale complicating chronic bronchitis and emphysema. Lancet 1:681–686, 1981.

38. Stokes DC, Wall MA, Erba G, et al.: Sleep hypoxemia in young adults with cystic fibrosis. Ann J Dis Child 134:741–743, 1980.

39. Guilleminault C, Challamel MJ: Congenital central hypoventilation syndrome (CCHS): Independent syndrome or generalized impairment of the autonomic nervous system?, in Guilleminault C, Korobkin R (eds): Progress in perinatal neurology (vol 1). Baltimore: Williams and Wilkins, 1981, pp. 197–215.

40. Richter T, West JR, Fishman AP: The syndrome of alveolar hypoventilation and diminished sensitivity of respiratory center. N Engl J Med 256:1165–1170, 1957.

41. Mendelson WB, Garnett D, Gillin C: Flurazepam induced sleep apnea syndrome in a patient with insomnia and mild sleep related respiratory changes. J Nerv Ment Dis 169:261–264, 1981.

42. Guilleminault C, Ariagno R, Korobkin R, et al.: Sleep parameters and respiratory variables in "near miss SIDS" infants. Pediatrics 68:354–360, 1981.

43. Tilkian AG, Guilleminault C, Schroeder JS, et al.: Hemodynamics in sleep induced apnea: Studies during wakefulness and sleep. Ann Int Med 85:714–719, 1976.

CHAPTER 15

Patterns of Disturbance

ARCHIE F. WILSON

INTRODUCTION

Pulmonary function tests allow assessment of physiologic processes; these tests also often allow deduction of abnormal anatomy and identification of specific disease entities. The deductive and identification processes are considerably facilitated if a classification of abnormal pulmonary function test patterns is utilized. Several classifications have been developed; three of these are presented in Table 15-1. The similarities and differences between the three classification schemes are evident from examination of Table 15-1. The main categories are indicated by italics. The classification in column I is from Cotes and is originally attributed to Scadding.[1] The classification in column II is from Wanner.[2] I have used the classification in column III for some time; this classification will be utilized in this discussion. Terms are repeated throughout for clarity.

Obstructive refers to airway narrowing sufficient to cause a measurable decrease of airflow not due to restriction. *Restrictive* refers to disease of the lungs, pleura, chest wall, or respiratory neuromuscular apparatus severe enough to cause reduction of vital capacity (VC) and total lung capacities (TLC). *Vascular* refers to primary diseases of the pulmonary circulation of sufficient severity to cause reduction in single-breath D_{LCO}. Further subdivision of abnormalities is possible depending upon either anatomic lesion and or pathophysiologic mechanism, e.g., obstructive can be subdivided into bronchoconstriction, dynamic airway compression, and upper airway and small airways obstruction. Although many clear-cut examples of each disease category exist, frequently, individual patients will have more than one type of process; hence, classification must allow for such overlap.

PULMONARY FUNCTION TESTING
INDICATIONS AND INTERPRETATIONS

Table 15-1 Three Classifications of Abnormal Pulmonary
Function Patterns

I	II	III
Obstructive ventilatory defect	*Obstructive lung disease*	*Obstructive*
Reversible	Asthma (chronic bronchitis)	Bronchoconstriction
Nonreversible	Emphysema (chronic bronchitis)	Dynamic airway compression
Nonreversible	Upper airway	Upper airway
Small airways syndrome	Chronic bronchitis	Small airways
Non obstructive ventilatory defect	*Restrictive lung disease*	*Restrictive*
Restrictive	Restrictive lung disease	Parenchymal removal/destruction
Restrictive	Restrictive chest bellows disease	Parenchymal infiltration
		Extrapulmonary deformity
	Restrictive chest bellows disease	
Hypodynamic	Restrictive chest bellows disease	Reduced force generation
Alveolar hypoventilation	*Disorders of ventilatory regulation*	Reduced force generation
	(Restrictive lung disease)	
Defect of gas transfer	*Pulmonary Vascular Disease*	*Vascular*

OBSTRUCTION

All types of obstructive pulmonary disease have the essential characteristic of airway narrowing. The major differences between subtypes is the nature and site of narrowing. Often, characteristic differences exist during forced expiration (Chapter 2 this volume). In Table 15-2, the types of obstructive disease, the sites of anatomic lesions, and the usual causative disease processes are listed. A mixed type is added to the categories identified in Table 15-1; this additional category was added because of the common finding of several types of obstructive processes (bronchoconstriction, small airways narrowing and dynamic airway compression) in COPD.

Bronchoconstriction is characterized by airways obstruction reversible by bronchodilator administration (Table 15-2). Bronchoconstriction may predominantly effect either large or small airways;[3] frequently, airways of all sizes are involved. Associated pulmonary function abnormalities include elevated lung volumes, abnormal distribution of ventilation, ventilation/perfusion mismatching, and elevated or normal DL_{CO}[4] (Table 15-3).

Dynamic airway compression occurs to a limited degree during forced expiration as a normal phenomenon (Chapter 2 this volume). In the presence of increased large airway deformability due either to loss of pulmonary parenchymal support of airways (emphysema) or destructive bronchitis-bronchiectasis and, frequently, severe small airways obstruction (bronchitis), increased airway compression during forced expiration of a degree severe enough to cause brief total collapse of large airways may occur.[5] When airway collapse occurs, a characteristic pattern may be noted[5] (Chapter 2 this volume); typically, peak inspiratory flow is greater than peak expiratory flow; other associated abnormalities (Table 15-4) include low DL_{CO} and high lung volumes (evidence of emphysema) plus abnormal distribution of ventilation and $\dot{V}/\dot{Q}$ mismatch. Because of increased central airways deformability and collapse during forced expiration, bronchodilatation may be difficult to assess by forced expiratory maneuvers; usually, in these circumstances, in response to bronchodilators, airway resistance declines and forced vital capacity (FVC) increases relatively more than forced

Table 15-2 Types of Obstructive Disease

Type	Anatomic Lesion(s)	Usual Diagnostic Term(s)
Bronchoconstriction	Contraction and inflammatory edema of large and/or small airway walls	Asthma (bronchitis)
Dynamic airway compression	Compliant large airways (+ small airway obstruction)	Emphysema (bronchitis)
Upper airway	Narrowing of extrathoracic trachea, larynx or pharynx	Tracheal, laryngeal stenosis, obstructive sleep apnea
Small airways	Edema and inflammation producing diffuse narrowing of small airways	Bronchitis (bronchiolitis, asthma)
Mixed	Variable combination of edema, inflammation, contraction and increased compliance of large and small airways	COPD

Table 15-3 Characteristics of Types of Obstruction

Type	Expiration at High Lung Volumes	Expiration at Low Lung Volumes	Pattern of Obstruction During: Inspiration	Airway Resistance	Bronchodilator Improvement
Bronchoconstriction	Yes (continuous)	Yes (continuous)	Yes	High	Yes
Dynamic airway compression	Yes (collapse) (pattern)	Yes (unevaluable)	Relatively normal	Normal	Nil
Upper airway	Yes	Normal	Yes (pronounced)	High	Nil
Small airways	Nil	Yes	Nil	Normal	Nil
Mixed	Variable	Yes	Variable	High	Variable

Table 15-4 Associated Abnormalities with Obstruction

	TLC and FRC	RV and CV	Distribution of $\dot{V}$	$\dot{V}/\dot{Q}$	DL_{CO}
Bronchoconstriction	High	High	Often abnormal	Often abnormal	Normal
Dynamic airway compression	High	High	Abnormal	Variable	Low
Upper airway	Normal	Normal	Normal	Normal	Normal
Small airways	Normal	High	Often abnormal	Often abnormal	Normal
Mixed	High	High	Abnormal	Abnormal	Low

expiratory flow (FEV_1) improves.[5,6] If density dependence of airflow is studied with HeO_2 mixtures, it is evident that a significant amount of small airway constriction is present[7] (Chapter 4 this volume).

Upper airway obstruction is produced by either localized marked narrowing or increased deformability of the trachea or larynx. When the orifice is narrowed to a critical point, characteristic patterns of airflow are noted during both forced inspiratory and expiratory airflow (Chapter 2 this volume). Typically, orifice-type flow is observed, particularly during recording of flow-volume curves; inspiration is relatively more affected than expiration if the narrowing is extrathoracic. If a portion of the upper airways is more deformable than normal (tracheomalacia, vocal cord paralysis), particularly when associated with more proximal airway narrowing (e.g., tracheal stenosis), maximal inspiratory flow rates may be much more severely reduced than expiratory flow rates. This type of variable or dynamic inspiratory extrathoracic obstruction is somewhat similar to the dynamic airway compression that occurs in intrathoracic airways during expiration but, because of differences in the pressure outside of the airways (positive pleural pressure in intrathoracic airways during expiration and positive ambient—in relationship to airway—pressure in extrathoracic airways during inspiration), airway narrowing occurs during inspiration rather than expiration.

Recently, it has been shown that many patients with obstructive sleep apnea have a form of variable extrathoracic obstruction that is maximal during sleep but may be partially manifest while awake.[8-10] The monitoring of physiologic changes during sleep was discussed in the previous chapter. In the awake patient, obstruction may be demonstrated in the pulmonary function laboratory by analysis of maximal flow-volume curves; many patients with obstructive sleep apnea show a characteristic saw-tooth pattern particularly during expiration, and, decreased maximal inspiratory rates while maximal expiratory rates are relatively normal.[9] Additionally, transrespiratory and transpulmonary resistances measured by the pulse-flow technique, at the end of expiration, are elevated in these patients.[10]

We have noted an unusual two-compartment pattern during the forced expiration associated with stenosis of one of the two mainstem bronchi; this pattern differs from the airway collapse pattern, which is a marked decline in airflow rate leading to an abrupt change usually within 400 ml to TLC, in that expiratory flow abruptly declines near mid-VC.

Small airways obstruction is usually characterized by essentially normal measures of airflow except for decreased forced expiratory flow at low lung volumes.[11] The bronchodilator response is usually not marked.[12] Very pronounced diffuse small airways obstruction will produce increased airway resistance and generalized decrease of airflow during spirometry. Diffuse, severe, small airways obstruction is probably an important factor in large airways collapse. Small airways obstruction may (or may not) be associated with abnormal distribution of ventilation and $\dot{V}/\dot{Q}$ mismatch.[12]

Mixed obstructive patterns are characteristic of chronic obstructive pulmonary disease (COPD), i.e., COPD may be considered a disease syndrome characterized by the presence of variable amounts of chronic bronchitis, emphysema, and bronchospasm. Although individual patients may have little cough and hypoxemia (pink puffers) and others suffer from productive cough, heart failure, and hypoxemia (blue bloaters),[13] most COPD patients have combined manifestations. Pink puffer patients usually have pulmonary function suggestive of emphysema (high lung volumes, low DL_{CO}, and fairly normal $\dot{V}/\dot{Q}$ matching); their pulmonary function also usually demonstrates abnormal distribution of ventilation, little reversibility with bronchodilator, and, frequently, severe dynamic airway compression and/or large airway collapse.[10] Blue bloater patients often demonstrate pulmonary function manifestations of chronic bronchitis (slightly elevated lung volumes, mismatched $\dot{V}/\dot{Q}$, hypoxemia, and only slightly reduced DL_{CO}.[13] Frequently, much of the airways obstruction is reversible with bronchodilator therapy, particularly with time. However, most COPD patients have mixed pictures with some hypoxemia, some lowering of DL_{CO}, some bronchodilator response, and so forth, indicating the coexistence of several disease entities.

RESTRICTION

As noted earlier, restrictive lung disease is characterized by a reduction of TLC and VC. Four subtypes of restrictive lung disease may be recognized (Table 15-5): parenchymal removal/destruction, parenchymal infiltration, extrapulmonary deformity, and reduced force generation. Because of the reduced VC, measures of airflow during forced expiration may be reduced. Under those circumstances, the possible presence of a complicating obstructive problem can be conveniently evaluated from the FEV_1/FVC ratio, which corrects FEV_1 values for reduction in VC. Except for some cases of reduced force generation, FEV_1/FVC values are normal or high in restrictive lung disease that is not complicated by airway disease (Table 15-6).

The parenchymal removal/destruction subtype of restrictive lung disease is caused by either surgical removal or localized postinflammatory obliteration of lung tissue or alveolar filling or collapse. In each instance a significant quantity of lung is permanently or temporarily not inflatable. Hence, all lung volumes and DL_{CO} are reduced but FEV_1/FVC is normal (Table 15-6). Because the remaining lung is normal, the distribution of ventilation and $\dot{V}/\dot{Q}$ are also normal (Table 15-7).[14]

Parenchymal infiltration or interstitial lung disease occurs when either inflammatory or fibrotic tissue appears in the interstitium of the lung. All lung volumes and DL_{CO} are reduced. Additionally, because of increased elastic recoil, FEV_1/FVC is either normal or increased (Tables 15-6 and 15-7). Because these

Table 15-5 Types of Restrictive Disease

Type	Location of Anatomic Lesion	Pathologic Condition
Parenchymal removal/destruction	Pulmonary parenchyma	Surgical removal, atelectasis, alveolar filling, postinflammatory obliteration
Parenchymal infiltration	Pulmonary parenchyna	Interstitial inflammation or fibrosis
Extrapulmonary deformity	Chestwall, pleura	Chest wall deformity, pleural disease, obesity
Reduced force	Peripheral and central nervous system, respiratory muscles	Poor cooperation, pain, neuromuscular disease including respiratory center disorders

processes are diffuse but also focal, i.e., they tend to affect local areas in a patchy fashion; maldistribution of ventilation (Chapter 7 this volume) and ventilation/perfusion mismatching are common (Chapter 11 this volume).[15]

Extrapulmonary deformity may be caused by such conditions as kyphosis, scoliosis, pectus excavatum, spondylosis, pleural effusion or thickening, and obesity (Table 15-5). Characteristically, chest expansion is limited and TLC is low. In conditions due to chest wall abnormality, chest deflation is also limited, hence RV is high.[16] In conditions due to pleural disease and obesity, chest deflation and RV are relatively normal.[17] When chest expansion is more limited on one side than the other or in discrete areas of the lung, distribution of ventilation and $\dot{V}/\dot{Q}$ may be abnormal. When chest expansion is equally abnormal on both sides of the thorax, distribution of ventilation and $\dot{V}/\dot{Q}$ are normal.[16] Because, in patients not complicated by airway or parenchymal disease, the underlying lung is normal, DL_{CO} values are usually normal (Tables 15-6 and

Table 15-6 Characteristics of Types of Restriction

Type	TLC	FRC	RV	Distribution of $\dot{V}_A$	$\dot{V}/\dot{Q}$	DL_{CO}
Parenchymal removal/destruction	Low	Low	Low	Normal	Normal	Low
Parenchymal	Low	Low	Low	Abnormal	Abnormal	Low
Extrapulmonary deformity	Low	Low	Variable	Variable	Variable	Normal
Reduced force generation	Low	Normal	High	Normal	Normal	Normal

Table 15-7 Summary of Usual Pulmonary Function Findings

Type	Airflow	Lung Volumes	DL_{CO}
Obstructive			
Bronchoconstriction	Reversible obstruction	All high	Normal or high
Dynamic airway compression	Collapse pattern	All high	Low
Upper airway	Inspiration worse	Normal	Normal
Small airways	Reduced at low lung volumes	CV & RV high	Normal
Mixed (COPD)	Collapse, some reversibility	High	Low
Restrictive			
Parenchymal removal destruction	Normal FEV_1/FVC	All low	Low
Parenchymal infiltration	High FEV_1/FVC	All low	Low
Extrapulmonary deformity	Normal FEV_1/FVC	Low TLC, high RV	Normal
Reduced force generation	Reduced	Low TLC, high RV	Normal
Vascular			
Occlusion	Normal	Normal	Low

15-7). With obesity and ascites, FRC is reduced and expiratory reserve volume (ERV) is usually also low;[18] many patients with obesity and ascites have virtually normal pulmonary function except for high closing volume and consequent hypoxemia.[18]

Reduced force generation occurs because of respiratory muscle weakness, poor patient cooperation due to pain with forced breathing, inadequate understanding, and/or less than maximal effort. Experienced technicians usually immediately recognize the technical problems. Patients with neuromuscular disease affecting the respiratory muscles or nerves also may not generate enough force to fully expand and deflate the chest. The magnitude of the reduction of force generation may be assessed by the measurement of maximal airway pressures (Chapter 9 this volume) and lung volumes (Table 15-6). Patients with hemiplegia and high paraplegia have predominant abdominal muscle weakness and consequent difficulty with exhalation;[19,20] characteristically, residual volume (RV) is high and ERV is low. Patients with more generalized weakness from such causes as myasthenia, polyneuropathy, and muscular dystrophy frequently have equal difficulty with inspiration and expiration; in these patients, TLC is low and RV is high.[21] In these conditions, the underlying lung and airways are normal, hence, prior to the development of complicating events such as bronchitis and pneumonia, the distribution of ventilation, $\dot{V}/\dot{Q}$, and DL_{CO} are normal. In many of the conditions that cause reduced force generation, alveolar hypoventilation with consequent increase $PaCO_2$ and decreased PaO_2 may occur. When alveolar hypoventilation occurs in the face of normal lung, airways, chest wall, and neuromuscular apparatus, primary hypoventilation, a disease of the respiratory center is present[22] (Chapter 13 this volume).

VASCULAR

Diffuse pulmonary vascular occlusion with normal airways, parenchyma, chest wall, and neuromuscular structures may occur as a consequence of multiple pulmonary emboli or primary disease of the pulmonary vasculature. The major pulmonary function abnormality of pulmonary vascular disease is the decrease of DL_{CO};[23] other pulmonary function measurements are usually normal, thereby eliminating such diseases as emphysema, resectional lung surgery, and parenchymal infiltration. In these later conditions, other pulmonary function tests such as lung volumes and/or airflow are abnormal.

COMBINED OBSTRUCTION AND RESTRICTION

Not infrequently, patients may suffer from either one or a combination of lung diseases that may produce both obstruction and restriction. Potential examples of diseases that may caused combined obstruction and restriction include heart failure (case 3, Chapter 6 this volume), sarcoidosis (typically associated with small airway obstruction and parenchymal infiltration), and far-advanced cystic fibrosis. More commonly, a combination of pulmonary diseases are responsible for combined obstruction and restriction. Patients with COPD who subsequently develop lung cancer may also become restricted because of pleural effusion (extrapulmonary deformity), pain (reduced force generation), surgical resection (parenchymal removal), or radiation pneumonitis (parenchymal infiltration). Patients with neuromuscular and chest wall disease frequently develop bronchitis with consequent small airways obstruction and, possibly, bronchospasm.

Usually, the clinical problem suggests the probability of the combined presence of obstruction and restriction. Pulmonary function findings that should suggest this combination include (1) smaller than expected lung volumes in the presence of significant airway obstruction, (2) low FEV_1/FVC ratio in the presence of significant restriction, and (3) an elevated RV/TLC ratio in the presence of parenchymal restrictive diseases.

CONTROVERSIES

In the introduction to this section, it was pointed out that pulmonary function tests allow the assessment of physiologic processes but do not necessarily imply the presence of specific pathology or disease processes. Therefore, although it may be suggested that the interpretation of pulmonary function tests should not proceed beyond listing the physiologic derangements of pulmonary function tests, it should also be pointed out that the pulmonary function characteristics of certain disease entities, such as small airway obstruction, upper airway obstruction and asthma, are well established whereas the characteristics of others, such as pulmonary vascular occlusion and emphysema, are somewhat less well-agreed upon. Hence, until more studies comparing pulmonary function and pathology are reported, the interpreter of pulmonary function tests probably should liberally use the phrase "consistent with."

SUMMARY

Pulmonary function abnormalities can be conveniently classified into several categories by fairly simple tests; airflow (spirometry and/or flow/volume), lung volumes (VC and TLC), and DL_{CO}. The categories identified suggest disordered physiology; they do not usually unequivocally identify disease entities. Further, in certain categories, such as COPD, the quantification and identification of specific pathologic entities (emphysema, bronchitis) is difficult, even with postmortem examination.[24] In these cases, pulmonary function tests may provide the best assessment of the nature of the intrapulmonary abnormalities. Although specific diseases may often not be clearly identifiable by pulmonary function tests alone, certain conditions such as asthma, simple bronchitis, panlobular (dry) emphysema, pulmonary vascular disease, and so forth, have patterns so well defined that clinical impressions may be adequately confirmed; at the least, diagnostic possibilities should be sharply defined.

REFERENCES

1. Cotes JE: *Lung Function: Assessment and Application in Medicine* (ed 4). Blackwell, Oxford, 1979, p. 388.
2. Wanner A: Interpretation of Pulmonary Function Tests, in Sackner MA (ed): *Diagnostic Techniques in Pulmonary Disease*, Part I. New York, Dekker, 1980.
3. Fairshter RD, Wilson AF: Relationship between the site of airflow limitation and localization of bronchodilator response in asthma. Am Rev Respir Dis 122:27–32, 1980.

4. Weitzman R, Wilson AF: Diffusing capacity and overall ventilation/perfusion in asthma. Am J Med 57:767–774, 1974.

5. Healey F, Fairshter RD, Wilson AF: Small airways obstruction and large airway collapse. Chest 85:476–481, 1984.

6. Ramsdell JW, Tisi GM: Determination of bronchodilatation in the clinical pulmonary function laboratory. chest 75:622–628, 1979.

7. Fairshter RD, Wilson AF: Relationship between sites of airflow limitation and severity of chronic airflow obstruction. Am Rev Respir Dis 1213:3–7, 1981.

8. Surrat PM, Dee P, Atkinson RL, et al.: Fluorscopic and computed ttomographic features of the pharyngeal airway in obstructive sleep apnea. Am Rev Respir Dis 127:487–492, 1983.

9. Tammelin BR, Wilson AF, Borowiecki B, et al.: Flow volume curves reflect pharyngeal airway abnormalities in sleep apnea syndrome. Am Rev Respir Dis 128:712–715, 1983.

10. Surrat PM, Wilhoit, SC, Atkinson, RL: Elevated pulse flow resistance in awake obese subjects with obstructive sleep apnea. Am Rev Respir Dis 127:162–165, 1983.

11. Fairshter RD, Wilson AF: Relative sensitivities and specificities of tests for small airway obstruction. Respiration 37:301–308, 1979.

12. Wilson AF, Fairshter RD: Relative effect of oral and inhaled bronchodilators in *Small Airways* in Sadoul P, Milic-Emili J (eds): Health and Disease. Amsterdam Excerpta Medica, 1979.

13. Mitchell RS, Silvers GW, Dart GA, et al.: Clinical and morphological correlations in chronic airways obstruction. Am Rev Respir Dis 97:54–62, 1968.

14. Kallquist I: Pulmonary resection in middle-aged and elderly patients. Am Rev Tuburc 73:40, 1956.

15. Gibson GJ, Pride NB: Pulmonary mechanics in fibrosing alveolitis: the effects of lung shrinkage. Am Rev Respir Dis 116:637–647, 1977.

16. Gacad GJ, Hamosh P: The lung in ankylosing spondylitis. Am Rev Respir Dis 107:286–289, 1973.

17. Barrera F, Reidenberg MM, Winters WL: Pulmonary function in the obese patient. Am J Med Sci 254:785–796, 1967.

18. Bedell GM, Wilson WR, Seebohm PM. Pulmonary function in obese persons. J Clin Invest 37:1049, 1958.

19. Fluck DC: Chest movements in hemiplegia. Clin Sci 31:383–388, 1966.

20. Fugl-Meyer AR, Linderholm H, Wilson AF: Restrictive ventilatory dysfunction in stroke: its relation to locomotor function. Scand J Rehab Med 9 (Suppl):118–124, 1983.

21. Harrison BDW, Collins JF, Brown KGE, et al.: Respiratory failure in neuromuscular diseases. Thorax 26:579–584, 1971.

22. Zwillich CW, Suton FD, Pierson DJ, et al.: Decreased hypoxic ventilatory drive in the obesity-hypoventilation syndrome. Am J Med 41:440–447, 1966.

23. Nadel, JA, Gold, WM, Jennings, DB, et al.: Unusual disease of pulmonary arteries with dyspnea. Structure-function relationships. Am J Med 41:440–447, 1966.

24. Thurlbeck WM: *Chronic Airflow Obstruction in Lung Disease*. Philadelphia, Saunders, 1976.

CHAPTER 16

Computers in Pulmonary Medicine

JOHN G. MOHLER
GARY A. WOLFF

Miniaturization of electronics has made computers, and their component parts and attachments smaller and less expensive. As a result, this technology has spread into almost every facet of life in technology-oriented societies. The purpose of this chapter is to provide a short introduction to the use of computers in a pulmonary medicine environment. As is true with any new technology or process, distinctive words are used that utilize meanings that are variations of common usage. We attempt to minimize such jargon but because certain ideas are best described by these words, they are defined as they are introduced. We outline the uses of a computer in a laboratory, discussing the steps from test to report. We give some description of component configuration. We show a detailed example of how the computer can be used to write an interpreted report and how statistical methods are used to generate a decision process. Finally, we give some case examples to demonstrate the procedure.

There are, of course, some obvious advantages along with some disadvantages to automation of any medical service, particularly in a pulmonary laboratory. Some advantages are obvious: fast return of results, accuracy of calculation, simplification of complicated maneuvers, and consistency of results. It is not always clear, however, that automation is cost effective. Several factors must be considered in each case before such a decision can be made. One must consider the cost of acquiring and maintaining the equipment, its through-put (how much and how fast the output is ready from the time the patient is tested), and how frequently the machine will be used. One must also weigh the value of the tests that can be added by the automation that are not available without it. Computerized systems that allow the computer to be used for other jobs such as bookkeeping, scheduling, and even word processing increase cost effectiveness. Turn-key (or black box) systems are weak in this regard, they are dedicated to

PULMONARY FUNCTION TESTING
INDICATIONS AND INTERPRETATIONS

single tasks and so are often designed to do just one job most effectively. One must be very cautious not to count on substantial reduction in personnel costs to offset the automation. The rule is that the more sophisticated the equipment, the more sophisticated the technologist must be to make it work properly. Therefore, it is unwise to reduce the competence of the technical staff to reduce salary costs.

The major disadvantage of automation is most painfully obvious when technical failure occurs. When planning to automate, it is important to plan for significant periods of down-time; this means redundancy. One must be prepared to use standard manual methods or have available back-up methods or equipment that will keep one operating for a week or more. This is especially true for those complicated, sophisticated, dedicated units that do not have stand-alone computers, but rather dedicated built-ins (black box or turn-key systems). In short, it is not advisable to throw away the functional and reliable devices upon changing to automated equipment. Of course, a good approach is to adapt microprocessors or minicomputers to old equipment so that when the processors misfunction, the manual methods can be easily restored to use.

A computer system can be procured as a turn-key package with all instrumentation, computer hardware, and software bundled together. The advantages of the turn-key system include single-vendor support, clearly stated costs, and a user community that may already be developed. The disadvantages include the lack of ability to modify the testing procedures and reports, upgrade components of the system, and perform new tests.

An in-house–developed system on the other hand is an integration of instrumentation, computer hardware, and software that has been developed under the direct guidance of the laboratory staff.

Using computers tends to de-skill laboratory technologists because they do not do the routine calculations and do not make the routine decisions regularly; hence, they may have to go through a short period of retraining to restore service during down-time. For this reason, personnel utilizing the system should include the most skilled and knowledgeable persons available. This may seem a paradox because the automated machine makes testing so easy one is tempted to use less expensive and less skilled technicians. The other side of the skill issue is that laboratory personnel should become skilled in the operations of the laboratory computer. Otherwise, the laboratory is at the mercy of strange people and strange machines.

FUNCTIONS OF A COMPUTER

DATA ENTRY

Some types of data are most effectively entered into the computer by typing using the keyboard. This type of entry is referred to as *manual entry*. The keyboard is connected to a video screen. This combination is often called a *video display terminal* (*VDT*). These, in turn, are connected to the computer which must deal with the information. Blood-gas data, for example, may be best handled in such a manner. The millimeter measurements taken from a spirogram for forced vital capacity (FVC) or one second forced expiratory volume (FEV₁), for example, could be entered with other data such as temperature, barometric pressure, bell factor, data, and time, which would be used by the computer to calculate the corrected results and produce a printed report. The printed report would be no different than if the data were transferred directly from the measuring device (spirometer) to the computer; this is called *on-line*. Most often, in pulmonary systems combinations of manual and on-line entry are usefully applied; manual entry is used for patient demographics and data are acquired online from the measuring device.

Batch loading by tape, discs, or machine-readable punched cards are seldom used for the purposes covered here. Hollerith developed the punch-card system in the late 19th century for the United States Census Bureau, thus, the card carries his name: the Hollerith card; "IBM card" is technically improper although common in usage.

One of the first steps in designing an automated system is to describe the input formats. To understand and communicate, one must become familiar with the terminology used in such an input design. Most commonly, data are grouped into *fields* such as weight, name, and hospital number. A collection of fields is a *record*. The values entered at the display terminal form a record. An example is the record of an analysis of a single blood-gas sample (Table 16-1). Note the fields; the whole page represents the record.

DATA STORAGE

A collection of records is called a *file*. To store the results of the analyses done in the laboratory, the system must be designed to store records in files in an inexpensive and readily retrievable manner. A file may be printed reports that go into a file cabinet to be manually retrieved. This is cheap, but slow. More commonly, the data are stored on some electronic media such as paper tape (slow and seldom used), magnetic tape (slow, but faster and more reliable than paper), floppy disks (fast, more commonly used, easily stored), hard-surface disks (very fast and more costly), or in the memory itself (fastest retrieval, costly, and very limited in number of files that can be stored). A storage and retrieval system must be chosen based upon the need for rapid retrieval, available money, and cost effectiveness. The most common system is the use of a floppy disk that can be easily stored and manually inserted when the data are needed. Many predesigned package systems have no long-term storage or retrieval capacity.

DATA RETRIEVAL

A record can be retrieved from a file when information is given about which record to retrieve. This is analogous to giving a file clerk the assignment to

Table 16-1   Example of a Blood Gas Analysis Record

Field Number	Field Length # of Characters	Field Description
1	12	Patient's name.
2	10	Patient's hospital number.
3	1	Patient's sex, coded as M or F.
4	5	Patient's location.
5	10	Date and time sample was drawn, coded as MMDDYYHHMM for month, day, year, hours, and minutes.
6	3	Patient's temperature, F.
7	3	Measured PO_2, mm Hg.
8	3	Measured PCO_2, mm Hg.
9	3	Measured pH, coded without the decimal point. A pH of 7.41 becomes 741.
10	2	Measured hematocrit.
11	3	Measured hemoglobin.
12	1	Sample site, coded by a number. Example: 1 means sample site was arterial.
13	3	Fractional inspired O_2, coded without the decimal point. An FIO_2 of 0.21 becomes 21.
14	1	Patient's position, coded as a number. Example: 2 means patient was sitting while the sample was being drawn.

retrieve a set of data from the file folders. Using the blood-gas example, as in Table 16-1, the computer could retrieve and print a report for all blood-gas records with a given patient hospital number. A second example might be to retrieve and print a report containing all blood-gas results that were drawn between two given dates for which a PCO_2 is in excess of some limit value. The first example of retrieval might be easy for a file clerk to perform if the data were filed by patient hospital number. The second example, however, would require a search of the entire file cabinet and each blood-gas report within each file folder, a task that might take someone hours or days; a computer can accomplish each task usually within minutes if the file system is properly set up.

CONTROL OF LABORATORY EQUIPMENT

The computer is capable of sending signals to equipment within the laboratory to cause test conditions to change or to facilitate the gathering of data. As an example, a signal can be sent to close the mouth shutter as part of a body plethysmograph procedure. Another example would be the switching of a valve that directs gas into a gas analyzer. The computer can also produce analog signals using a digital-to-analog converter (D-A) that can be used to drive X-Y recorders and oscilloscopes.

The use of feedback becomes possible with a computer (Fig. 16-1). When a computer sends signals back to modify the test conditions, the computer becomes part of a closed-loop test procedure. An example of a closed-loop procedure is in exercise testing when the measurements are used to control the test conditions of inspired gas concentration, workload, or both.

REPORT GENERATION

As with the input requirements for field definitions, the output requires rigid definitions. This process of field definition and structure of an output report is often tedious, frustrating, and most difficult. This process is the first step in a system design, even before the equipment is purchased because without it one cannot be sure of the real needs. Once the design is specified, the output needs, questions such as what to buy, what configurations are needed, and how much of

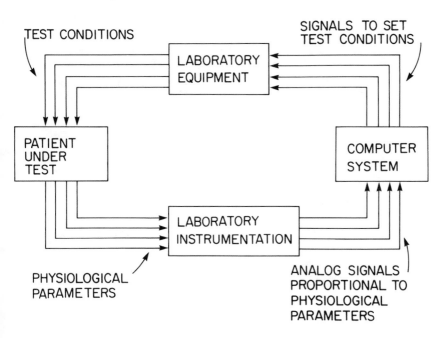

Figure 16-1. Computer in a closed-loop test procedure.

what kind of storage is needed, became much easier to answer. The output should be designed to be readable as well as functional. Because a computer can calculate many values quickly and cheaply, one must evaluate the utility of each result to avoid loading a report with so much data that it is unreadable. Such sensory overload is the most common error of an output format. If many values are needed, they should be divided into several logical report formats, and reiterated as needed. The use of graphics is an excellent way to communicate the relationships among data. An example of this is the flow-volume loop plotted on an absolute volume scale with a corresponding predicted or reference loop.

COMPUTER COMPONENTS

HARDWARE CONFIGURATION

A computer system is composed of several major components that define its hardware configuration. Fig 16-2 shows the interconnection of these components. The input/output (I/O) interfaces allow the computer to communicate with its environment. The interfaces convert the digital signals within the computer to

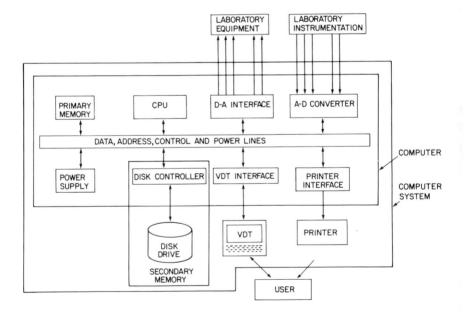

Figure 16-2. Major components of a computer system.

signals that can be utilized by laboratory equipment and computer terminals. Computer terminals are devices that allow the computer user to communicate with the computer. The VDT displays readable characters and graphic representations on a screen. A keyboard or some other mechanism allows the user to enter data. Another type of interface allows signals from laboratory instrumentation to be converted to digital signals within the computer. This type of interface is known as *analog-to-digital converter* (A-D).

Memory is used to store computer instructions and data. The smallest element of memory is the *bit*. A bit can represent a quantity with two possible values such as 0 or 1, on or off, or yes or no. Bits are combined in groups of eight to form *bytes*. Bytes are usually combined in groups of two to form *words*. A 16-bit word can then represent a quantity with 2^{16} or 65,536 possible values. For example, a word can represent an integer in the range $-32,768$ to $+32,767$. *Primary memory,* often referred to as *random-access memory* (RAM), provides very fast access to the values which are stored. Primary memory is usually expensive and limited to several thousand to a million or so bytes per computer system. Secondary memory, encompassing disk and tape subsystems, provides slower access to the values stored but is usually less expensive for a given amount of storage compared to primary memory.

The *central processing unit* (CPU) controls the transfer of data within the computer system, performs arithmetic computations, and performs logic functions. The CPU can, for example, direct the transfer of data from primary memory to secondary memory, from the VDT interface to primary memory, and from the A-D converter to primary memory. The CPU can perform simple arithmetic computations such as addition and subtraction. The CPU logic functions include comparing two values and based on the outcome of the comparison an alternate sequence of instructions can be performed.

The *resolution* of a given A-D converter is determined by the number of bits that are used to represent the voltage that is to be converted. A-D converters typically are either 8, 10, or 12 bits with a corresponding resolution of 1 in 256, 1 in 1024, or 1 in 4096, respectively. The output of the instrument that is being converted should be matched closely to the input of the A-D converter. For example, if a spirometer produces a voltage of 0 to 10 volts to reflect a spirometer volume of 0 to 7 liters, and if the A-D converter was designed to produce a converted value of 0 in response to 0 volts and a value of 255 in response to 10 volts, then the overall resolution would be 0.027 liters in 7 liters. If the instrument output range and the A-D converter input range do not match closely enough, given the desired overall resolution, then a signal conditioner must be used between the instrument and the A-D converter.

The *sampling rate* is the number of A-D conversions done on one signal per unit of time. The sampling rate must be high enough to prevent *aliasing*, which is a phenomenon that causes frequency components of a signal that are higher than one half of the sampling rate to appear as frequencies that are less than one half of the sampling rate. An example of this is that a frequency that is exactly the sampling rate will appear as a DC offset, i.e., a constant rather than rapidly changing signal. Because of aliasing, the sampling rate must be greater than twice the highest frequency component that is present in the signal at the A-D converter input. All frequency components must be considered in the signal—the noise as well as the desired signal. If the sampling rate is limited due to the computer memory that will be storing the converted values or due to the converter itself, then signal conditioning in the form of a low-pass filter must be placed before the A-D input.

SOFTWARE CONFIGURATION

Software controls the hardware in such a way that the computer system performs a useful task. The software ultimately interfaces with the hardware by providing instructions that perform operations. Software can be analyzed as a hierarchy of components. The basic software components are the operating system and the application software. The *operating system* (OS) is a set of instructions that allows the application task and the hardware components to communicate. The OS manages the hardware components so that two or more application tasks can share the computer at the same time. The OS also provides a filing structure that treats the secondard memory devices (disk and tape) as volumes, each volume containing files, and each file containing records. This file structure is analogous to a filing cabinet drawer (volume) which contains file folders (files); each folder, in turn, contains sheets of paper with information (records). The OS often provides software drivers that interface the A-D converters with the application task. This relieves the application task of having to deal with the problems associated with CPU and A-D converter communications. If the driver is not part of the OS, then the application task is responsible for issuing the appropriate instructions to cause the A-D converter and the CPU to work together to sample a signal. The OS is usually provided by the vendor of a computer system; however, special-purpose operating systems are available from third-party vendors.

The application software is the software component that makes the computer system perform a specific task, such as pulmonary function testing or computing the Fourier transform of a time sequence of data. Although the OS needed to support these applications could be the same, the application software will be very different for each task. The application software can be written in assembly language which resembles the hardware instructions. a high-level language such as FORTRAN, BASIC, COBOL, FORTH, or PASCAL is generally easier to program because these languages offer the syntax and data structures that are more closely related to the application. For example, the FORTRAN statement that could be used to correct a PCO_2 reading from a blood-gas analyzer to the patient's temperature is one statement: $PCO_2C = PCO_2M * 10 ** (0.019 *$

DELTAT). The equivalent assembly language statement would be many statements long, and the written code would be less obvious to read. Another advantage of using a high-level language is that the resulting programs can be more easily run on different hardware without being completely rewritten. Assembly language, by comparison, is usually specific to a particular computer type. Application software can be purchased with the hardware or from a vendor other than the hardware vendor or can be written by the user of the computer system. Often a combination of the three is used.

Software components, whether OS or application, must be implemented properly or the computer hardware will fail to perform the tasks accurately and reliably. The implementation should follow these four steps: identification of requirements, design, construction, and operation/maintenance. Verification and testing should be performed at each stage of the implementation. The identification of requirements includes a written description of what the task is to do, the format and units of the input data, what formulae are needed, the accuracy of the computations, and how the user will interact with the computer system. The design includes a description of the principle data structures, algorithms, basic program organization by subdivision into modules, and a description of the hardware components needed. The construction is the actual coding using assembly language or a high-level language to implement the design. If identification of requirements and design have been done carefully, the construction stage is straightforward. The techniques of structured programming greatly simplify this stage and make the code reliable and easy to modify. The operation/maintenance is the actual running of the application, correcting errors that escaped the verification, and testing and modifying the program to adjust to changing user needs and to add extensions to the program as needed.

COMPUTER INTERPRETATIONS

Few have dared to venture far from the original interpretative methods of Hutchinson,[1] who introduced the percent-of-predicted technique for comparing patient data to normals in the mid-1800s. Computer permit rapid solutions of complex equations not known to Hutchinson. These equations were not used until the computer was developed because hand solutions were so tedious and difficult. The current use of computers has taken away much of the tedium and, thus has opened new methods of routine data evaluation which are used widely, except in pulmonary testing interpretations. Lung mechanics lends itself well to automated analysis and multidimensional interpretation. As described by Dawson and Mohler,[2] on-line measurements of vital capacity (VC), inspiratory and expiratory flows can be rapidly and accurately done by computers. These results can be readily evaluated statistically, in considerable depth, very rapidly, and new information not achieved by hand methods is revealed.

STAGES OF DECISION MAKING

The interpretation of laboratory results has three stages leading to a conclusion: (1) statistical; (2) pattern reading; and (3) clinical. The use of computers to do the first stage (statistical) and parts of the second (patterns), is reasonable in developing interpretations of medical information. Computers probably should not be used to perform medical consultations. In general, computers are not programmed to approach diagnosis in the same manner as a clinician (i.e., achieving a clinical impression, and then performing laboratory tests to obtain agreement with the clinical impressions). The computer is unbiased, permitting fast, reliable access to the first and second steps of statistical analysis and pattern reading. The clinician may choose to correct (or be corrected by) the computer's calculations, statistical analyses, and tests for certain patterns, then add or substitute his or her clinical interpretation to the comments selected by the computer.

USE OF STATISTICAL MATRICES

The approach to the first (statistical) step by computer is to calculate the Z and P values; i.e., the numbers relating to SD and statistical significance. These are standard calculations found in any statistical text; the specific approach here is shown in the attached prediction equations (Table 16-2) and the map for

Table 16-2

Prediction Equations	1 SD	Reference #
Males: (Age $\geq$ 18)		
$IVC = .113 \times HT - .032 \times Age - 1.86$	0.50	†
$FVC = 0.148 \times HT - 0.025 - Age - 4.241$	0.74	4
$FEV_1 = .092 \times HT - .032 \times Age - 1.26$	0.55	4
$FEV_3 = .98 \times IVC$ Predicted	$0.06 \times IVC$	
$FEV_1/FVC = FEV_1$ Predicted/FVC Predicted $\times$ 100	8.10	†
$MEFR = .183 \times HT - .0717 \times Age - 1.63$	1.67	†
$MMF = .047 \times HT - .045 \times Age + 2.513$	1.12	4
$FEF_{25} = 3.689 - .039 \times Age$	0.58	5
$FEF_{50} = 7.012 - .033 \times Age$	1.25	5
$FEF_{75} = 8.170 - .009 \times Age$	1.82	5
$MIFR = .238 \times HT - .05 \times Age - 7.7$	1.67	†
$TLC = .239 \times HT - .015 \times Age - 9.167$	0.75	6
$RV = .06858 \times HT + .015 \times Age - 3.447$	0.53	6
$FRC = .129 \times HT - 5.1614$	0.50	6
$MVV = .048 \times HT - .03 \times Age + .7167$	0.444	†
Females: (Age $\geq$ 18)		
$IVC = .1 \times HT - .012 \times Age - 2.8$	0.40	†
$FVC = .115 \times HT - .024 \times Age - 2.852$	0.52	4
$FEV_1 = .089 \times HT - .025 \times Age - 1.932$	0.47	†

Prediction Equations	1 SD	Reference #
$FEV_3 = .98 \times IVC$ Predicted	$0.06 \times IVC$	
$FEV_1/FVC = FEV_1$ Predicted/FVC predicted $\times$ 100	6.40	†
$MEFR = 1158 \times HT - .026 \times$ Age $- 1.23$	1.167	†
$MMF = .06 \times HT - .03 \times$ Age $+ .551$	0.80	4
$FEF_{25} = 2.413 - .022 \times$ Age	0.43	5
$FEF_{50} = 5.059 - .026 \times$ Age	1.00	5
$FEF_{75} = 6.646 - .035 \times$ Age	1.38	5
$MIFR = .7 \times MEFR$ Predicted	1.167	†
$MVV = .019 \times HT - .0093 \times$ Age $+ 1.08$	.038	†
$TLC = .20066 \times HT - .008 \times$ Age $- 7.49$	0.70	6
$RV = .08128 \times HT + .009 \times$ Age $- 3.9$	0.40	6
$FRC = .11938 \times HT - 4.853$	0.40	6
Males: (Age < 18)		
$IVC = 4.4 \times 10^{-6} \times HT \ (cm)^{2.6727}$	13.0%	
FVC use IVC		
$FEV_1 = .86 \times IVC$ Predicted	10.0%	7
$FEV_1/FVC = 86$	.7	7
$MEFR = .188 \times HT - 6.83$	$.05 \times HT - 2.03$	‡
$MMF = .0447 \times HT - .067$	$.022 \times HT - .55$	‡
$MIFR = .06 \times HT \ (cm) - 5.26$	23.0%	7
$MVV = .054 \times HT - 1.67$	21.0%	7
$TLC = 5.6 \times 10^{-6} \times HT \ (cm)^{2.6691}$	11.6%	7
$RV = 4.41 \times 10^{-6} \times HT \ (cm)^{2.4101}$	22.8%	7
$FRC = 7.5 \times 10^{-7} \times HT \ (cm)^{2.9173}$	18.8%	7
Females: (Age < 18)		
$IVC = 3.3 \times 10^{-6} \times HT \ (cm)^{2.7294}$	13.0%	7
FVC use IVC		
$FEV_1 = .86 \times IVC$ Predicted	10.0%	7
$FEV_1/FVC = 86$	7	7
$MEFR = .154 \times HT - 5.15$	$.054 \times HT - 2.15$	‡
$MMF = .055 \times HT - .367$	$.032 \times HT - .67$	‡
$MIFR = .06 \times HT \ (cm) - 5.26$	23.0%	7
$MVV = .054 \times HT - 1.67$	21.0%	7
$TLC = 4 \times 10^{-6} \times HT \ (cm)^{2.7302}$	11.6%	7
$RV = 4.41 \times 10^{-6} \times HT \ (cm)^{2.4101}$	22.8%	7
$FRC = 1.78 \times 10^{-6} \times HT \ (cm)^{2.795}$	18.8%	7

The above volumes are in liters, the flows in liter/sec. Age is in years. Height is inches unless noted by (cm), which indicates centimeters. SDs are absolute unless indicated as % of mean predicted.

† Armstrong, BW: Data collected during Veteran's Administration study. Unpublished.

‡ Wiseman, D.: Personal communication. Jan. 1977.

spirometric and lung volume interpretations (Table 16-3). VC and inspiratory and expiratory flow are single-tailed tests; that is, such values are abnormal only if they are below the mean of the referent value by some measure. The 95% confidence band for these variables is $Z = -1.64$, and the 99% band is $Z = -2.3$. Thus, if the VC and flows of a particular patient are below the referent mean, but within the 95% confidence band, the patient data cannot be rejected as belonging to the data of a healthy population on statistical grounds. If, however, the pattern of the variations in the data or the clinical information supports

Table 16-3　Map for Spirometric and Lung Volume Interpretations

Definitions: I: Prefix for integer number. The expression on the right of the equal sign is evaluated and all decimal digits truncated. Do not round off; P: Prefix for predicted value; SD: Prefix for standard deviation; Z: Prefix for Z score; E: Suffix for estimated value.

EQUATIONS

1. $Z\,VC = (P\,VC - VC)/SD\,VC$
2. $Z\,MBC = (P\,MBC - MBC)/SD\,MBC$
3. $I\,VC = Z\,VC + 1$ (Truncated)
4. $I\,MBC = Z\,MBC + 1$ (Truncated)
5. $Z\,TLC = (TLC - P\,TLC)/.7$
6. $Z\,RV = (RV - P\,RV)/SDVC$
7. $Z\,MMF = (P\,MMF - MMF)/SD\,MMF$
8. $I\,MMF = Z\,MMF + 1$ (Truncated)
9. $MBC\,E = (MEFR \cdot MIFR)/(MEFR + MIFR)$
10. Airways resistance is about equal to $P\,MBC/MBC$
11. Lost volume $= P\,VC - VC$ or $P\,TLC - TLC$ taken to the nearest half liter

SDs

	SD VC	SD MBC	SD MMF
1. Boys (less than 18 years)	13%	21% of mean predicted	12.8% of mean predicted
2. Girls (less than 18 years)	13%	21% of mean predicted	12.8% of mean predicted
3. Men	.50	26.6	67.2
4. Women	.40	23.0	48.0

Age Correction: $SD = SD \times (1.5 - (Age \times 0.01))$
(Adults Only)

QUALITATIVE MODIFIERS

Spirometry	Lung Volume
Z Value $= 0-1$ blank (if needed, use slightly)	If $Z\,RV$ or $Z\,TLC$ is positive, use increase
1−3 moderate or moderately	If $Z\,RV$ or $Z\,TLC$ is negative, use decrease
4−5 marked or markedly	Z Value $= / 1 /$　slightly or slight
6　severe or severely	$/ 2 / - / 3 /$ moderately or moderate
	$/ 4 / - / 5 /$ markedly or marked
	$/ 6 /$　severely or severe

another interpretation, then the latter supercedes the former. The final and clinical level of judgement is assisted by computers but done by physicians, who must have the final word regarding the clinical interpretation.

Total Lung Capacity (TLC) and Residual Volume (RV) may be increased or decreased with disease, especially the TLC. However, a particular disease should change TLC in only one direction. TLC is commonly increased in emphysema, for example, and is decreased in fibrosis. Thus, these tests are also one tailed, and the Z values for confidence bands are the same as noted for VC, except positive or negative. The computer can easily calculate probabilities and develop analyses in three, four, or more dimensions. An example of three-dimensional lung mechanics, flow-volume pressure, is shown by the three-dimensional lung model of Fry et al.[3] Similar abstractions in multidimension are possible for intrepretation as well, with the limitation that these dimensions are still statistical and not clinical. The final stage, the clinical information, is best layered into the final interpretation by the clinician. Table 16-4 is a map of the four-quadrant matrix for lung volumes (Table 16-4) and Table 16-5 is a map for the two-quadrant matrix for FVC and flow.

The calculation for Z, TLC, and P, RV, is shown in Table 16-3. In each cell in Table 16-6 is an index to the sentence library, which is the statistical interpretation. One may of course, chose one's own prose. The problem is greater with spirometry alone because one must distinguish between obstructed airway disease, unobstructed diseases, and those that show no apparent problem. We use one of the four criteria (Table 16-5) shown to select the second, the obstructed matrix; all others default to the first unobstructed matrix. Because VC and flow are abnormal only below the mean, the Z value is calculated as positive for convenience. The I (integer) value is calculated by adding one and truncating all the decimal places of the Z value (interger values are not rounded off). The I (VC) and the I (Flow) are then used in the selected matrix to read the pointers to the library of sentences. Finally, certain tests, as shown, are used to modify the resultant interpretation, based on modifier words and sentences (Table 16-5).

Qualitative modifiers are arbitrarily selected but based upon several years of use in our laboratory. In our experience, about 20% of these statistical interpretations are changed during review by a physician, chiefly changing the use of these modifiers. As is evident in other chapters of this text, the criteria for the use of selected modifiers such as mild, moderate, and severe can be improved.

EXAMPLES

CASE 1

A 68-year-old, white woman underwent routine screening spirometry in a public screening program. She was active and apparently asymptomatic. She

Table 16-4 Lung Volume Matrix

Cells are grouped into four matrix fields. Each cell is identified by two integers, positive or negative. Calculate the Z value to one decimal place. Any number in the first decimal moves the reading to the next cell in sequence reading from the middle. 1.2 is in cell 2; −1.2 is in cell −2. Similarly 2.9 is in cell 3 and −2.9 is in cell −3. The numbers within the cells refer to statements (Table 16-5) to be utilized on the report.

Field Requirements

	TLC	RV
I	+	+
II	+	−
III	−	−
IV	−	+

Top labels: −TLC (left), IV, I, +TLC (right)

RV	−6	−5	−4	−3	−2	−1	+1	+2	+3	+4	+5	+6
+6 top	1 8 3	1 8 3	1 8 3	1 8 4	1 8 4	2 8	2 8	1 7	1 7	1 7	1 7	1 6
+6 bot	16 17	16 17	16 17	16 17	16 17	15	15	11	11	11	15	15
+5 top	1 8	1 8	1 8	1 8	1 8	2 8	2 8	1 8	1 7	1 7	1 6	1 8
+5 bot	16 17	16 17	16 17	16 17	16	15	15	11	11	11	15	15
+4 top	1 8	1 8	1 8 4	1 8 4	1 8	2 8	2 8	1 7	1 7	1 6	1 8	1 9
+4 bot	16 17	16 17	9 17	9 17	9		15	11	11	15	15	15
+3 top	1 8	1 8	1 8	1 8	1 8	2 8	2 8	1 7	1 6	1 8	1 8	1 8
+3 bot	16 17	16	4 9	4 9	9		11	11	15	15	15	15
+2 top	1 8	1 8	1 8	1 8	1 8	2 8	2 8	1 6	1 8	1 8	1 8	1 8
+2 bot	16 17	3 12	3 12	4	14	14	11	15	15	15	15	15
+1 top	1 5	1 5	1 5	1 5	1 5	2 5	2 5	1 5	1 5	1 5	1 5	1 5
+1 bot	3 12	3 12	3 12	4 12	14	14	13	14	14		14 17	14 17
−1 top	1 5	1 5	1 5	1 5	1 5	2 5	2 5	1 5	1 5	1 5	1 5	1 5
−1 bot	3 12	3 12	3 12	4 12	14	13	14	14	14	14	14 17	14 17
−2 top	1 8	1 8	1 8	1 8	1 6	2 8	2 8	1 8	1 8	1 8	1 8	1 8
−2 bot	3 9	3 9	3 9	4 9	14	4 14	14	14	14	14	14	14 17
−3 top	1 8	1 8	1 8	1 6	1 7	2 7	2 8	1 8	1 8	1 8	1 8	1 8
−3 bot	12	12	3 9	4 9	9	4 12	14	14	16 17	16 17	16 17	16 17
−4 top	1 8	1 8	1 6	1 7	1 7	2 7	2 8	1 8	1 8	1 8	1 8	1 8
−4 bot	12 17	12 9	3 9	4 9	3	4	16 17	16	16 17	16 17	16 17	16 17
−5 top	1 8	1 6	1 7	1 7	1 7	2 7	2 8	1 8	1 8	1 8	1 8	1 8
−5 bot	9 17	9 17	3 9	4 9	3	4	16 17	16 17	17	16 17	16 17	16 17
−6 top	1 6	1 7	1 7	1 7	1 7	2 7	2 8	1 8	1 8	1 8	1 8	1 8
−6 bot	9 17	9 17	3 17	4 9	3	4	16 17	16 17	16 17	16 17	16 17	16 17

Bottom column labels: −6 −5 −4 −3 −2 −1 +1 +2 +3 +4 +5 +6

Bottom field labels: −TLC (left), III, II, +TLC (right)

Left/right margin RV labels: +RV (top), −RV (bottom)

I VC

I MBC	1	2	3	4	5	6
1	18	22	22	22	22	22
2	19	23	26	26	26	22
3	19	27	23	26	26	26
4	19	27	27	27	27	29
5	19,17	27	27	27	29	29
6	19,17	19,17	27	29	29	29

I VC

I MBC	1	2	3	4	5	6
1	33	33	21	21	21,17	21,17
2	20	24	24	24	21	21,17
3	20	30	28	32	32	32,17
4	31	25	28	28	30	32
5	31	25	28	28	28	29
6	31	28	28	28	29	29

Figure 16-3. Requirements for Spirometry Matrices: If any of the following statements are true, use matrix two, otherwise use matrix one. The numbers within the matrices refer to statements to be utilized on the report. (1) MEFR/MIFR less than 0.7; (2) MEFR/MIFR less than 1.0 and FEV_1/FVC greater than 1 SD from mean normal ratio; (3) $FEV_1/$ FVC greater than 1.7 SD from mean normal ratio; (4) If I MEFR is 3 or more and the I MIFR is 3 or more; (5) If I MMF is 3 or more. **A:** Matrix 1; **B:** Matrix 2.

Table 16-5 (continued)   TLC Statements

1. The total ventilable lung volume is (increased, decreased) about (lost volume) L.
2. The total ventilable lung volume is about the mean value of a comparative population.
3. This loss of total ventilable lung volume most commonly results from (adj) (I TLC) diffuse fibrosing alveolitis, pleural thickening with retraction, parenchymal replacement, or crowding due to mass lesions.
4. This loss of total ventilable lung volume is commonly associated with early or slight loss of parenchyma, or pulmonary circulatory plethora.

RV STATEMENTS

5. However, the RV is not significantly different than the mean value of a comparative population.
6. However, the RV is (increased, decreased) commensurately.
7. However, the RV is (increased, decreased) relatively more than the TLC.
8. However, the RV is (adj) (I RV) (increased, decreased).

HENCE

9. Hence, the observed parenchymal volume loss is most commonly due to surgery, destructive or constrictive lesions of the parenchyma or pleura, or combinations of these. Pulmonary compliance determinations would be helpful for further differentiation.
10. Hence, the increase of parenchymal volume almost surely is due to diffuse destructive diseases of the pulmonary parenchyma producing an increased pulmonary compliance.
11. Hence, the VC has been (adj) (I RV) reduced due to compensatory mechanisms commonly seen in parenchymal destructive diseases and obstruction to airflow in the major airway or both.
12. Hence, the ratio of RV/TLC does not confirm obstruction to air flow due to airways disease. Because a normal thoracic wall may preserve the RV with advancing parenchymal contraction due to fibrosis, airways disease must be demonstrated by other confirming tests, if suspected.
13. Thus, evidence of structural changes in the lung parenchyma is not seen.
14. These lung volume findings may represent a normal variation in the distribution of volume compartments or may suggest early changes of the parenchyma, airways, or both.
15. These findings suggest parenchymal destruction as seen in emphysema which can be further described by an increased pulmonary compliance.
16. The mechanism for this change is obscure but arterial O_2 transfer may be impaired.

MATRIX SENTENCES

17. This is an unusual combination of values.
    Results confirmed: PPT _____ Date _____
18. There is no evidence of ventilatory insufficiency.
19. This patient has (adj) (Z MBC) reduced flows, but the VC compares favorably with a normal population. As physiological evidence for tracheobronchial airways disease is not evident, diseases of the parenchyma or of the small airways or of neuromuscular origin or poor effort or combinations of these must be present.
20. There is no evident loss of ventilable lung volume, but the flows are moderately impaired. The shape of the tracings suggests that these findings are due to moderate obstructive pulmonary disease.
21. This patient has lost (lost volume) L of ventilable lung volume, which is much greater than might be expected for this limited evidence of obstructive bronchopulmonary disease. It is not possible from these tracings to completely evaluate the obstructive component. If indicated, further tests may help clarify the functional state.

22. This patient has lost (lost volume) L of ventilable lung volume. Because flows compare favorably with a normal population, this loss may be a normal variant or may be due to diffuse interstitial disease, parenchymal replacement or loss.

23. This patient has lost about (lost volume) L of ventilable lung volume, and the flows are reduced commensurately. The shape of the tracings suggests that these findings are due to diffuse interstitial disease or parenchymal replacement rather than obstructive bronchopulmonary disease.

24. This patient has lost about (lost volume) L of ventilable lung volume. This may account for the moderate reduction of flows, but the shape of the tracings suggests that there is moderate obstructive disease.

25. This patient has lost about (lost volume) L of ventilable lung volume. More important, there seems to be definite evidence of moderate to severe obstructive bronchopulmonary disease as shown by the shape of the tracings and the flows, which are reduced relatively more than the VC.

26. This patient has lost about (lost volume) L of ventilable lung volume. Because the shape of the tracings does not suggest obstructive bronchopulmonary disease, the moderately impaired flows almost surely are due to loss of ventilable lung volume.

27. This patient has lost about (lost volume) L of ventilable lung volume. The shape of the tracings suggests that diffuse interstitial disease or parenchymal replacement rather than obstructive disease probably accounts for the (adj) (Z MBC) subnormal flows.

28. This patient has lost about (lost volume) L of ventilable lung volume. More important, there is (adj) (Z MBC) reduction of flows which is probably due to obstructive bronchopulmonary disease. Hence, the observed reduction of VC is almost surely secondary to the increased RV.

29. This patient has severe ventilatory insufficiency.

30. This patient has lost about (lost volume) L of VC and the flows are (adj) (Z MBC) impaired. The shape of the tracings suggests that these findings are due to moderate to severe obstructive bronchopulmonary disease.

31. There is no evident loss of ventilable lung volume, but the flows are (adj) (Z MBC) impaired. The shape of the tracings suggests that these findings are due to moderately severe obstructive airway disease.

32. This patient has lost about (lost volume) L of VC. This may account for some of the reduction of the flows, but the shape of the tracings suggests that there is marked obstructive bronchopulmonary disease present.

33. The VC and flows compare favorably with a normal population. However, the shape of the tracings suggests that this patient may have obstructive bronchopulmonary disease.

OTHER SENTENCES IF APPLICABLE

Diagnostics

D-1. The low MBC value is due to submaximal effort and should be ignored. A more meaningful value of (MBC E) is estimated from the MEFR and MIFR. (This statement is used if I MBC is less using the MBC E instead of the measured MBC.)

D-2. Note: the VC is reduced relatively more than the flows. Conditions other than obstructive bronchopulmonary disease may account for some of the loss of ventilable lung volume. (This statement is written when statement 24 or 32 of matrix two is used: I VC is greater than I MBC.)

D-3. There is some evidence that terminal airflow may be impaired, suggesting disease of the small airways. Further evaluation of closing volumes or gas exchange (alveolar-arterial oxygen difference) is indicated. (Statement made if I MMF greater than 1 SD and only following spirometry sentences of matrix One or sentences in matrix Two when I MBC = 1, and I VC = 2, 3 or 4.)

Table 16-5   TLC Statements

Bronchodilator Notes

B-1.   None of this patient's spirometric values increased appreciably after giving nebulized bronchodilator.

B-2.   The following measurements increased appreciably after giving nebulized bronchodilator—(measurement list).

Upper Airways Disease Sentences (Matrix One Only)

U-1.   Assuming optimum test performance, there is (Z MBC) (adj) evidence that obstruction to inspiratory airflow is present. Evaluation for diseases of the thoracic inlet is indicated. (This statement used if 1.5 < MEFR/MIFR < 1.8 and MEFR > −1.5 SD)

U-2.   The observed reduction in inspiratory flow and the necessarily accompanying loss of exercise tolerance are almost surely due to obstruction to airflow in the thoracic inlet. Direct visualization of the upper airways is indicated. (This statement used if MEFR/MIFR > 1.8 and MEFR > −1.5 SD)

Reversible Airways Disease

R-1.   An improvement of one half a SD of the population confirms the impression of reversible airways obstructive disease. (Use Matrix Two if MEFR or FEV_1 or MBC impaired one half SD or more).

R-2.   Reversible obstruction to inspiratory and expiratory airflow is confirmed. These findings that suggest parenchymal loss are also compatible with asthma, bronchitis, or some stages of pulmonary congestion and congestive heart failure. (Use Matrix One after sentences 23 and 27 and if MEFR and MIFR increase by one half SD or more or if MBC increases by one half SD or more.)

For Fair Patient Performance

Note: The above interpretation must be tempered by the less than optimal performance of this patient in doing the tests.

For Poor Patient Performance

This patient either could not, or would not, perform the tests such that values for vital capacity and flows could be accurately determined.

smoked cigarettes, one pack per day for 40 years. She reported a minimal morning cough. Her test results are shown in Table 16-6.

Using Hutchinson's percent of predicted approach, the FVC is 83% of predicted, the $FEV_{1.0}$ sec is 77%, and the maximum voluntary ventilation (MVV) is 60%. From this one would conclude that this patient has significant obstructive airways disease. When analyzed statistically, the Z value for FVC is −0.96, well within the 95% confidence band of Z = −1.64. The Z for $FEV_{1.0}$ sec is (1.7–2.2/0.47) −1.06. The Z for MVV is −1.7. The $FEV_{1.0}$ sec is also within the 95% band. Only the MVV is outside the normal limits. The pattern of flows and volumes, and the clinical history of 40-pack years of cigarette smoking cause one to favor an interpretation of chronic obstructive pulmonary disease (COPD), but this patient has no exertional dyspnea and a minimal cough. The percent-of-predicted method would have this patient clearly obstructed, but the statistical method is much less convincing for the obstruction and is in better agreement with the clinical state of the patient.

Table 16-6 Case 1

Test	Observed Value	Referent Value (White)	± SEE
Inspiratory VC	2.7	3.0	0.4 liter
Forced VC	2.5	3.0	0.52 liter
$FEF_{(200-1200)}$	160	260	100 liter/min
$FEF_{(25-75\%)}$	80	135	48 liter/min
$FEV_{1.0}$ sec	1.7	2.2	0.47 liter
FEV_1/FVC	68	73	6.4 %
$FEV_{3.0}$ sec	2.4	2.8	0.5 liter
$FIF_{(25-75\%)}$	170	185	70 liter/min
MVV	60	100	23 liter/min

CASE 2

A 40-year-old, black male was studied repeatedly by many physicians for a denied disability claim. He was a heavy manual laborer (hod carrier) who reported marked exertional dyspnea during climbing of stairs and ladders. He had no cough and did not smoke. Test results are shown in Table 16-7.

Because he was a large, muscular man and his chest X ray was clear, the patient was repeatedly denied disability. His spirometric values were 118% of predicted for VC and the effort-dependent flows seemed to confirm the clinical impression of health. His complaint of dyspnea was never challenged with exercise testing. When viewed statistically, the Z for FVC is clearly well within the 95% band. The Z for $FEV_{1.0}$ sec is 0.5, also within the 95% limit. In addition, the Z for his TLC is +1.7, above the 95% band. The pattern of airway

Table 16-7 Case 2

Test	Observed Value	Referent Value (Black)	± SEE
Inspiratory VC	5.2	4.4	0.5 liter
Forced VC	4.9	4.4	0.7 liter
$FEF_{(200-1200)}$	410	540	100 liter/min
$FEF_{(25-75\%)}$	205	255	67 liter/min
$FEV_{1.0}$ sec	3.2	3.5	0.55 liter
$FEV_{3.0}$ sec	3.8	4.2	0.55 liter
$FIF_{(25-75\%)}$	460	475	100 liter/min
MVV	100	184	27 liter/min
FEV_1/FVC	65	79	8.1 %
TLC	9.2	7.9	0.75 liter
RV	4.0	2.2	0.5 liter

obstruction is confirmed by the FEV_1/FVC ratio of 65%, beyond the 95% limit, $(FEF_{(200-1200)}/FIF_{(25-75\%)}$ of 0.67 (below the 0.7 seen in early to moderate airways obstruction), and an RV/TLC ratio of 49%. These data now support the patient's clinical complaints of airways disease. Exercise testing supported his complaint of inappropriate dyspnea and his disability was granted.

REFERENCES

1. Hutchinson J: On the capacity of the lungs, and on the respiratory functions, with a view of detecting disease by a spirometer. Med Clin Trans 2(11):137–252, 1846.
2. Dawson A, Mohler JG: Microprocessor-assisted spirometry, in J Clausen (ed): Pulmonary Function Testing: Guidelines and Controversies. New York, Academic Press, 1982.
3. Fry DL, Ebert RV, Stead WW, et al.: The mechanics of pulmonary ventilation in normal subjects and in patients with emphysema. Ann J Med 16:87, 1954.
4. Goldman HI, Becklake MR: Respiratory function tests: Normal values at medium altitudes of the prediction of normal results. Am Rev Tuberc 79, 1959.
5. Morris J, Koski A, Johnson LC: Spirometric standards for healthy nonsmoking adults. Am Rev Respir Dis 103, 1971. Polgar G, Promhdhat V: Pulmonary Function Testing in Children. 1971.
6. Kory RC: The Veterans Administration Army, cooperative study of pulmonary function I. Am J Med 30, 1961.
7. Black LF, Offord K, Hyatt RE: Variability in the maximal expiratory flow curve in asymptomatic smokers and in nonsmokers. Am Rev Respir Dis 110, 1974.

CHAPTER 17

Pulmonary Function Testing in Pediatric Patients

ARNOLD C. G. PLATZKER
THOMAS G. KEENS

In the child younger than 7 years old, it is usually not feasible to obtain comprehensive pulmonary function tests in the adult-oriented laboratory. The reliability of pulmonary function tests in childhood, especially in the younger groups, are suspect, because the measurements are fraught with poor patient cooperation and difficulty in obtaining reproducible results. Children younger than 6 years old are usually unable to inspire to total lung capacity (TLC), exhale to residual volume (RV), or produce maximal inspiratory effort on request.[1] These problems are compounded by a general lack of pulmonary function equipment miniaturized to the patient. Implicit in normal pulmonary function test data in childhood (most prominent in the younger age groups) is the broad distribution of values around the mean for each test. Thus, expressing pediatric values as a percentage of the mean is less revealing than comparing the patient's performance with respect to the 95% confidence limits, for an age-matched control population. It is for this reason that it is advisable for each laboratory to develop its own normal values using its own equipment, even though normal pediatric pulmonary function data are available for most tests that are commonly performed.[2-9]

In order to achieve reasonable success in obtaining pulmonary function tests in children, factors that are usually not important in testing the adult patient must be considered. These include the technician/nurse staff, the pulmonary function equipment, and the laboratory facilities (e.g. the laboratory reception area, dressing area, procedure area, pulmonary function testing cubicles, and toilet facilities). Because children are fearful of the unknown, they need an informative, reassuring, but honest introduction to the pulmonary laboratory. The technician who will perform the study should take the child and the parents on a tour of the laboratory and explain, in language that even the smallest child can understand, the tests that are conducted in each area of the laboratory. In effect, the technician will be quieting the parent's fears as well as those of the patient. It is advisable to work with the pre-teen and the parent as a unit. For the teenager, the approach must be individualized. A teenager may or may not wish to have a parent in attendance during the tour and during the tests, especially if arterial blood is to be drawn.

The laboratory must be designed carefully so that the patient will not be overwhelmed by a noisy laboratory and an overpowering amount of equipment. One solution to this problem is to carpet the floor and to arrange the laboratory in specialized testing areas, separated with moveable sound-conditioning partitions. The ceiling of the laboratory should also be covered by sound-conditioning tiles. Areas that are partitioned by moveable dividers are better than individual rooms or cubicles, because they give the laboratory an open feeling and the size of each area can be modified by rearranging the partitions. Separate areas may be utilized for (1) spirometry, dilutional lung volumes, and diffusion capacity; (2) body plethysmography; (3) exercise; (4) special procedures (e.g. arterial puncture and cannulation, respiratory muscle strength); and (5) blood-gas analysis. A sleep laboratory requires a separate, sound-proofed suite with one study room and an adjoining second control room (a large one-way mirror between the rooms permits continual observation of the patient during the study); the recording equipment is located in the second room.

Prior to the scheduled appointment, the physician and technician should review the request for pulmonary function studies, review the accompanying history and physical findings, and then define the pulmonary function tests desired. This plan may have to be modified or revised at the clinic after the patient is examined by the pulmonologist and the child's capacity to cooperate and his or her mental and physical limitations are defined. In the initial pulmonary function session with the younger or handicapped child, it may only be possible to introduce the mouthpiece and noseclip used in the studies and begin to train the child to perform the pulmonary function maneuvers. Frequently, it is advisable to send the patient home with a mouthpiece and to reschedule the desired study at a later date. The parent is instructed in the use of the mouthpiece and is asked to work with the child on its use for at least ten minutes, twice daily prior to the scheduled study.

INDICATIONS FOR PERFORMING PULMONARY FUNCTION TESTS IN CHILDREN

The major clinical indications for performing pulmonary function tests are as follows.

1. *To define the type and severity of and determine the magnitude of the physiologic abnormality.* Though pulmonary function tests are not diagnostic for a specific disorder, they define whether the functional impairment is consistent with clinical diagnosis.

2. *To monitor the course of lung function impairment.* In pediatric patients, pulmonary function tests often provide more sensitive, objective, and quantitative information concerning changes in lung function than patient history, physical examination, and chest roentgenograms.

3. *To determine the effectiveness of therapy.* Pulmonary function tests are particularly helpful in determining the acute and long-term effectiveness of aerosol bronchodilator therapy in airway obstructive disease, steroids or antimetabolites in interstitial lung disease, and methylxanthines in respiratory control disorders, because they are objective and quantifiable measures of lung function.

4. *To assist both in the preoperative planning of general anesthesia and in anticipating the need for postoperative O_2 and/or assisted ventilation.* Preoperative pulmonary function evaluation is particularly important in patients with chest wall deformities such as scoliosis, collagen vascular disorders, sickle cell disease, neuromuscular disorders, and in infants with a history of neonatal respiratory problems, especially those who were premature and were treated with O_2 or assisted ventilation.

METHODOLOGY

SELECTION OF PULMONARY FUNCTION TESTS

Unless a specific physiologic abnormality has already been documented by previous pulmonary function studies or suggested by history, physical findings, and other studies, the child is studied to characterize: (1) lung volumes, (2) lung mechanics (maximal air flow and airways resistance), (3) distribution of ventilation, and (4) gas exchange.

Further studies, such as provocation tests (e.g., aerosol bronchodilators, histamine or methacholine aerosols, or exercise), ventilatory response to exercise, and respiratory muscle strength may also be indicated as discussed later.

Studies of ventilatory control are generally reserved for infants and children with a history of documented or suspected apnea, a newborn infant with a sibling who died of sudden infant death syndrome, or an infant or child with or without upper airway obstruction who is thought to have an irregular respiratory pattern during sleep.

Lung volumes

Although measurement of lung volumes requires cooperation of the patient and thus is not often feasible in children younger than 6 years of age, there are methods that permit the measurement of lung volumes in even the newborn period. The methods used are body plethysmography,[10-12] nasal pneumotachyography[13] (because infants less than 6 months old are obligate nasal breathers), or respiratory induction plethysmography.[14-15] These methods are impracticable for use in the general pulmonary function laboratory due to the cost of the equipment and the bioengineering and pediatric support personnel required to perform these studies.

Spirometry. Spirometry is performed with the child in a seated position; the torso must be erect. The patient should use nose clips and the patient must be closely observed to assure that there is no leak around the mouthpiece. The use of a wedge, rolling-seal, or water-filled spirometer is preferable to a pneumotachygraph for the measurement of lung volumes. The results should be recorded and measured on a polygraph or other graphic device rather than having the calculation results only presented on the digital display of the spirometer.[16] The best of at least three efforts is used; in children less than 10–12 years old, more than three trials may be required to obtain the child's best possible effort. Both the slow and forced VC maneuvers should be performed. The standard regression equations (for each test) for children and the reference for each test is found in the Table 17-1.

Derived lung volume. Functional residual capacity (FRC) can be measured by the helium dilution (single-breath or steady-state), nitrogen wash-out, or body plethysmographic methods.[2] However, body plethysmography is the method of choice for both procedural and technical reasons. The young child has a short attention span and, when breathing through a mouthpiece, may have a rapid respiratory rate while tending to have a breath-by-breath change in the FRC. Thus, with the gas dilution methods, it is difficult to catch the patient at the end-tidal respiratory point for measurement of FRC. With the rapid, electrically activated, mouth shutter used in plethysmography, it is possible to obtain the measurement of thoracic gas volume (TGV) at FRC. It is also possible to repeat this measurement until a *consistent minimal value* for the patient is determined. In the child with a very short attention span it may be essential to perform spirometry as well as TGV in the plethysmograph. Spirometry in the plethysmograph is obtained either by integration of the mouth-shutter pneumotachygraph signal or by connecting the mouthpiece to a wedge or rolling-seal spirometer.

Table 17-1

Pediatric Pulmonary Function Studies
TABLE OF SUMMARY EQUATIONS

STUDY	SUMMARY REGRESSION EQUATION	%SD	REFERENCES
LUNG VOLUMES			
VC (Boys)	log VC(ml) = -2.3554 + 2.6727 x log Ht.(cm)	13	2 (p. 100)
VC (Girls)	log VC(ml) = -2.4756 + 2.7194 x log Ht.(cm)	13	2
FRC (Boys)	log FRC(ml) = -3.1274 + 2.9173 x log Ht.(cm)	18	2 (p. 109)
FRC (Girls)	log FRC(ml) = -2.8622 + 2.795 x log Ht.(cm)	18	2
RV (Boys & Girls)	log RV(ml) = -2.355 x 2.4101 x log Ht.(cm)	22.8	2 (p. 123)
ERV (Boys)	ERV = FRC (Boys) - RV	22.8	2 (p. 123)
ERV (Girls)	ERV = FRC (Girls) - RV	22.8	2 (p. 123)
IC (Boys)	IC = VC (Boys) - ERV (Boys)	22.8	2 (p. 123)
IC (Girls)	IC = VC (Girls) - ERV (Girls)	22.8	2 (p. 123)
TLC (Boys)	log TLC(ml) = -2.2469 + 2.6691 x log Ht.(cm)	11.6	2 (p. 131)
TLC (Girls)	log TLC(ml) = -2.388 + 2.7302 x log Ht.(cm)	11.6	2 (p. 131)
%RV/TLC (Boys)	%RV/TLC = 100 x RV(ml)/TLC (Boys)(ml)	22.8	2 (p. 131)
%RV/TLC (Girls)	%RV/TLC = 100 x RV(ml)/TLC (Girls)(ml)	22.8	2 (p. 131)
LUNG MECHANICS			
FEV1.0 (Boys & Girls)	log FEV1.0(ml) = 2.6781 + 2.7986 x log Ht.(cm)	8.8	2 (p. 130)
FEV1.0/VC (Boys)	%FEV1.0/VC = 100 x FEV1.0(ml)/VC (Boys)(ml)		
FEV1.0/VC (Girls)	%FEV1.0/VC = 100 x FEV1.0(ml)/VC (Girls)(ml)		
PEFR (Boys & Girls)	PEFR (L/min) = -425.5714 + 5.2428 x Ht.(cm)	13	2 (p. 183)
MIFR (Boys & Girls)	MIFR (L/min) = -349 + 3.8 x Ht.(cm)	23	2 (p. 211)
MMEFR (Boys & Girls)	MMEFR (L/min) = -207.7 + 2.62 x Ht.(cm)	32	2 (p. 211)
Vmax 60% TLC			
(Boys & Girls)	0.86	0.25	25
Vmax 70% TLC			
(Boys & Girls)	1.10	0.26	25
Vmax 80% TLC			
(Boys and Girls)	1.29	0.25	25
MVV (Boys & Girls)	MVV (L/min) = -99.507 + 1.276 x Ht.(cm)	21	2 (p. 153)
RAW (Boys & Girls)	Average of:	28	
	RAW(cm H20/L/sec) = 1/(-.3819 + .00472 x Ht.(cm))		17
	RAW(cm H20/L/sec) = 16.936 - 0.089 x Ht.(cm)		18
CL (Boys & Girls)	Average of:	26	
	log CL(ml/cm H2O) = 2.78 + 2.18 x log Ht.(cm)		19
	log CL(ml/cm H2O) = 4.61 + 3.03 x log Ht.(cm)		20
	log CL(ml/cm H2O) = -4.47 + 2.951 x log Ht.(cm)		21
DISTRIBUTION OF VENTILATION			
CV*			
(Boys & Girls) (L)	pred CV/VC x pred CV		24
CV/VC			
(Boys & Girls)(%)	-1.25 Age-26.12 (if Age = 17 or over)		24
CC/TLC			
(Boys & Girls)(%)	(pred CV - pred RV)/pred TLC		24
40 breath N2			
(Boys & Girls)(%)	1.5		2 (p. 55)
GAS EXCHANGE			
Single Breath DLCO(SB)			
(Boys & Girls)	log DLCO(ml/min/mmHg) = 0.308 + 0.00656 x Ht.(cm)	17.6	22
Steady State DLCO(SS)			
(Boys & Girls)	DLCO(ml/min/mmHg) = 19.075 Ht.(cm) - 1332.8	19.3	23
DLCO/VA	DLCO/L = 5.50	1.5	CHLA data

*CV also known as phase IV
Age = age in years

The lung mechanics, e.g., maximal air flow and airways resistance (R_{AW}), are also measured. If the child is fearful of being confined alone in the plethysmograph, the study can be performed with the child seated in the plethysmograph on a parent's lap. In this instance, the parent is instructed not to close his or her glottis when the patient is performing the TGV or R_{AW} maneuver, but can continue to breathe in and out slowly without affecting the measurement.

FRC by the helium dilution method is less reliable because it requires more patient cooperation to perform the test and does not measure poorly ventilated or nonventilated lung compartments. When the FRC from the helium dilution method is compared with the TGV, it provides a rough index of the volume of trapped gas. The TGV must exceed the FRC (HE) by more than 400 ml to be interpreted as significant gas trapping. In children, FRC (HE) often exceeds TGV, indicating failure of the child to maintain a tight seal around the mouthpiece.

Lung volume measurement provides a useful guideline for planning postoperative care. In a child who will undergo a major surgical procedure, e.g., scoliosis, pectus excavatum repair, major upper abdominal, or chest surgery, inspiratory capacity (IC) might fall as much as 50–70% in the postoperative period. The patient with a postoperative IC of significantly greater than 15 ml/kg will probably not require assisted ventilation. Thus, a preoperative IC of 30 ml/ kg may be required (as long as other parameters of lung function are within normal limits) to provide assurance that the child will not have the need of assisted ventilation following surgery. However, in major cardiothoracic surgical procedures in children, the FVC has been reduced by 60% for as long as four days following surgery.

Lung Mechanics

Air flow.   In childhood, the mid-maximal expiratory flow rate is the most reliable and reproducible index of airway function. While the young child (7 years or younger) may not inspire to total lung capacity (TLC) or exhale to residual volume (RV), valuable and reproducible information concerning airway function in this age group can be obtained by a partial flow-volume curve measuring maximal expiratory flow at FRC.[1] With this study it is often possible to study children as young as 4 years old and as small as 96 cm tall. Children older than 7 years should be able to perform maximal expiratory flow from TLC. At least three trials are required with each maximal expiratory or inspiratory flow maneuver to increase the potential of obtaining an accurate estimate of airway function. Because the level of the lung volume at which the maximal expiratory flow is initiated will affect the test result, it is helpful to determine whether the patient is at TLC when the maximal expiratory flow rate is initiated.[2,16] Analysis of the contour of the maximal expired flow-volume (MEFV) curve, as in adults, provides important qualitative information concerning the level of the airways responsible for limitation of expired airflow. Sequential studies of MEFV are helpful in determining when, in the child with tracheal stenosis, tracheal dilatation needs to be repeated.

Airways resistance.   Airways resistance, although technically an easy test for a child to perform, is a less sensitive test for determination of limitation of expired flow.[17,25] The equations for these studies are listed in the Table 17-1.

Distribution of Ventilation

Single breath. The most sensitive test of the uniformity of ventilation is the slope of phase III of the single-breath N_2 wash-out curve. When elevated above 2.5% N_2/L2, it indicates nonuniform distribution of ventilation.

Although in childhood, the closing volume (CV)[24] reflects the elastic properties of the lung, CV is only an index of small airway function when maximal expiratory flow rates are within the normal range. With a steep slope of phase III, measurement of phase IV (i.e., CV) is, at best, imprecise.

40 breath nitrogen wash-out. The forty-breath N_2 wash-out curve[2] and the single-breath O_2 test, when elevated, indicate nonuniform distribution of ventilation. Analysis of the slope of phase III in the single-breath test is the more sensitive of the two tests. The 40-breath test, although more fraught with technical artifact (e.g., occasional air-leak around the mouthpiece diluting the O_2 the patient breathes with air), can provide important data concerning the size of the poorly ventilated lung compartment.

Gas Exchange

Blood-gas analysis. Arterial blood-gas analysis provides the most sensitive index of lung function (e.g., O_2 uptake and alveolar ventilation) in infants and children. Measurement of arterial blood gases during exercise further increases the sensitivity of this test. (See the section on exercise testing.)

The arterial O_2 tension is generally the most sensitive index of lung disease in pediatric patients. It is the test that is most likely to be abnormal in patients with apparently minimal lung disease. The right radial and temporal[59] arteries are the most accessible superficial arteries in newborn infants; whereas the radial artery is often most accessible in children. Femoral artery puncture should be avoided and placement of an *indwelling* temporal artery catheter has been associated with focal brain necrosis. Local anesthesia with 0.5–1.0% lidocaine is indicated to reduce spasm of the radial artery. The Allen tests to determine ulnar artery patency should be performed prior to radial artery puncture. Polypropylene syringes may be used for collecting arterial blood. The volume of anticoagulant in the syringe should be less than 0.05 ml when a 0.5 ml blood sample is to be withdrawn.

Noninvasive. Although the diffusing capacity (DL$_{CO}$,[2.22]) was developed to assess pulmonary membrane gas transport, in practice it is a test of the pulmonary capillary blood volume. The DL$_{CO}$ is reduced in restrictive lung disorders but when normalized for patient's alveolar volume (V$_A$), the test may become normal. The DL$_{CO}$SB also requires optimal patient cooperation. The exhaled gas sample size required for gas analysis by some DL$_{CO}$ systems may preclude measurement of this parameter in the young child. The DL$_{CO}$SS test provides less information than the $DL_{CO}SB$ and is not useful unless the child has difficulty with breathholding required in the $DL_{CO}SB$ or the size of the gas sample precludes use of the single-breath method. With both of these tests, the results are normalized for the patient's lung volume (DL_{CO}/V_A). In contradiction to adults, the $DL_{CO}SB$ is relatively insensitive in children, and some pediatric pulmonary function laboratories do not even perform this test.

Arterialized capillary blood accurately reflects arterial pH and PCO_2 under good conditions: (1) when the skin is adequately prewarmed (e.g., 42°C for ten minutes;[3]) and (2) when the blood flow to the area is normal, and (3) when the proper technique is used for the collection of blood. However, arterialized samples do not approximate arterial PO_2 in neonates and infants. Recent advances in technology permit measuring transcutaneous O_2 and CO_2 tension.[38,60] These methods require warming of the skin to 42–45°C. Although they provide continuous assessment of transcutaneous O_2 or CO_2 tension, these values may not be accurate enough to be as synonymous with arterial values. Their approximation to arterial values are dependent on cutaneous blood flow, skin thickness, and technical factors such as the quality of the membrane and the seal of the electrode to the skin.

Provocation Testing

Nonallergic provocation tests are usually performed in children with respiratory symptoms to determine whether asthma is the underlying cause. Three types of provocation tests are generally used: bronchodilators, exercise, and histamine or methacholine. The selection of the provocation test used depends on facilities available, presentation of the patient, age, ability to cooperate, and specific questions to be answered. Children should not receive bronchodilator medications, antihistamines, and disodium cromoglycate 24 hours prior to provocation testing.

Bronchodilators—aerosol.   When airways obstruction is detected on routine pulmonary function tests, the response to bronchodilator aerosol is often measured routinely. Improvement in maximal expiratory flow rates of 15% or reduction in RV indicate a reduction in airways obstruction. In children, this is most often seen in asthma. Obstruction due to fixed anatomic obstruction, airway inflammation, or mucus plugging may not respond acutely to inhaled bronchodilators. Thus, some patients with chronic asthma may not acutely respond to bronchodilators in the pulmonary function laboratory, but may still have asthma as the etiology of their lung disease. Inhaled isoproterenol (0.5%), isoetharine (0.5%), metaproterenol (0.5%), or salbutamol may be used. We have found no difference in response whether five VC breaths of the full-strength bronchodilator aerosol solution are taken or the patient tidally breathes the diluted aerosol for ten minutes. Generally, a 15% change in pulmonary function parameter is required to define a response. However, it is more correct for each laboratory to define its own reproducibility or establish each patient's own standard.[26] Children with obstructive lung disease (OLD) have larger coefficients of variation for pulmonary function parameters than normal subjects.[26] One should be careful to consider changes in RV while interpreting flow rates before and after bronchodilators. A fall in RV, a positive response to bronchodilators in airway obstruction, may result in decreased flow rates due to the reduction in airway caliber with a fall in lung volume. We find the V_{max} 80% TLC, V_{max} 70% TLC, and V_{max} 60% TLC especially useful because the changes in lung volume are reflected in the measurement.[25] (See Table 17-2). If routine pulmonary function tests are normal, one may not see a response to bronchodilators, even with asthma.

Exercise. Virtually all asthmatic children will demonstrate exercise-induced bronchospasm (EIB) if subjected to strenuous exercise.[27] Thus, EIB should not be considered as separate from asthma, but rather as one of several nonspecific factors that will frequently precipitate exacerbation of bronchospasm in asthmatics. Exercise provocation testing is useful in evaluating a child with a history consistent with asthma but who presents with normal physical examination and resting pulmonary function tests. In this case, exercise may be used to provoke diagnostic bronchoconstriction. Certain forms of exercise are most successful at provoking EIB. Free running and uphill treadmill running are more likely to provoke EIB than bicycling and swimming.[28] Strenuous exercise is required to provoke EIB. Most investigators require six to eight minutes of exercise, preferably uphill treadmill running, which achieves a maximum heart

Table 17-2 Normal Pulmonary Function Values

Test	Unit	Equation	SD	Reference
V_{max}60% TLC		0.86	0.25	25
V_{max}70% TLC		1.10	0.26	25
V_{max}80% TLC		1.29	0.25	25
DL_{CO}SS	ml/min/mm Hg	$19.075H - 1.332.8$	19.3	
DL_{CO}SB	ml/min/mm Hg	$10^{(0.00656H + 0.308)}$	17.6	
DLV_A	DL_{CO}/liter	5.50	1.5	
CV/VC	%	$-1.25A - 26.12$ (if A 17) .56A $- 3.75$ (if A 16)		24
CV	Liters	pred CV/VC $\times$ pred VC		24
CC/TLC	%	(pred CV + pred RV)/pred TLC		24
40 breath N_2	%	< 1.5		2

All equations valid for both sexes.
H = height in centimeters.
A = age in years.

rate of 170–180 beats per minute.[27,29] It is frequently difficult to obtain adequate cooperation during exercise stress in children under 10 years of age, consequently, exercise provocation testing is most useful in adolescents.

Maximal expiratory flow rates are measured serially at 3,10, and 15 minutes after the completion of exercise and should be compared to pre-exercise baseline values. Because each pulmonary function parameter has unique variability, laboratories should establish their own normal values if possible.[26,27] Generally, a fall in the peak expiratory flow rate (PEFR) of 12.5%, in forced expiratory volume (FEV$_1$) of 10%, and/or in MMEF (maximum expiratory flow rate) of 26% following exercise, is diagnostic of EIB. PEFR and FEV$_1$ demonstrate diagnostic changes in 99% of EIB. Tests of small airway function are only abnormal when PEFR and/or FEV$_1$ are also abnormal. EIB is readily reversed by the inhalation of a bronchodilator aerosol. Once the diagnosis of EIB is made, exercise provocation testing can be used to determine the efficacy of various bronchodilator medications to prevent EIB. The bronchodilator can be administered 10–20 minutes prior to exercise and the response compared to the nonmedicated exercise test. These tests should be repeated on different days at the same time of day to be truly comparable. The disadvantage of exercise provocation testing is that children are often too short of breath or have too much bronchospasm to cooperate fully with postexercise measurements of expiratory flow rates.

Histamine/methacholine.   Virtually all asthmatic children will develop bronchoconstriction in response to inhaled histamine or methacholine.[30–32] These tests are useful also in the child with a suggestive history of asthma but with a normal physical examination and normal resting pulmonary function tests. During this test, the patient is challenged with one of the nonspecific stimuli (histamine or methacholine) to cause bronchoconstriction. Sensitivity to these stimuli are measures of the increased bronchial reactivity characteristic of asthma. However, children with severe OLD other than asthma may show increased bronchial reactivity due to airway injury.[33] In children with cystic fibrosis, this does not correlate with indices of atopy, but rather with abnormal baseline pulmonary function tests.[33] Thus, baseline pulmonary function tests must be normal in order to properly interpret histamine or methacholine challenge tests results.[30,32,33] The inhalation challenge for histamine or methacholine involves the serial inhalation of increasing concentrations of medication. Expiratory flow rates are measured following each inhalation. A 20% decrease in FEV$_1$ compared to baseline, indicates a positive response and no further testing is required. Normal subjects show no response to inhaled aerosol of histamine or methacholine aerosol up to a concentration of 10 mg/ml or 25 mg/ml respectively. Bronchospasm induced by histamine or methacholine is readily reversed by the inhalation of bronchodilator aerosol. Usually, children show the necessary bronchoconstriction for a positive response without any subjective feelings of distress. This is a distinct advantage over exercise provocation testing in children because they are able to complete testing without subjective wheezing or distress.[32] A comparative study of exercise and histamine provocation testing in asthmatic children reveals that histamine is more sensitive in the detection of asthma, it is more comfortable and safer, and all children with EIB are detected by histamine inhalation challenge.[32] Thus, we recommend histamine or methacholine inhalation as the routine provocation test for asthma in children with normal resting pulmonary function tests.

Exercise and Ventilation

Exercise stress testing is used in children primarily to provoke EIB, to uncover evidence of lung disease when resting pulmonary function tests are normal, to define the etiology of exercise limitation (i.e., heart versus lung) to monitor the course of disease, and to monitor the effectiveness of treatment in alveolar or pulmonary vascular disease. Exercise provocation testing for asthma has already been discussed. However, asthma remains the most common cause of exercise-related chest pain or shortness of breath in children and adolescents. Consequently, we routinely measure maximal expiratory flow rates before and after every exercise stress test regardless of the initial indication for testing.

The questions asked in an exercise stress test are (1) is there abnormal exercise limitation; (2) is exercise limited primarily by pulmonary or cardiovascular mechanisms; (3) is there evidence for lung disease; and (4) is there evidence of pulmonary vascular disease? A progressive exercise stress test with increasing workloads every minute until exhaustion is the format generally used to answer these questions. The details of exercise stress testing are discussed elsewhere, however, some general comments specific to children should be mentioned.

Few children will exercise maximally with an indwelling arterial or venous catheter in place. Consequently, in children, exercise stress tests are best accepted when they are bloodless.[34-37] Noninvasive measurement of gas exchange is obtained from analysis of expired gas during exercise. If a computerized system is not available for breath-by-breath analysis or analysis of timed mixed samples, data can still be calculated from time expired-gas samples in Douglas bags. We also use transcutaneous O_2 monitoring to assess oxygenation during exercise.[38]

Younger children are not as likely to exercise maximally as adolescents. Thus, it is extremely important to assess whether a given result truly represents maximal exercise. Maximal exercise performance is achieved when the respiratory quotient is greater than 1.1 and the maximal heart rate for age is obtained at the peak workload. In this case, exercise is limited by cardiovascular mechanisms, as in normal subjects. If the child has impaired pulmonary function, even maximal exercise may not be accompanied by maximal heart rate or an elevated respiratory quotient. However, one should see a fall in transcutaneous O_2 tension or other evidence of pulmonary limitation.

Younger children are not able to exercise maximally by following a voluntary target. Thus, an electronically braked bicycle ergometer, which keeps a constant workload regardless of pedalling frequency, is very useful. Unfortunately, some small children cannot fit on any commercially available ergometer. Treadmill running will result in a higher maximal oxygen consumption because of larger muscle mass involved in exercise, and thus is a better reflection of maximal exercise than a bicycle ergometer. It is also less dependent on technique, and more likely to provoke EIB than bicycling.

The selection of the protocol for increasing workloads is critical for children. The ideal progressive exercise stress test brings the subject to his or her maximal level after 8–12 minutes of exercise. This is long enough to allow aerobic metabolism to be fully operative yet short enough to prevent fatigue at submaximal exercise due to the sheer duration of exercise. Our protocol for the bicycle ergometer is 2 minutes of rest, 2 minutes of free pedalling against zero work, then increasing workloads by 50 to 150 kilopondmeters per minute, depending on size, until exhaustion. We then continue measurements three to five minutes into recovery.

The normal values for exercise in children are not generally available in the medical literature. Values differ for each laboratory depending on the methods of measurement and exercise protocol that are used. Thus, each laboratory must establish its own normal values.

Children have most commonly been referred for exercise stress testing to investigate complaints of exercise limitation either due to chest pain or shortness of breath. Cardiovascular versus pulmonary causes of exercise limitation can usually be easily distinguished. Pulmonary limitation may be accompanied by a decreased maximal O_2 uptake, fall in transcutaneous O_2 tension, failure of VC to increase with increasing minute ventilation (restriction), increased ventilatory equivalent for O_2, increased V_D/V_T (dead space/tidal volume) ratio, maximal minute ventilation equal to or greater than the resting maximal voluntary ventilation, and/or development of EIB. If the pulmonary disability has been a long-standing one, cardiovascular fitness may have decreased secondarily to the level of maximal exercise permitted by the lung disease. Thus, it is not unusual for a child with primary pulmonary limitation to have a respiratory quotient greater than 1.1 and maximal heart rate at peak workload. We have also found exercise stress testing to be a sensitive index of pulmonary vascular disease in children. Failure of the V_D/V_T ratio to fall on exercise is a sensitive index of deterioration in the condition of children with interstitial pneumonitis.

Respiratory Muscle Strength

Ventilatory muscle strength is measured as the most negative intrapleural pressure generated during inspiration against a near-total airway occlusion.[39-41]

This can be approximated by measuring mouth pressure. If inspiration against a complete airway occlusion is used, subjects can generate, artifactually, a higher mouth pressure using their cheeks. Consequently, a 14-gauge needle is used to provide a slow leak preventing this artifact.[41] The introduction of this leak does not affect the true maximal inspiratory mouth pressure generated by the inspiratory muscles.[41] Inspiration should begin at or near residual volume to give the maximal result. Maximal inspiratory pressure improves with practice so that 20 attempts should be used, and the best result taken. Normal values are greater than 60 cm H_2O for children and adolescents.[41]

Diaphragmatic strength is measured as the maximal transdiaphragmatic pressure (Pdi) generated during inspiration against an occluded airway.[42-45] Pdi is defined as the difference between intraabdominal and intrapleural pressures. Intrapleural pressure is measured by an intraesophageal balloon. Intraabdominal pressure is measured by an intragastric balloon subtracting a constant determined by comparing intragastric pressure with intrapleural pressure during complete relaxation of the diaphragm. This constant is affected by gastric tone and hydrostatic differences between the stomach and subphrenic region. Consequently, this constant is extremely sensitive to changes in body position. Maximal Pdi is obtained during inspiration from RV against an occluded airway. In infants, the highest values obtained during crying can be used. Normal values for infants are greater than 35 cm H_2O.[46] In older children, the values are somewhat higher.

Ventilatory muscle endurance is commonly measured as the maximal minute ventilation that can be sustained for ten minutes during isocapneic hyperpnea.[40,47] The technique requires a sophisticated apparatus not usually available outside the research laboratory. Normal values are approximately 60–70% of the 12-second maximal voluntary ventilation. This method is dependent on pulmonary mechanics in addition to ventilatory muscle endurance and has been measured as the maximal inspiratory pressure that can be generated on each inspiration for ten minutes.[41,48] Endurance of the diaphragm can be determined in a similar manner using Pdi instead of mouth pressure.[49]

Ventilatory Control

Unfortunately, there are no clinical tests of respiratory control available that directly measure the neural output of respiratory centers. Most tests measure only minute ventilation or V_T, which are also affected by pulmonary mechanics, chest wall mechanics, and ventilatory muscle function. Thus, results of tests of respiratory control must be interpreted in the light of any pulmonary, chest wall, or neuromuscular abnormalities.

Ventilatory response to CO_2. Minute ventilation increases linearly with increasing alveolar PCO_2. The ventilatory response to CO_2 tests both central and peripheral chemoreceptor function. Two methods are used: rebreathing and steady state. In older children, who will breathe through a mouthpiece, the rebreathing method provides a more accurate assessment of CO_2 response.[50] The subject rebreathes from a bag containing 70 ml/kg of 95% O_2 and 5% CO_2. The 95% O_2 is used to ensure that the results are not influenced by a hypoxic ventilatory response. The test is usually continued until an end-tidal PCO_2 of 65–70 mm Hg is achieved. Minute ventilation is plotted against end-tidal (alveolar) PCO_2. The slope of the regression line through those points (V_E/P_ACO_2) is the measure of the CO_2 response. For children, the results are divided by body weight. Normal values differ between studies, but are in the range of 63.1 $\pm$ 19.1 (SD) ml V_E/kg/mm Hg P_ACO_2. In infants, it is often easier and more reproducible to perform a steady-state CO_2 response. Minute ventilation is measured after five minutes of breathing room air, 2% and 4% CO_2. Clearly, the ventilatory response is dependent on pulmonary mechanics, chest wall mechanics, and ventilatory muscle function, as well as respiratory control.

In an attempt to bypass these mechanical influences of the CO_2 ventilatory response test, the measurement of mouth pressure at 100 msec after airway occlusion (by mouth shutter) has been advocated as a more direct reflection of respiratory center output.[51] This can be used in conjunction with either rebreathing or steady-state CO_2 response tests. The airway is occluded at end-expiration and the mouth pressure is generated 100 msec after the beginning of inspiration is measured (P0.1 or P100). The subject does not react to airway occlusion before about 200 msec, thus P0.1 is a reflection of respiratory center output. Because no change in lung volume occurs, pulmonary mechanics do not influence the test. P0.1 increases linearly with increasing alveolar PCO_2. The normal value for the slope of P0.1 plotted against alveolar PCO_2 is 0.51 $\pm$ 0.25 (SD) cm H_2O P0.1/mm Hg P_ACO_2. Alterations in the diaphragm muscle length will alter the tension generated for a constant neural output according to the length-tension curve of the muscle. Thus, the P0.1 response is altered by changes in lung volume, reflecting changes in ventilatory muscle function, and may be decreased in the presence of hyperinflation.

Ventilatory response to hypoxia.   Minute ventilation increases exponentially with decreasing PaO_2 or linearly with decreasing O_2 saturation of hemoglobin.[52,53] The ventilatory response to hypoxia tests the peripheral chemoreceptor function, but may be complicated by depression of central respiratory neurons in newborn infants. As with the CO_2 response, the test may be performed by rebreathing or steady-state methods. When performing the rebreathing method, a CO_2 absorber must be placed in the circuit to prevent contamination of the results with a ventilatory response to rising inspired CO_2 tension (P_ICO_2).[53] O_2 saturation can be monitored using an ear oximeter and PaO_2 may be monitored by a transcutaneous O_2 electrode. With the rebreathing method, the ventilatory response to hypoxia is expressed as the slope of minute ventilation plotted against O_2 saturation (V_E/SaO_2; normal values are 1.09 to 4.90 liter/min/% SaO_2 for adults), or the parameter A in the exponential equation:

$$V_E = \frac{A}{1/(PaO_2 - 32)} \quad \begin{array}{l} \text{(normal value } 90 \pm 60 \text{ for} \\ \text{A/body surface area).} \end{array}$$

With the steady-state method, the hypoxic response is the change in minute ventilation occurring at a specified reduced PaO_2. A 300% increase in ventilation normally occurs when inspired O_2 pressure P_IO_2 is reduced to 80 mm Hg. Mouth occlusion pressure (P0.1) can be used during a hypoxic response test to eliminate mechanical factors. Again, this will be affected by changes in lung volume.

Hypoxic and hypercapneic arousal responses. In young infants, it is often difficult to perform hypercapneic or hypoxic ventilatory response tests. A screening test of chemoreceptor function can be obtained by measuring arousal responses to reduced P_IO_2 and elevated P_ICO_2 during sleep.[54] The infant is studied during quiet sleep under a head hood. For the hypoxic arousal response test, N_2 is mixed with air in increasing concentrations until the transcutaneous O_2 tension drops 25 mm Hg and P_IO_2 has fallen to 80 mm Hg, or until the infant shows behavioral signs of arousal (agitation, restlessness, eye opening, and crying). Failure of the infant to arouse from quiet sleep when exposed to this degree of hypoxia for 3 minutes on two consecutive challenges is interpreted as an abnormal arousal response to hypoxia.[54] The hypercapneic arousal response test is performed by introducing 10% CO_2 and 90% O_2 into the head hood until the end-tidal CO_2 is elevated to 60 mm Hg. Failure to arouse from quiet sleep with this hypercapneic stimulus is an abnormal arousal response to CO_2.[54] These tests should be performed during quiet sleep because arousal responses are normally decreased during active sleep.

Pediatric pneumogram. During wakefulness, the cerebral cortex has a stimulatory influence on central respiratory centers. Consequently, many respiratory control disorders are primarily manifest during sleep. Thus, quantitation of the ventilatory pattern during sleep is useful in the diagnosis of respiratory control disorders, especially in the evaluation of infants with apnea. The chest wall impedance and ECG are recorded for 12 hours overnight.[55-57] There is no significant difference in the amount of information obtained during a 24-hour recording versus 12 hours if the recordings both include overnight sleep. Only the ventilatory pattern during sleep is scored. All apneas over 15 seconds are abnormal (prolonged apneas). HRs below 80 up to 3 months of age, below 70 from 3 to 6 months of age, and below 60 over 6 months of age are abnormal if sustained for ten seconds (bradycardia). Any apnea with bradycardia or cyanosis is abnormal. Periodic breathing is defined as three or more respiratory pauses over 3 seconds each interrupted by not more than 20 seconds of normal breathing. It is timed from the onset of the first pause to the end of the last pause in the series. Periodic breathing should not exceed 4% of the TST, except in preterm infants.[58] These constitute an abnormal ventilatory pattern during sleep which suggests a respiratory control disorder.

The pediatric pneumogram does not detect obstructive apneas nor hypoventilation. It does not differentiate the sleep state accurately. When more information is required, more sophisticated polysomnography measuring ventilation, EEG, EOG, and expired concentrations of CO_2 and O_2 as described previously are indicated.

REFERENCES

1. Taussig LM: Maximal expiratory flows at functional residual capacity: A test of lung function for young children. Am Rev Respir Dis 116:1031–1038, 1977.
2. Polgar G, Promodhat V: Pulmonary function testing in children: techniques and standards. Philadelphia, WB Saunders Co, 1971.
3. Binder RD, Mitcheli AC, Schoenberg JB, et al.: Lung function among Black and White children. Am Rev Respir Dis 114:955, 1976.
4. Hsu KHK, Jenkins DE, Hsi BP, et al.: Ventilatory functions of normal children and young adults—Mexican-American, white and black. II. Wright peak flowmeter. J Pediatr 95:192, 1979.
5. Liang A, Pulley B, Salive HT, et al.: Spirometric standards from 387 healthy New Zealand children. Aust NZ J Med 5:260, 1975.
6. Michaelson ED, Watson H, Silva G, et al.: Pulmonary function in normal children. Bull Physiopathol Respir 14:525, 1978.
7. Pistelli G, Paci A, Dalle Lucne A, et al.: Pulmonary volumes in children. II. Normal values in female children 6 to 15 years old. Bull Physiopathol Respir 14:513, 1978.
8. Warwick WJ: Pulmonary function in healthy Minnesota children. Minn Med 6:435, 1977.
9. Taussig LM, Harris TR, Lebowitz MD: Lung function in infants and young children. Am Rev Respir Dis 116:233, 1977.
10. Cross KW: The respiratory rate and ventilation in the newborn baby. J Physiol 109:459, 1949.
11. Cross KW, Oppe TE: The respiratory rate and volume in the premature infant. J Physiol 116:168, 1952.
12. Klaus M, Tooley WH, Weaver KH, et al.: Lung volume in the newborn infant. Pediatrics 30:111, 1962.
13. Gregory GA, Kitterman JA: Pneumotachygraph for use with infants during spontaneous or assisted ventilation. J Appl Physiol 31:766, 1971.
14. Kattan M, Miyasaka K, Volgyesi G, et al.: A respiratory jacket for ventilatory measurement in children. J Appl Physiol 45:630, 1978.
15. Duffty P, Spriet L, Bryan H, et al.: Respiratory induction plethysmography (Respitrace): An evaluation in infants. Am Rev Respir Dis 123:542, 1981.
16. Taussig LM, Chernik V, Wood R, et al.: Standardization of lung function testing in children. J Pediatr 97:668, 1980.

17. Zapletal A, Montoyama EK, Vonde Woestigne KP, et al.: Maximum expiratory flow curves and airway conductance in children and adolescents. J Appl Physiol 26:308, 1969.

18. Weng TR, Levison H: Standards of pulmonary function in children. Am Rev Respir Dis 99:879, 1969.

19. Helliesan PJ, Cook CD, Friedlander L, et al.: Studies of respiratory physiology in children. I. Mechanics of respiration and lung volumes in 85 normal children 5 to 17 years of age. Pediatrics, 22:80, 1958.

20. Engstrom I, Karlberg P, Swarts CL: Respiratory studies in children. IX. Relationships between mechanical properties of the lungs, lung volumes, and ventilatory capacity in healthy children 7 to 15 years of age. Acta Paediatr Scand 51:68, 1962.

21. Kamel M, Weng TR, Featherby EA, et al.: Relationship of mechanics to lung volumes in children and young adults. Scand J Respir Dis 50:125, 1969.

22. Bucci G, Cook CD, Barrie H: Studies of respiratory physiology in children. Part V. Total lung diffusion, diffusing capacity of pulmonary membrane, and pulmonary capillary blood volume in normal subjects from 7 to 40 years of age. J Pediatr 58:820, 1961.

23. Strang LB: Measurements of pulmonary diffusing capacity in children. Arch Dis Child 35:232, 1960.

24. Mansell A, Bryan C, Levison H: Airway closure in children. J Appl Physiol 33:711, 1972.

25. Cooper DM, Cutz E, Levison H: Occult pulmonary abnormalities in asymptomatic asthmatic children. Chest 71:361, 1977.

26. Nickerson BG, Lemen RJ, Gerdes CB, et al.: Within-subject variability and percent change for significance of spirometry in normal subjects and in patients with cystic fibrosis. Am Rev Respir Dis 122:859–866, 1980.

27. Kattan M, Keens TG, Mellis CM, et al.: The response to exercise in normal and asthmatic children. J Pediatr 92:718–721, 1978.

28. Godfrey S: Exercise Testing in Children. London, W.B. Saunders, 1974.

29. Silverman M, Anderson SD: Standardization of exercise tests in asthmatic children. Arch Dis Child 47:882, 1972.

30. Chai H, Farr RS, Froelich LA, et al.: Standardization of bronchial inhalation challenge procedures. J Allergy Clin Immunol 56:323, 1975.

31. Laitinen LAI: Histamine and methacholine challenge in the testing of bronchial reactivity. Scand J Respir Dis 86(suppl):33, 1974.

32. Mellis CM, Kattan M, Keens TG, et al.: Comparative study of histamine and exercise challenges in asthmatic children. Am Rev Respir Dis 117:911–915, 1978.

33. Mellis CM, Levison H: Bronchial reactivity in cystic fibrosis. Pediatrics 61:446–450, 1978.

34. Astrand PO, Rodahl K: Textbook of Work Physiology. New York, McGraw-Hill, 1970.

35. Jones NL, Campbell EJM, Edwards RHT, et al.: Clinical Exercise Testing. Philadelphia, W.B. Saunders, 1975.

36. Wasserman K, Whipp BJ: Exercise physiology in health and disease. Am Rev Respir Dis 112:219–249, 1975.

37. Godfrey S: Physiologic response to exercise in children with heart or lung disease. Arch Dis Child 45:534–538, 1970.

38. Schonfeld T, Sargent CW, Bautista D, et al.: Transcutaneous oxygen monitoring during exercise stress testing. Am Rev Respir Dis 121:457–462, 1980.
39. Black LF, Hyatt RE: Maximal static respiratory pressures in generalized neuromuscular disease. Am Rev Respir Dis 103:641–650, 1971.
40. Leith DE, Bradley M: Ventilatory muscle strength and endurance training. J Appl Physiol 41:508–516, 1976.
41. Nickerson BG, Keens TG: Measuring ventilatory muscle endurance in humans as sustainable inspiratory pressure. J Appl Physiol 52:768–772, 1982.
42. Campbell EJM, Agastoni E, Newsom-Davis J: The Respiratory Muscles: Mechanics and Neural Control (ed 2). Philadelphia, W.B. Saunders, 1970.
43. Agostoni E, Rahn H: Abdominal and thoracic pressures at different lung volumes. J Appl Physiol 15:1087–1092, 1960.
44. Agostoni E: A graphical analysis of thoracoabdominal mechanics during the breathing cycle. J Appl Physiol 16:1055–1059, 1961.
45. Loh L, Goldman M, Newsom Davis J: The assessment of diaphragm function. Medicine 56:165–169, 1977.
46. Scott CB, Nickerson BG, Sargent CW, et al.: Developmental pattern of diaphragm strength in infancy. Pediatr Res 17:707–709, 1983.
47. Keens TG, Krastins IRB, Wannamaker EM, et al.: Ventilatory muscle endurance training in normal subjects and cystic fibrosis patients. Am Rev Respir Dis 116:853–860, 1971.
48. Roussos C, Fixley M, Gross D, et al.: Fatigue of the inspiratory muscles and their synergistic behavior. J Appl Physiol 46:897–904, 1979.
49. Roussos CS, Macklem PT: Diaphragmatic fatigue in man. J Appl Physiol 43:189–197, 1977.
50. Read DJC: A clinical method for assessing the ventilatory response to carbon dioxide. Australas Ann Med 16:20–32, 1967.
51. Cosgrove JF, Neuburger N, Bryan MH, et al.: A new method of evaluating the chemosensitivity of the respiratory center in children. Pediatrics 56:972–980, 1975.
52. Rebuck AS, Campbell EJM: A clinical method for assessing the ventilatory response to hypoxia. Am Rev Respir Dis 109:345–350, 1973.
53. Rebuck AS, Woodley WE: Ventilatory effects of hypoxia and their dependence on PCO_2. J Appl Physiol 38:16–19, 1975.
54. Hunt CE: Abnormal hypercarbic and hypoxic sleep arousal responses in near-miss SIDS infants. Pediatr Res 15:1462–1464, 1981.
55. Stein IM, Shannon DC: The pediatric pneumogram: a new method for detecting and quantitating apnea in neonates. Pediatrics 55:599–603, 1975.
56. Stein IM, White A, Kennedy JL Jr, et al.: Apnea recordings of healthy infants at 40, 44, and 52 weeks postconception. Pediatrics 63:724–730, 1979.
57. Stein IM: Patterns of the pediatric pneumogram. Med Instrum 13:177–180, 1979.
58. Kelley DH, Shannon DC: Periodic breathing in infants with near-miss sudden infant death syndrome. Pediatrics 63:355–360, 1979.
59. Schlueter MA, Johnson BB, Sudman DA, et al.: Sampling from scalp arteries in infants. Pediatrics 51:120–122, 1973.
60. Peabody JL, Gregory GA, Willis MM, et al.: Transcutaneous oxygen tension in sick infants. Am Rev Respir Dis 118:83–87, 1978.

CHAPTER 18

Bedside Pulmonary Function and ICU Monitoring: Indications and Interpretation

ROBERT J. FALLAT

In *Pulmonary Function Testing: Guidelines and Controversies,*[1] the methods used in respiratory intensive care units (RICU) were discussed in two chapters: Chapter 24 on bedside testing of pulmonary function, which included both pulmonary mechanics and gas exchange, and Chapter 25 on hemodynamic monitoring. The methods discussed for monitoring the respiratory rate, tidal volume (V_T), airway pressure, and gas exchange are considerably different depending on whether the patient is spontaneously breathing or endotracheally intubated. Similarly, the gas exchange and hemodynamic monitoring techniques discussed in those chapters are considerably different depending upon the number of invasive, intravascular catheters used. Because of these factors, this current chapter discusses monitoring for three separate clinical conditions. (1) Early monitoring of the spontaneously breathing patient who may have a high potential for respiratory problems. The emphasis is on the prevention of respiratory failure and the decision to employ more invasive treatment modalities. (2) Monitoring of the more severely, acutely ill patient who has already required endotracheal intubation and some form of catheterization. The emphasis is on monitoring to provide optimization of ventilator management, prevention of complications, and indication of prognosis. (3) Monitoring of the recuperating patient who is in transition from mechanical to spontaneous ventilation. The emphasis is on monitoring to prevent exacerbation, to optimize management during recovery, and on predicting the eventual outcome. Several areas are not covered in this chapter. Arterial blood gases (ABG) are discussed extensively in Chapter 11 of this volume, and are therefore only referred to as an adjunct to noninvasive blood-gas measurements or hemodynamic monitoring. Similarly, spirometry is presented fully in Chapter 2; hence, this chapter is limited to discussion of spirometry in its simplest form as used at the bedside, i.e., forced vital capacity (FVC) and forced expiratory volume in one second (FEV_1). Hemodynamic monitoring is, of course, an extensive area; its multiple indications and interpretations are limited only to those problems frequently associated with acute respiratory failure (ARF), such as the differential diagnosis of pulmonary edema and O_2 transport. Finally, extensive discussion of noninvasive monitoring associated with sleep apnea and pediatric or neonatal monitoring are not included here because this material may be found in Chapters 14 and 17.

INDICATIONS

Indications for various bedside tests are summarized in Table 18-1. The disease groups listed are those that occur frequently in a RICU. The tests or variables monitored are divided according to the mode of ventilation and whether they are manual or automated. The + and − indicate the frequency or degree of importance of the variable for the given disease state. Clearly, this grading system is quite arbitrary and depends more on the severity of the condition rather than on the category.

EARLY MONITORING: SPONTANEOUSLY BREATHING PATIENTS

For the spontaneously breathing patient, monitoring is largely manual and intermittent. Routine, manually obtained vital signs (temperature, pulse, blood pressure, and respiratory rate), arterial blood gas (ABG), and chest X rays should be included as monitoring variables because they are frequently the only monitoring done on a patient not in the intensive care unit (ICU).

The importance of the simple measurement of respiratory rate (RR) cannot be overemphasized because it is a harbinger of respiratory failure. Automation of the variable is possible, but is not frequently done in the spontaneously breathing patient. Once EKG monitoring is indicated, RR can be monitored using the same electrodes to measure chest impedance changes. Because EKG monitoring systems offer this option, such continuous RR monitoring should become more frequent in the future. Many other methods to monitor RR, including nasal temperature or CO_2 changes, laryngeal sounds, magnetometers, and electromyograms[2,3] have been used, but to a limited extent and largely in research settings.

Spontaneous or Mechanical Ventilation / Mechanical Ventilation Only

Disease	Manual Tests			Automated or Continuous					Mechanical Ventilation Only					
	RR	ABG	Spirometry	EKG (RR)	Arterial Catheter	PA Catheter	O_2 Cutaneous or Ear	CO_2 Cutaneous or Airway	V_T/V_E	PS/C	P_{max}/P_{aw}	ECO_2	VO_2/VCO_2	V_D/V_T
COPD														
Asthma	+	+	+	+	±	±	+++	+++	+++	+	++	+	−	±
Bronchitis	+	++	++	+	+	±	+++	+++	+++	++	+++	++	−	±
Emphysema	+	+++	+++	+	+	±	+++	+++	+++	±	+	++	−	+
RLD														
Pneumonia and/or interstitial lung disease	+++	+++	+	+	+	+	+	±	+	++	+	+	+	±
Pleural/chest wall	+++	+	+	±	±	−	+	+	+	++	±	±	−	−
ARDS/Pulmonary Edema														
High Probability	+++	+++	+	+	+++	+++	+	++	++	++	±	±	+	+
Low Probability	+	++	±	+	+	±	+	±	++	++	−	−	−	+
Overdose														
Coma, absent gag	+++	+++	±	+	+	±	+	++	+	+	+	+	−	−
Stupor, gag present	+++	+++	±	++	−	−	+	++	+	±	±	++	−	−
Postanesthesia or surgery	+++	+++	+	+	+	−	+	+	++	±	±	+++	−	−
Neuromuscular disease	+++	++	+++	+	±	−	+	+	++	+	±	+	−	−
Emboli	+	++	+	+	+	+++	+++	±	++	++	+	+	+	+

The + and − indicate the frequency or degree of importance of the variable for the given disease state. Clearly this grading system is quite arbitrary and depends more on the severity of the condition rather than on the category.

Many methods have been used in pediatric or neonatal monitoring, particularly for sleep apnea studies; these methods are described in Chapter 14 of this volume. Except for chest impedance, most methods to continuously monitor the RR rate are experimental and not applicable for a routine, long-term monitoring of an adult spontaneously breathing patient.

Lung Mechanics

Spirometric monitoring in the nonintubated patient is the simplest way to monitor lung mechanics and should probably be done more frequently than is current practice. Certainly, in the patient with chronic obstructive pulmonary disease (COPD), FEV_1/FVC is probably as valuable and is certainly less invasive than ABGs. FEV_1 has been shown to be a good indicator of severe functional derangement of ABGs; e.g., PCO_2 elevations are seldom seen in asthmatics until FEV_1 is less than 25% of predicted.[4] The use of ABGs and chest X rays in acutely ill patients could possibly be reduced if more spirometry were performed. Perhaps more important, respiratory distress or impending respiratory failure may be detected and prevented, not only in COPD patients, but in other patients likely to develop ARF if FVC measurements were commonly done.

Continuous monitoring of V_T or FVC in the nonintubated patient is more difficult. Chest impedance and magnetometer methods have been tried but are not reliable due to the complex configuration of the chest and the changing contribution of chest wall and diaphragmatic contractions to tidal breathing with changes in position.[5] Measuring the changing inductance of chest and abdomen using two separate, insulated wire coils held in place by a mesh suit has been reported to be a reliable method for monitoring V_T in the spontaneously breathing patient.[6] This method measures thoracic gas volume and, therefore, differs from exhaled volume measurements due to the intrathoracic gas compressibility and blood volume fluctuations. The recommendation of widespread clinical use of this device in the ICU awaits further clinical experience.

Maximum inspiratory and expiratory pressure (MIP, MEP) are other measures of respiratory sufficiency. These tests may be more sensitive indicators of respiratory failure, particularly in patients with neuromuscular disease,[7] but they are not sufficiently different from FVC measurements to necessarily warrant obtaining both types of measurement.

Maximum voluntary ventilation (MVV) measurements are also recommended as a bedside test, particularly for preoperative neuromuscular disease patients. The measurement of MVV does require more voluntary effort, and is not feasible in many of the more ill patients in the Respiratory Intensive Care Unit (RICU). Some investigators have argued that because MVV is dependent upon patient effort, this test not only measures mechanical performance but also the ability of patient to cooperate and do well following surgery. In neuromuscular disease patients, particularly those with myasthenia gravis, MVV may be a more sensitive test than FVC for detecting early disease.[7]

Gas Exchange

Arterial blood O_2, CO_2, and pH have become the sine qua non of respiratory failure, and therefore have played a predominant role in the monitoring of the respiratory patient. The severity of the respiratory failure dictates the frequency of the arterial samples needed and the necessity for the placement of an arterial line. Noninvasive monitoring of blood gases using skin electrodes has been used with increasing frequency and success, particularly in the neonatal and infant populations. Problems with variable gradients between gas concentrations in the blood and at the skin surface have limited their use in adults.[1] In the future, such monitoring will undoubtedly be used more frequently in place of, or as a supplement to, arterial gas sampling.

Ear oximetry is a particularly useful adjunct in monitoring oxygenation. Currently, the use of O_2 is largely based on arterial blood sampling. Ear oximetry provides an easy way to optimize O_2 usage and provides a noninvasive means for indicating when arterial blood samples may be needed as O_2 saturation falls.

CO_2 may be monitored either by nasal cannula[8] or cutaneously. The skin gradient problems for CO_2 are not as great as for O_2 in the adult population because CO_2 electrodes or the infrared analyzers used do not consume CO_2 and therefore do not require a continuous flux of CO_2 through the skin. Monitoring the CO_2 tensions should be particularly useful in COPD and drug overdose patients as is indicated in Table 18-1; the clinical experience with their use, however, is still limited.[10,11]

Hemodynamics

EKG monitoring is indicated in many of the diseases listed in Table 18-1, but is usually obtained primarily to provide information about cardiac complications such as arrhythmias rather than as part of the monitoring of the primary pulmonary disease process. However, because any respiratory patient with disease severe enough to produce hypoxia or respiratory acidosis is a candidate for an arrhythmia, these patients should have EKG monitoring. Once EKG monitoring is initiated, chest impedance measurements can also readily be obtained to monitor respiratory rate, as mentioned earlier.

An arterial line is indicated when arterial blood gases are severely abnormal or are changing rapidly and therefore require frequent sampling. Using a small, number 23–25 gauge needle, three to five arterial punctures a day are probably not too traumatic for the patient or the artery. If more than five punctures a day are needed, or if several days of monitoring are anticipated, an arterial line is probably indicated. Even when arterial blood gases are stable and not grossly abnormal, an arterial line may be indicated because of hemodynamic instability. Blood pressure fluctuations are often pronounced particularly in patients with sepsis, severe pneumonia, drug overdose, and particularly in patients with severe acute respiratory distress syndrome (ARDS) who require positive pressure breathing (PPB) as discussed below.

Cardiac complications rather than the pulmonary disease are usually the indications for a pulmonary artery catheter. Two possible exceptions to this statement are the diagnosis of pulmonary emboli and differential diagnosis of pulmonary edema. The diagnosis of pulmonary emboli may be difficult because lung scans and other noninvasive diagnostic studies may be nonspecific and pulmonary angiography may be necessary. If pulmonary emboli or pulmonary hypertension is found, continuous monitoring with a pulmonary artery line may be necessary. O_2 transport analysis is also possible when both lines are present, and is frequently needed in the more acutely ill patients as discussed in the next section. The differential diagnostic separation between cardiogenic pulmonary edema and alveolar-capillary leak (noncardiogenic pulmonary edema) often requires a pulmonary artery catheter. When both peripheral arterial and pulmonary arterial lines are available, a diagnostic decision tree may be followed as is shown in Figure 18-1 taken from an article by Stevens.[9]

ACUTELY ILL, MECHANICALLY VENTILATED PATIENTS

Lung Mechanics

When a patient has become ill enough to warrant endotracheal intubation, the potentials for respiratory monitoring increase considerably. Now RR, V_1,

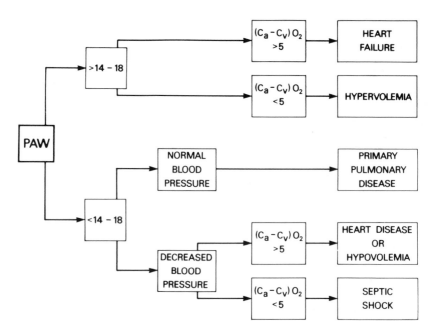

Figure 1.   Scheme for assessment of cardiac versus pulmonary causes of lung edema. Adapted from Stevens.[9] With permission.

expired volume per minute (V_E), and more precise measures of pulmonary mechanics (maximum inspiratory pressure) (P_{max}), static pressure (P_{ST}), compliance (C), and pulmonary (lung and chest wall) resistance (R_p) are all possible. If the patient is continuously mechanically ventilated, all of these variables can be manually measured and recorded at least every four hours or when changes are made in the ventilator. Only C and Rp are derived variables, while the RR, V_T, P_{ST}, and P_{max} are basic measurements which allow monitoring the respiratory status of a ventilated patient.

The calculation of compliance and resistance is relatively easily obtained from basic measurements.

Static C of the lung is defined as:

$$C = V_T \div P_{ST} - PEEP$$

where P_T = static or no flow airway pressure at end inspiration, and PEEP = positive and expiratory pressure.

Resistance is a flow-dependent characteristic and is more difficult to measure. The difference between the P_{max} and P_{ST} is one estimate of airway resistance.

$$R_p = P_{max} - P_{ST} \text{ flow,}$$

where flow is measured at the time of P_{max}.

In automated systems as detailed in other references,[1,8] pulmonary mechanics can be monitored at more frequent intervals. The usefulness and indications for such systems to continuously and automatically monitor respiratory mechanics remains to be established. The measurement of P_{ST}, C, and airway resistance (R_{aw}) are not easily or routinely done manually because they depend on the visualization of a single point with considerable chance for signal noise and error. Because automated systems utilize all the pressure (P) and flow data throughout the breathing cycle, these systems provide more precise information about ventilatory mechanics. When it is important to follow respiratory variables accurately, automation does have a rational basis.

As shown in Table 18-1, P_{ST} and C measurements are of most importance in ARDS and pneumonia patients with severe oxygenation problems requiring PEEP. The initial determination of "optimum PEEP" may be made on the basis of C measurements as suggested by Suter et al.[14] Table 18-2 lists some of the general factors that may indicate the need for more frequent measurements of P_{ST} and C.

The measurement of Rp and C provides a means for differentiating between potential sources of pressure requirements of the mechanically ventilated patient. A rise in Rp indicates airway problems such as bronchospasm or secretions whereas a rise in C points toward parenchymal problems such as atelectasis, consolidation, or pulmonary edema.

Table 18-2   Indications for Measurement of Compliance and Resistance
on Mechanical Ventilator

---

1. High airway pressures
   ($P_{st} > 40$ cm H_2O, $P_{max} > 50$ cm H_2O)
2. PEEP > 5 cm H_2O
3. Rapidly changing pressures or volumes
4. Severe hypoxemia
   ($PaO_2 < 60$ mm Hg or $FIO_2 > .50$)
5. Unstable hemodynamics
6. Progressive or prolonged disease

Gas Exchange

The adequacy of ventilation is most readily defined by PCO_2 and pH. Arterial PCO_2 and pH can only be effectively measured from blood samples, although tissue probes and skin sensors have been utilized in research settings. The partial pressure of CO_2 may readily be monitored via the airway and skin sensors that are currently being clinically evaluated.[10] Airway PCO_2 has been monitored by infrared spectrophotometers and mass spectrometers. Most of these devices sample gas from the airway, which is passed through the instrument located several feet away. Newer units utilize miniaturized infrared units that are fitted into the airway or on the skin and thereby obviate the problems of gas sampling.[10] The Severinghaus electrode used for blood CO_2 measurement has been adopted for transcutaneous use and is much more reliable than an O_2 electrode in the adult.[11]

End-tidal CO_2 (ECO_2) is an approximation of $PaCO_2$. In normal subjects, ECO_2 is 1–4 torr below $PaCO_2$. As the distribution of ventilation becomes more uneven, as in obstructive airways disease or other lung pathology such as emboli, this gradient can increase to 10 torr or more. Some researchers have argued that the ECO_2 is of little value because of this large and potentially variable gradient. However, as a trend monitor it can be extremely valuable. When changes occur it is indicative either of a change in the $PaCO_2$ or in the gradient, both of which are useful to know in optimally managing patients on a ventilator. A rebreathing technique can be used to make a more accurate assessment of blood CO_2 and has recently been advocated strongly by Campbell and associates.[12]

O_2 monitoring currently is performed largely by blood sampling. Most ventilators monitor O_2 only in a gross manner by sensing that the O_2 intake chamber is filling or by using in-line O_2 sensors that have a slow time response and, therefore, give mean values of airway O_2 to $\pm$ 5%. Mass spectrometers have a rapid time response and have been advocated for monitoring both CO_2 and O_2. Because O_2 concentration on some ventilators may vary widely during a breath, the continuous measurement of O_2 is difficult and is currently limited to research rather than clinical uses.

Batch collections of expired gas can be made and both CO_2 and O_2 can be measured by a variety of less expensive, slow-response sensors. When coupled with minute volume measurements, O_2 consumption, CO_2 production, and RQ can be calculated. Several automated units are available, used primarily in exercise studies, but can monitor patients on a ventilator. When combined with arterial and venous blood gas measurements, one can calculate output by the Fick method. Such metabolic information may be essential to correctly interpret hemodynamic changes occurring in the ARDS patient. Recent studies have shown that patients on hyperalimentation may produce excess CO_2 which limits their ability to be weaned from the ventilator.[13] CO_2 production measurements are needed to document this, but when weaning is difficult and is not explained by poor ventilatory mechanics, simple assessment of the caloric intake by hyperalimentation may give the answer. By current practice, the measurement of O_2 consumption and CO_2 production in the ICU is limited to research or referral centers; automated measurements of these complex parameters can now be done at the bedside, but should be validated by manual laboratory methods.

Wasted ventilation, V_D, or the ratio of V_D to V_T, i.e., the V_D/V_T ratio, has been suggested as a useful monitoring parameter for acutely ill patients. V_D and V_D/V_T are invariably higher than normal on mechanically ventilated patients, particularly in patients on PEEP, in whom values of V_T/V_T may be as high as 90%. The measurement of V_D/V_T is technically difficult requiring either a batch collection or continuous monitoring of the CO_2 and airway flow. In my view, it is a physiologic curiosity that becomes useful only in unusual situations to explain the difficulty in weaning some severely compromised COPD or ARDS patients. Like O_2 consumption and O_2 production, the frequency of use is limited as is indicated in Table 18-1.

Hemodynamics—O_2 Transport

All of the indications mentioned previously for the spontaneously breathing patients apply to the more acutely ill, mechanically ventilated patient. In addition, because acutely ill patients are frequently significantly hypoxic, hemodynamic measurements become critical for the optimum analysis of O_2 delivery to tissues. To perform analysis of O_2 delivery some estimates of O_2 content of the blood (CaO_2 and $C\bar{v}O_2$) and cardiac output ($\dot{Q}t$) is needed.

The drop in $\dot{Q}t$ that occurs with positive pressure breathing (PPB) and in particular when PEEP is used, is well recognized. Although levels of PEEP, V_T, and P_{ST} can be initially optimized using mechanical measurements,[14] the ultimate decision regarding proper ventilation must rest with adequate oxygenation. An improvement in PaO_2 may be associated with an even greater fall in $\dot{Q}t$ and a fall in the net O_2 delivery and a fall in $C\bar{v}O_2$ and $\dot{Q}t$. The content of O_2 (CO_2) is calculated from the saturation (SO_2), and PaO_2 and hemoglobin (Hgb) by the following equation:

$$CaO_2 = 1.34 \times \% \ SO_2 \times Hgb + (.003 \times PaO_2) = \text{content of } O_2 \text{ in arterial}$$
blood and

$$C\bar{v}O_2 = 1.34 \times \% \ SO_2 \times Hgb + (.003 \times P\bar{v}O_2) = \text{content of } O_2 \text{ in venous blood.}$$

Thus, because O_2 delivery is directly proportional to hemoglobin (Hgb), the importance of monitoring Hg in acutely hypoxic patients is emphasized. Not all circulating Hgb even in acutely hypoxic patients is utilized: carboxyhemoglobin and methemoglobin are two abnormal Hgb's that may be found in blood under some unusual toxic circumstances. The factor 1.34 is based on normal Hg. Some patients may have an abnormal Hgb that has a lower O_2 capacity, but these conditions are rare and not generally measured or recognized. Of greater importance is the O_2-Hgb desaturation curve which relates the percent saturation to PO_2. In critically ill patients, many factors alter this curve so that saturation calculated from PO_2 may be inaccurate. This is particularly true on the steep portion of the curve, when PO_2 is below 50 torr. When PO_2 is below 50, as it almost always is in mixed venous samples, the percent saturation or content should be measured directly and not obtained from PO_2.

Numerous methods to estimate $\dot{Q}t$ are available by the analysis of expired CO_2 or the use of soluble gases such as N_2O or acetylene, but these are not generally available and the accuracy and reliability markedly diminishes as $\dot{V}/\dot{Q}$ abnormalities increase (as is common in critically ill patients).

Measurement of $\dot{Q}t$ is most readily and commonly performed by thermal dilution via the PA catheter as described in *Pulmonary Function Testing: Guidelines and Controversies*.[1] When a thermodilution catheter is not in place, $\dot{Q}t$ can be calculated by the Fick equation:

$$\dot{Q}t = (CaO_2 - C\bar{v}O_2)/VO_2,$$

where $\dot{V}O_2$ = minute O_2 consumption.

A mixed venous blood sample is required and O_2 consumption must be measured. In critically ill patients, FIO_2 is often in excess of 50% O_2 and the measurement of $\dot{V}O_2$ becomes difficult if not impossible because of the error introduced by the small difference in large numbers (e.g., FIO_2 may be 82% and FEO_2 may be 80%). There are two alternatives to combat this problem. (1) Because there is no CO_2 in inhaled gas, $\dot{V}CO_2$ can be measured accurately by collecting exhaled gas and $\dot{V}O_2$ can be approximated by assuming a normal expiratory quotient of 0.8. (2) Another common alternative used in clinical situations is to use the arterial-venous O_2 difference as an estimate of $\dot{Q}t$ and assume that $\dot{V}O_2$ does not change. The use of this alternative implies that the physician has accepted the proposition that mixed venous O_2 is the primary determinant of O_2 transport. If any change in ventilatory or other management (e.g., use of PEEP, fluids, diuretics, or cardiotonic drugs) causes a fall in $C\bar{v}O_2$, the overall effect is detrimental, even if PaO_2, CaO_2, and $CaO_2 \times \dot{Q}t$ all increase. However, it is important to recognize that any increase in activity, even mild exercise in a normal individual, may cause a widening of the arterial-venous difference and a lowering of $C\bar{v}O_2$. Hence, it may be very misleading to make decisions on $C\bar{v}O_2$ alone unless the patient is kept in a sedated baseline state and other metabolic factors such as temperature do not change.

To summarize, the indications for more extensive measurements of O_2 transport depend on the severity of the hematologic, cardiovascular, and respiratory abnormalities. Severe hypoxemia ($PaO_2 < 50$) and depressed cardiac output in a mechanically ventilated patient usually require both peripheral and pulmonary arterial catheterization. The details of interpretation of these data will be discussed later.

MONITORING THE RECUPERATING OR WEANING PATIENT

As patients recover from acute respiratory failure (ARF) and ventilatory demands decrease, major respiratory and hemodynamic changes can occur that require careful monitoring.

Reducing the airway pressures or PEEP too rapidly may cause pulmonary edema because the volume load in the peripheral vascular bed shifts to the central blood pool. Pulmonary congestion should be followed by monitoring with a pulmonary artery catheter. If a pulmonary artery line is not available, a fall in C or PaO_2 can be expected if pulmonary congestion occurs.

Intermittent mandatory ventilation (IMV) may be the mode of weaning or might even be used throughout the management of the intubated patient. V_t and RR in such a system may vary considerably and it may be difficult to assess what is adequate for patients. Reduction in the mandatory volume or rate usually is monitored by arterial blood sampling. During weaning, ECO_2 can be quite useful as a supplement to the arterial blood gas. Spontaneous V_t may be too low to adequately clear dead space during IMV, and an erroneously low ECO_2 may be obtained. However, ECO_2 values during mandatory, mechanical breath should accurately reflect the mean alveolar CO_2 and adequacy of ventilation.

In the transition from ventilator to spontaneous ventilation via a T piece, there is invariably a decrease in V_t and an increase in RR. Such a trial should not be instituted until at least two questions have been answered. (1) Is the PaO_2 adequate on an FIO_2 compatible with weaning (usually 40%)? (2) Is the FVC at least 10 ml/kg? Other measurements used by some investigators include MIF, which should be over 20 cm/H_2O, and MVV, which should be twice the resting ventilation.

Not uncommonly, patients who are being weaned are not fully cooperative and do not give maximal effort, thereby invalidating the measurement of FVC, MIF, and MVV. Under these circumstances, a C measurement may be used instead. If the C is over 25 ml/cm H_2O, the patient may be weanable. Because C is size dependent, the expected value must be properly adjusted in infants or very small or very large adults. In the absence of neuromuscular disease or emphysema, a transpulmonary pressure of 30 cm H_2O should be possible. Therefore, the measured compliance multiplied by 30 should equal the FVC requirement of 10 ml/kg. For example, a compliance of 30 means that 900 ml may be generated with 30 cm H_2O transpulmonary pressure (i.e., $V = C \times P = 30$ ml/cm $H_2O \times$ 30 cm $H_2O = 900$ ml). Nine hundred milliliters is an adequate VC for weaning a 50-kg person but may be too low for a 110-kg, 6'7" basketball player.

Ultimately, during the T-piece trial, arterial blood analysis will be the determining factor in the success of weaning. In this situation, ECO_2 may be a very useful monitor to detect early decompensation before serious respiratory acidosis and patient distress occur. It might be expected that a large change in the ECO_2-$PaCO_2$ gradient would occur in shifting from mechanical ventilation to T piece. This has not been observed in a series of weaned patients, with the exception of those patients whose V_t markedly decreased close to the V_D.[10]

Ear oximetry might also be used to monitor patients as they are being weaned from the ventilator, particularly when altering PEEP and F_IO_2. Generally, in ARF patients ventilatory changes during weaning are made slowly over a period of hours and ABG monitoring is adequate.

After the patient is extubated and no longer maintained on positive pressure, progressive atelectasis may occur. The incentive spirometer may be useful both as a monitor of VC and as a treatment modality. Daily measurements of VC are probably the simplest means of monitoring the recovery of ARF patients. Changes in FVC or other routine vital signs are an indication for other more invasive or costly studies such as ABG or chest X rays.

INTERPRETATIONS AND LIMITATIONS OF TESTS

The interpretation of the commonly used tests in bedside and ICU monitoring are summarized in Table 18-3. The values given are useful only for adults and may need adjustment for the elderly (e.g., O_2 tension in the range of 60–70 mm Hg may be normal) or the extremes of size where predicted normals may not be accurate.

RESPIRATORY RATE

The (respiratory rate), simple and basic, is probably the most useful of monitoring variables. Low RRs of < 10 are found either in severe obstructive airways disease (OAD), particularly in emphysematous patients with prolonged expiration times or in hypoventilating patients such as postanesthesia or drug overdose patients. Restrictive lung disease (RLD) patients characteristically have high RRs; when RRs are over 30, respiratory failure becomes more likely. Adults should not be expected to maintain RRs of over 40 for long before ventilatory assistance may be required.

Table 18-3 Interpretations of Tests Degree of Disease

	Normal	Mild	Moderate	Severe
1. RR	10–20	< 10	20–30	> 30
2. Spirometry				
FVC (% predicted)	> 80	60–80	40–60	< 40
FVC (ml/kg)	> 40	20–40	10–20	< 10
$FEV_1/FVC \times 100$ (%)	> 75	60–75	40–60	< 40
MIP (cm H_2O)	> 100	50–100	20–50	< 20
3. Ventilator-mechanics				
P_{max}	< 30	30–40	40–60	> 60
P_{st}	< 20	20–30	30–40	> 40
C	> 40	30–40	20–30	< 20
4. O_2				
PaO_2 (Torr)	> 80	60–80	50–60	< 50
O_2 Sat, Art (%)	> 95	90–95	80–90	< 80
O_2 Sat, Ven	> 70	60–70	50–60	< 50

	Mild to Moderate		Severe	
	Acidosis	Alkalosis	Acidosis	Alkalosis
5. CO_2 (Torr)				
$PaCO_2$	35–40	45–60	20–35	> 60	< 20
ECO_2	35–45	30–55	20–35	> 55	< 20
$TCCO_2$	40–55	55–75	25–40	> 75	< 25

SPIROMETRY

The FVC will vary widely depending on age, gender, and size and there-fore, is presented as a percentage of predicted. It provides an objective guide to the degree of RLD though the cause for reduction is frequently OAD. High or even normal FVC values in the ICU patient should not be expected. Values of FVC based on weight are frequently used to determine the ability to wean. Both RLD and OAD can be expected to give low values of FVC as indicated in Table 18-3. The FEV_1/FVC ratio does normalize for size and provides a measurement of OAD in the presence of RLD. Bedside measurements frequently are compli-cated by poor patient effort; therefore, a reduction in FEV_1, FVC or FEV_1/FVC may not reflect changes in the lung or chest wall but in the patient's cooperation and mental status. This will be evident from examination of the spirometry curves and is the reason why a written record of the spirometric traces is neces-sary for bedside tests.

The ratio of FEV_1/FVC may be misleadingly high when done at bedside if a full FVC is not obtained. In this instance, the degree of airway obstruction might be underestimated. Conversely, poor effort may result in a low FEV_1/FVC ratio in the absence of significant OAD. Experienced personnel are necessary to exhort patients to maximal efforts and the ability to critically review the shape of spirometry curves is necessary to detect these efforts. The use of bedside flow-volume loops showing the curvature may be helpful.

VENTILATOR MECHANICS

The measurement of pulmonary volume-pressure relationships at the bedside is limited to mechanically ventilated patients. The measurements of C and Rp detailed previously are of necessity, those of the lung and chest wall combined, since pleural pressure measurement by esophageal balloons or directly, are generally not available for routine bedside use.

Airway pressures may be markedly changed by altering the V_t and flow rates by the ventilator. Assuming the usual 10–15 ml/kg V_t and normal flow of 0.5 to 1.0 liter/sec, ranges of P_{max} and P_{ST} are given in Table 18-3.

C values vary considerably depending on the size of the individual. Size normalization may be obtained by dividing C values by functional residual capacity (FRC); unfortunately, however, the FRC is not generally known in RICU patients. The values given in Table 18-3 are for an average 70-kg patient being ventilated with 800 ml V_t. A 6'4" male will have a normal C of as high as 100 ml/cm H_2O, whereas a 5' person may be as low as 40 ml/cm H_2O. Even in these extremes of size, the P_{ST} will be similar.

Rp normal values are not given because of the very large effect produced by endotracheal tubes and airway adaptors. Characteristically, Rp values of 5–15 cm H_2O/liter/sec are measured in mechanically ventilated patients, whereas only about 10–20% of those values may be due to intrinsic airway resistance.[15] In addition, large changes in airway resistance can be induced by changes in ventilator flow rates. Just as measurement of P_{ST} provides normalization to the wide variations in compliance with size, the measurement of P_{max} gives a guide to excess airway resistance. The difference between P_{max} and P_{ST} is generally less than 10 cm H_2O, even in a severely obstructed patient who requires higher airway pressures. A change in the difference, $P_{max} - P_{ST}$, is perhaps the best indicator of significant Rp changes.

GAS EXCHANGE

Standard interpretations of ABGs have been extensively reviewed and presented in another chapter in this volume. A brief range of values for O_2 tension and saturation and CO_2 tensions are given in Table 18-3.

In the acutely ill ICU patient, supplemental O_2 is common, so the value of the arterial O_2 must be related to estimated inspired O_2. Precise measurement of $(A-a)O_2$ is possible only when breathing room air; breathing air $(A-a)O_2$ should be less than 20 torr. With the use of supplemental O_2, and in the clinical setting, with attendant less accurate estimates of inspired O_2, a gradient of less than 50 torr is acceptable. A gradient of over 300 torr indicates a severe oxygenation problem requiring more than 50% O_2 and therefore, requiring some closed system of ventilation. If ear oximetry comes into more common usage, SO_2 may be utilized to estimate the severity of hypoxemia as indicated in Table 18-3. Mixed venous O_2 should be the best indicator of adequate oxygenation.[16] Levels below 50% saturation or $P\bar{v}O_2$ less than 30 mm Hg are associated with poor prognosis.[17]

The adequacy of ventilation is best estimated by $PaCO_2$ values. The separation of acid/base problems into acute or chronic and respiratory or metabolic acid requires analysis of pH and HCO_3 as discussed in Chapter 11. As shown in Table 18-3, a $PaCO_2$ of more than 43 torr indicates hypoventilation. However, a PCO_2 value of over 60 torr may be an acceptable and even desirable value in a chronically obstructed patient with a pH of 7.40. On the other hand, acute intubation may be indicated in an asthmatic with PCO_2 rising from 30 to 40 torr and pH falling from 7.40 to 7.30. Arterial pH and $PaCO_2$ must be interpreted together to determine the clinical meaning.

The values for ECO_2 are usually less than $PaCO_2$; the gradient is determined primarily by the inequality of ventilation and perfusion. Rough guidelines for interpretation of this and other measurements are suggested in Table 18-3; it is important to note that the gradient must be determined for each patient by obtaining an arterial sample. Similarly, transcutaneous CO_2 values will be higher than arterial, as indicated in Table 18-3. A change in either the ECO_2 or transcutaneous CO_2 ($P_{TC}CO_2$) in any given patient should serve as an alarm to check an ABG to verify either a true change in the CO_2 or a change in the gradient. In the case of $P_{TC}CO_2$, hemodynamic factors may produce major changes in the gradient and limit the usefulness of this modality in patients with compromised cardiovascular systems; because of this sensitivity of $P_{TC}CO_2$ to cardiovascular function, $P_{TC}CO_2$ may ultimately find use as a monitor of the degree of cardiovascular insufficiency.

CONTROVERSIES

The major controversy in bedside monitoring probably lies in two areas; the use of continuous, computerized monitoring systems and the use of noninvasive blood-gas sensors.

In the spontaneously breathing patient, little is available for continuous respiratory monitoring beyond chest impedance for respiratory rate and cutaneous O_2 and CO_2 monitoring. These measurements have been extensively utilized in the pediatric setting. It is probable that these modes will find increasing use in adult ICU patients who are recognized to have a higher incidence of respiratory failure.

In the mechanically ventilated patient, monitoring is rapidly becoming more sophisticated as newer ventilators are developed with more sensors. It was emphasized earlier both in this chapter and in a previous publication,[1] that measurements of mechanics can be accomplished manually, easily, and with a frequency compatible with most clinical changes. However, ECO_2, cutaneous CO_2 or O_2, or ear oximetry all present new bedside methods formerly available only intermittently from ABGs in a remote laboratory. Changes in CO_2 and O_2 can occur rapidly and frequently require acute changes in management. It therefore seems desirable, and likely, that these newer methods find increasing use. However, it has yet to be shown that automated or continuous measurements of pulmonary mechanics or noninvasive blood-gas analyses are either cost effective or save lives.

An even more controversial future development to look forward to will be the age of interactions with "smart computers." Currently, alarm systems are limited to bells and lights. With the increased amount of physiologic data available, particularly on the mechanically ventilated patient, it is only rational to use computer technology to analyze the physiologic trends and provide algorithms for interaction with the nurse and physician to optimize patient management. One day, some might argue that we can close the loop and let the computer make the management decisions, and write this chapter.

REFERENCES

1. Fallat RJ: Bedside testing and intensive care monitoring of pulmonary function, in Clausen J (ed): Pulmonary Function Testing: Guidelines and Controversies. New York, Academic Press, 1981.
2. Krumpke PE, Cummiskey JM: Use of laryngeal sound recordings to monitor apnea. Am Rev Respir Dis 122:797, 1980.
3. Polgar, G: Comparison of methods for recording respiration in newborn infants. Pediatrics 36:861, 1965.
4. McFadden ER, Jr, Lyons HA: Arterial-blood gas tensions in asthma. N Engl J Med 278:1027, 1968.
5. Ashutosh K, et al.: Impedance pneumograph and magnetometer methods for monitoring tidal volume. J Appl Physiol 37:964, 1974.
6. Cohn MA, et al.: A transducer for non-invasive monitoring of respiration, in Stott FD, Raftery EB, Sleight P, et al. (eds): ISAM Proceedings of the Second International Symposium on Ambulatory Monitoring. London, Academic Press, 1975.
7. Fallat RJ, Jewitt B, Bass M, et al.: Spirometry in amyotrophic lateral sclerosis. Arch Neurol 36:74–80, 1979.
8. Fallat RJ, Osborn JJ: Patient monitoring techniques, in Burton GG, Hodgkin JE (eds): Respiratory Care: A Guide to Clinical Practice. Philadelphia, J.B. Lippincott, 1977.
9. Stevens PN: Assessment of acute respiratory failure: cardiac versus pulmonary causes. Chest 67:1, 1975.

10. Fallat RJ, Roebkin C, Hershon J, et al.: Non-invasive CO_2 monitoring. Am Rev Respir Dis 123 (abstract):93, 1981.

11. Severinghaus JW: A combined transcutaneous PCO_2 electrode with electrochemical HCO_3 stabilization. J Appl Physiol 51:1027–1032, 1981.

12. Powles ACP, Moran Campbell EJ: How to be less invasive. Am Med 67:98–104, 1979.

13. Covelli HD, et al.: Respiratory failure precipitated by high carbohydrate loads. Ann Int Med 95:579–581, 1981.

14. Suter PM, Fairly HB, Isenberg MD: Optimum end pressure in patients with acute pulmonary failure. N Engl J Med 292:284–289, 1975.

15. Mitchell RR, Fallat RJ: Non-invasive parameters in a patient monitoring system. Innovations in Medicine: San Diego Biomedical Symposium, February, 1974.

16. Tenney SM: A theoretical analysis of the relationship between venous blood and mean tissue oxygen pressures. Respir Physiol 20:283, 1974.

17. Springer RR, Stevens PM: The influence on survival of patients in respiratory failure. Am J Med 66:196, 1979.

CHAPTER 19

Preoperative Evaluation

MYRON STEIN

HISTORIC DEVELOPMENT

Postoperative pulmonary complications have been recognized for many years. In 1843, Chevers[1] observed that 56% of postoperative deaths were due to pulmonary complications. Subsequent studies including recent ones have indicated continuing morbidity and mortality due to postoperative pulmonary complications.

Prior to the early 1900s, postoperative pulmonary complications were considered to be misfortunes of the patient and/or acts of God. In 1927, the introduction of pulmonary physiologic studies postoperatively suggested that the complications did not occur de novo. Churchill and McNeil[2] demonstrated dramatic decreases in vital capacity (VC) to 25% of the preoperative value following cholecystectomy. A few years later, Beecher[3,4] demonstrated the rapid, shallow breathing and decreases in functional residual capacity (FRC) and total lung capacity (TLC) associated with smaller decrements in (RV) postlaparotomy; these were classic observations that would be reconfirmed frequently in ensuing years.[5-8] Although overlooked for many years, these postoperative decrements in lung volumes have been linked to pulmonary complications.

During the past 20 years, there have been intensive efforts to classify the presurgical patient in terms of risk for postoperative pulmonary complications and to provide therapy to prevent and/or alleviate these complications. Studies demonstrating the pulmonary physiologic alterations induced by anesthesia, surgery, and the postoperative state have augmented the ability to classify the patient into pools of risk (good or poor). In 1908, Pasteur[9,10] made bedside observations indicating an increase in postoperative pulmonary complications

PULMONARY FUNCTION TESTING
INDICATIONS AND INTERPRETATIONS

following surgery near the diaphragm, an observation verified by numerous investigators.[11-14] Also, factors such as age, obesity, gender, and cigarette smoking have been recognized as contributory to the postoperative pulmonary complication. In recent years, multiple studies of pulmonary function have also been utilized to evaluate the risk preoperatively.[13-18] Generally, but not specifically, the more severe the preoperative pulmonary impairment (see the "Controversies" section at the end of this chapter), the more likely the complications, particularly after thoracic or abdominal surgery.

REVIEW OF METHODS

The pulmonary preoperative evaluation should have specific goals. These may include: (1) selection of candidates at high risk to be given pulmonary therapy designed to reduce the frequency and severity of pulmonary complications;[19,20] (2) preoperative pulmonary evaluations to predict the need for extended postoperative intubation and ventilation;[21,22] and (3) more recently, preoperative pulmonary studies in thoracotomy patients to predict their ability to withstand resection of lung tissue, e.g., the compatibility of remaining lung with an acceptable clinical status and lifestyle.[23-26]

The prevention of postoperative pulmonary complications can only be accomplished by recognition of preoperative risk factors. A list of factors that may increase risk is included in Table 19-1 and when available, data indicating the increased risk are provided. Some risk factors can be determined by simple but careful history taking or physical examination. Others may require semi-skilled or skilled technology.

Predictive thinking allows the physician to make inferences regarding the future course of diseases and is basic to decision making regarding diagnosis, prognosis, prophylaxis, and therapy. The physician may utilize the multiple factors listed in Table 19-1 for the predictions. However, individual factors vary in their predictive values. As shown in Figure 19-1, an ideal predictor would (1) render an accurate prediction (100% correct predictions) and (2) achieve the prediction quickly with minimal financial, personnel, and time expenditure, e.g., line 1 in Figure 19-1. At the other extreme, a prediction may not be possible despite intensive investigation (line 4, Figure 19-1). Once the plateau is reached, additional study can be costly and time consuming.[44] As suggested by Bendixen,[45] a simple history and physical examination in a young, nonsmoking adult with no previous history of cardiac or pulmonary disease having elective surgery on an extremity, will indicate an extremely low risk of a postoperative pulmonary complication. Similarly, history and physical examination will suggest great risk of developing a serious pulmonary complication after thoracic or abdominal surgery in an aged patient with a long history of smoking and respiratory distress on minor exertion. Pulmonary complications need not be limited to patients with severe respiratory distress preoperatively (Table 19-2). Recently,

Table 19-1 Factors Utilized for Preoperative Evaluation

Factor	Increase in Risk × 1	Reference #
Acute or chronic pulmonary disease	3–4	27–29
Abnormal pulmonary function	20	13, 15–18, 30
Cigarette smoking (> 10 cigarettes/day)	2–7	27, 31
Age (> 60 yr)	2–3	27, 32, 33
Sepsis	3	27, 34
Male Sex	2	27
(corrected for smoking)	1	
Cytologic changes (bronchial epithelium)	5	35
Chest film		36
Auscultation, abnormal findings		
Dynamometry (decreased strength, hand grip)	7	37
Sputum volume (> 2 oz/day)		22
Respiratory rate, postoperative increase		38
Preoperative anxiety		39
Breath holding		
Match test		
Stair climbing		40
Pulmonary hypertension (cardiac catheter)		41
Ventilation/perfusion studies (radionuclide)		25, 26, 42, 43
Obesity (> 30% above ideal weight)	2	27

the patients listed in Table 19-2 were observed postoperatively over a period of one month on the Surgical Intensive Care Unit (SICU) of a community hospital. The vast majority of patients who had prolonged stays in the SICU due to postoperative pulmonary complications had been passed for surgery on the basis of the clinical examination. Only two patients among those who had postoperative pulmonary complications had preoperative pulmonary function studies. Anecdotal communications suggest that the data described in Table 19-2 are representative occurrences in many institutions. As suggested in Table 19-1, pulmonary function studies are the most efficient preoperative indicators of postoperative complications and are most likely to fulfill the requirements of line 1, Figure 19-1. Furthermore, as mentioned above, pulmonary function studies have been used to indicate the need for preoperative intubation and ventilation. Also, when utilized in combination with radionuclide studies of ventilation and/ or perfusion, they may prognosticate future clinical hazards following lung tissue resection.

SPECIFIC METHODS

Careful history and physical examinations may render semiquantitative evaluations (Table 19-1). Bedside findings of acute or chronic pulmonary disease

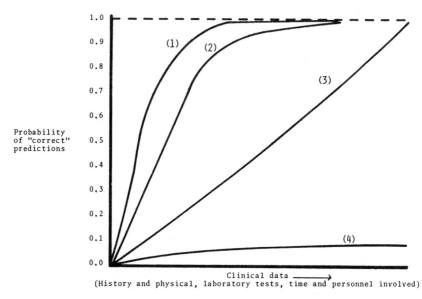

Figure 19–1.   Efficiency of predictors. Line 1 indicates test with most efficient predictive value. Line 2 suggests an increasing number of tests and time without enhancing predictive value. Line 3 indicates that a high level of prediction is attained by performing many studies. Line 4—inaccurately performed tests, false positive tests, and/or studies with low predictive values. Tests performed above shoulders or curves (lines 1 and 2) add to expense without augmenting prediction.

Table 19-2   SICU Admissions over a Period of 31 Days in a Community Hospital

	Pulmonary Complications	No Pulmonary Complications
Number of patients	21	10
Age	64	69
Surgical incisions		
Thoracic	9	1
Upper abdominal	7	1
Other	5	8
Smoking history	12	1
Length of stay, SICU days	5.4	2.4
Deaths	0	0
Preoperative evaluation (pulmonary function)	2	0

suggest an increased risk of postoperative pulmonary complications, particularly following thoracic or abdominal surgery. The need for performing the pulmonary function studies described below is enhanced in these patients.

Tisi[19] has recently reviewed the role of simple spirometric studies in preoperative evaluations. VC, various portions of the timed VC,[12,46,47] $FEF_{200-1200}$,[13] $FEF_{25-75\%}$,[22,48] N_2 meter single-breath test,[13] maximal breathing capacity,[15,16] RV/TLC ratio,[13] and arterial blood gases[13,49] have been utilized as preoperative screening tests. The performance, quality controls, analyses, significance, and interpretations of these studies are discussed in *Pulmonary Function Testing: Guidelines and Controversies.*

Assignment into pools of risk prior to surgery

Simple spirometric studies can be utilized to place patients into good- and poor-risk groups (pools), separating patients into risk groups indicating those more and less likely to develop pulmonary complication.[13,19,20,46] The risk assignment may be accomplished by simple screening studies, e.g., FEV_1, $FEV_{1.0\%}$, $FEF_{200-1200}$, $FEF_{25-75\%}$, and MVV (Fig. 19-2). These studies of lung spirometry cannot indicate the pulmonary outcome in the individual patient—they place the patient into classifications of greater and lesser risk of postoperative pulmonary complication. However, when the risk of postoperative pulmonary complication is considered on the basis of preoperative lung function (Fig. 19-2) and the location of the surgery (Fig. 19-3), the frequency of adverse effects may increase markedly. In a recently study, Lockwood[50] demonstrated that the addition to those described above of multiple studies of pulmonary function—TLC, RV, and diffusion study—did not enhance the preoperative assessment in patients undergoing thoracotomy. Furthermore, data are lacking at the present time to indicate that screening studies of small airways function[19,50]

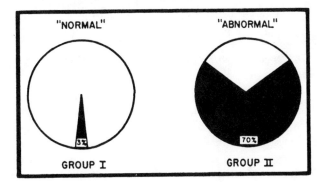

Figure 19–2. Postoperative percent of pulmonary complications in patients with normal (3%) and abnormal preoperative lung function studies (70%). (Reprinted with permission.)[13]

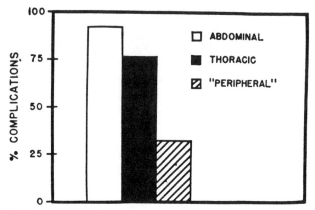

Figure 19–3.   Postoperative pulmonary complication rate for abdominal, thoracic, and "other" types of surgery in high-risk patients. (Reprinted with permission.)[19]

would be helpful in further delineating the risk when compared to the simple spirometry tests described above.

In some patients, preoperative evaluations tailored to a suspected abnormality may be helpful, e.g., preoperative assessment of the physiologic dead space in an individual with suspected pulmonary vascular obstruction: flow-volume loops when upper airways obstruction is suspected; nocturnal studies in patients suspected of sleep apnea; CO_2 response studies in patients with possible respiratory control problems; and arterial blood gases (ABGs) when the forced expiratory volume in one second (FEV_1) is markedly decreased[49] or there is suspicion of blood gas abnormalities (preoperative assessment of blood gases may relieve concerns raised by postoperative observations of abnormal values—at times a continuation of a preoperative abnormality). Furthermore, a preoperative PaO_2 < 50 mm Hg and/or $PaCO_2$ elevation should cause a reconsideration of the possible risk and benefits of the contemplated surgery.

Indicate the need for postoperative intubation and ventilation (delayed weaning)

Peters, Brimm, and Utley[21] performed VC, FEV_1, $FEF_{50-75\%}$, FEF_{75-85}, and maximal inspiratory (MIP) and maximal expiratory pressures (MEPs) on 49 adult patients undergoing elective cardiac surgery for coronary artery disease, valvular corrections, or combinations. The patients were observed independently for successful weaning within 24 hours postoperatively. Those who could not be weaned from the ventilator had significantly lower values for VC, FEV_1, $FEF_{50-75\%}$, FEF_{75-85}, MEP, and MIP. However, there was great overlap in that many patients who were weaned successfully had abnormal values and many of those in whom weaning was unsuccessful had normal values on one or more tests. The application of techniques of discriminant analysis demonstrated that the combination of MEF_{75-85} and MEP predicted failure or success of weaning in

90% of the patients studied. At the present time, the application of these data to patients having other types of surgery is unknown. Gracey, Divertie, and Didier[22] observed that preoperative values of $FEF_{25-75\%}$ and maximum voluntary ventilation (MVV) of $<$ 50% of predicted after pulmonary therapy were associated with frequent and prolonged requirements for mechanical ventilation. Recent studies have indicated that the routine use of prophylactic intubation and ventilation in pulmonary high-risk patients may be unnecessary and even harmful (see following discussion).[51]

Prediction of ability to withstand lung tissue resection

Differential bronchospirometry,[24] temporary occlusion of a single pulmonary artery produced by ballon occlusion,[23,52] right heart catheterization,[41] lateral decubitus studies of pulmonary function,[53] and radionuclide tests of ventilation and/or perfusion have been utilized to assess the physiologic function of lung tissue to be removed versus that projected to remain. As discussed by Tisi,[19] tests of regional lung function may be used qualitatively or quantitatively. For the latter purpose, ventilation and/or perfusion studies will suffice. The VC, FEV_1, or MVV is measured preoperatively; an independent preoperative study of ventilation and/or perfusion is performed and the proportional radioactive counts to the contralateral (nonoperated) lung is calculated; predicted postoperative VC, FEV_1, or MVV would equal the preoperative value multiplied by the percent of perfusion or ventilation to the lung that will remain.[54,55] The preoperative spirometric study must represent an accurate assessment of the patient's function if the prediction is to be valid.[52] MVV of $<$ 50% of predicted

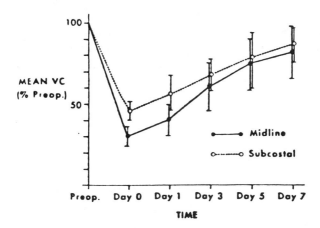

Figure 19–4. Comparison of postoperative changes in vital capacity, VC, following midline and subcostal incisions. Data are represented as percent of the preoperative measurements.[65]

or FEV_1 < 2.0 liter would be indications for performance of the radionuclide test preceding pneumonectomy. Predicted postoperative MVV < 20 liter/min or FEV_1 < 0.8 liter are considered to be contraindications to pneumonectomy. These data and the use of the scanning techniques prior to lobectomies are discussed in the "Controversies" section.

Radionuclide studies should not act as a substitute or replacement for the spirometric preoperative screening for postoperative complications. Boysen, Block, and Moulder [56] recently identified a high postthoracotomy incidence of lethal and morbid pulmonary complications in a group of patients with poor preoperative FEV_1 and MVV. They had been passed for surgery on the basis of the radionuclide studies.

Tisi[19] has also described preoperative performance of ventilation perfusion ratio ($\dot{V}/\dot{Q}$) studies in a qualitative manner. He described four patterns of $\dot{V}/\dot{Q}$ relationships in evaluations of lung tissue to be resected.[1] Lung tissue to be resected has similar $\dot{V}/\dot{Q}$ to remainder of the lung. The physiologic impact of resection is proportional to quantity of tissue removed.[2] The lung tissue to be resected has absent ventilation and perfusion in the preoperative study—in a sense, an autolobectomy has taken place. Resection of the tumor should have little or no long-term effect on lung function.[3] The lung tissue to be resected bears a major share of overall $\dot{V}/\dot{Q}$. As described by Tisi, a major postoperative deleterious effect on lung formation would occur.[4] There is perfusion, but absent ventilation of the lung tissue to be resected. In effect, a right-to-left shunt has occurred, e.g., an obstructive endobronchial lesion. Resection may improve lung hypoxemia.

The development of radionuclide scanning techniques has replaced the need for differential bronchospirometry and temporary unilateral pulmonary artery balloon occlusion studies in the preoperative evaluation. The ubiquitous use of scanning, the ease of performance, and the elective nature of the procedure should obviate any need for the lateral decubitus position test[53] even in smaller medical installations. Exercise studies of ventilation, gas exchange, and cardiac catheterization should be indicated only rarely in the preoperative evaluation, perhaps in unusual instances when clinical and pulmonary function findings are conflicting. In a few patients, confirmation of pulmonary hypertension may be required prior to thoracic or abdominal surgery due to the high associated mortality rate.

PATHOPHYSIOLOGICAL RATIONALE

Postoperative pulmonary complications include but are not limited to the following: bronchospasm, severe dyspnea not due to pulmonary embolism nor congestive heart failure, exacerbation of bronchitis with signs of airway obstruction, purulent sputum and fever, severe disabling cough, radiologic changes showing atelectasis and/or pneumonia, and pulmonary failure as indicated by postoperative alterations of blood gases. Postoperative pulmonary complications due to aspiration, pulmonary embolism, or bleeding disorders affecting the lung are not included in this discussion of preoperative evaluation of lung function.[45] Nevertheless, preoperative abnormalities of lung function may augment the effects of these complications, if they occur. Also, to diminish controversies regarding the presence and nature of postoperative pulmonary complications, they can be graded on a + to + + + + scale with + + + + being a lethal postoperative pulmonary complication and +, a transient episode with minor contributions to morbidity; + + and + + + complications would add to morbidity, length of stay, and possibly days on a SICU at times requiring prolonged intubation and ventilation. These gradings tend to distinguish the postoperative alterations in lung function that may be normal sequelae to surgery near the diaphragm or prolonged surgery from the more serious pathophysiologic alterations in lung function that alter the postoperative course.

The late postoperative complications that may occur following resection of lung tissue include severe dyspnea and/or pulmonary hypertension, cor pulmonale and cardiac failure, postoperative changes that may affect the prognosis and lifestyle as severely as an underlying malignancy.

The pulmonary responses to anesthesia, various operative procedures, and the postoperative state have been described in lucid detail by others[19,27,41,45,57-59] and are only presented briefly. It is suggested that the postoperative alterations in lung function that occur in many surgical patients with normal preoperative lung function are magnified in those who may enter surgery with compromised pulmonary function. Furthermore, when patients with abnormal lung function preoperatively undergo thoracic or abdominal surgery, the postoperative pulmonary complications can be severe and frequent (Fig. 19-3).

Alterations in pulmonary function may be induced by anesthesia; by the surgical procedure; and by the conditions, postures, and medications during the early postoperative state. Generally, there may be great difficulty in separating the contributing roles of each of the foregoing to the development of postoperative changes in lung function. Although the changes described below may occur in patients with normal preoperative lung function, they tend to be more severe and less easily reversible in subjects with preexisting lung diseases.

Preanesthetic medication and anesthesia produce multiple effects on lung function. In spontaneously breathing subjects during anesthesia, there is depression of respiratory control mechanisms.[60,61] Anesthesia is also associated with increases in physiologic dead space and (A-a) PO_2 difference, and a decrease in FRC, whether the subject is breathing spontaneously or on a ventilator.[60] Recently, Dueck et al.[62] using the multiple inert gas technique, have demonstrated profound increases in low $\dot{V}_A/\dot{Q}$ units, intrapulmonary shunts, or both in ten patients with a variety of preoperative pulmonary function abnormalities. Their studies also suggested that uptake of soluble anesthetic gases may have had a concentrating effect on alveolar PaO_2. Thus, the arterial PaO_2 may not be an accurate indicator of the development of low $\dot{V}_A\dot{Q}$ units during anesthesia. Anesthetic gases may also depress mucociliary clearance by decreasing ciliary activity.[61,63] Furthermore, there is a correlation between the duration of anesthesia and postoperative pulmonary complications,[63] e.g., anesthesia longer than three hours may be associated with an increase in pulmonary complications following abdominal surgery. The particular anesthetic agent employed does not appear to play an important role in the development of the postoperative complication. Arora and Gal[64] have recently studied the effects of d-tubocurarine on the cough mechanism of healthy subjects. They observed interference with effective cough related to expiratory muscle weakness, decreased airway compression, and reduced linear velocity of air flow. Thus, the cough would be less effective due to the diminished kinetic energy in the postsurgical patient recovering from anesthesia and muscle weakness.

The operative procedure may augment some of the alterations in pulmonary function described above. As stated previously, incisions in proximity to the diaphragm have a greater effect on pulmonary function. Transverse abdominal incisions are associated with smaller decrements in VC, FRC, and PaO_2 and a lower incidence of pulmonary complications when compared to midline incisions. Compression of the lungs by retraction may also contribute to postoperative difficulties. The attentive anesthetist will usually avoid the deleterious effects of rapid, shallow breathing on $\dot{V}/\dot{Q}$ relationships and lung surfactant.

During the immediate postoperative state, the mechanisms described above may be intensified. In subjects with normal preoperative lung function, there may be postoperative alterations in ventilatory function that mimic RLD, especially after thoracic or abdominal surgery. Surgical pain and diminished diaphragmatic motion result in the splinting of the respiratory apparatus with rapid, shallow tidal volumes, smaller end-tidal thoracic gas volume (FRC), TLC, inspiratory capacity (IC), and end-expiratory reserve volume. The normal breathing range may fall on or below the closing volume with resulting $\dot{V}/\dot{Q}$ abnormalities and a drop in arterial blood O_2 tension. The depression of cough and sighing enhances these physiologic changes. Narcotics may not be effective in relieving these conditions and may have deleterious effects on respiratory control, cough, sighing,[45] and mucus clearance.[48] A decrease in lung compliance usually associated with microatelectasis or macroatelectasis may occur. In the individual with healthy lungs, these alterations in lung function may reach a peak effect in 24–48 hours after surgery and resolve over a period of 1 or 2 weeks. The hypoxemia that may occur in patients with normal preoperative lungs is usually of no clinical significance.

PATHOPHYSIOLOGIC RATIONALE FOR POSTOPERATIVE
PULMONARY COMPLICATIONS

Patients with preoperative lung disease, especially chronic obstructive lung disease, may have more severe perioperative and postoperative alterations in lung function. Airway obstruction, decreases in air flow rates, and lung volumes and atelectasis may be more severe in these patients and retained pulmonary secretions may become infected. Postoperative sepsis,[45] anxiety, and pain may increase metabolic demands and the work of breathing, but the patient may not be able to accommodate the need for an increase in ventilation. Thus, pulmonary failure may occur. Postoperative abdominal distension and/or ileus may also interfere with ventilation. Improper fluid replacement may induce right and/or left heart failure, airway edema, and subsequent alterations in blood-gas exchange.

As the pathophysiologic process continues, events may become cyclical with reinforcement of the pulmonary complication. The intubated patient on a ventilator may become starved with impairment of ventilatory drive and breakdown of ventilatory muscle.[63] As increasing concentrations of O_2 are required to maintain arterial blood O_2, the injured lung may be more susceptible to O_2 toxicity. When observed and followed in the ICU, these patients frequently develop multiple organ failure. These postoperative sequelae may be similar in patients with other types of lung disease, neuromuscular diseases, heart disease, and so forth.

The pathophysiologic rationale related to the need for postoperative intubation and ventilation is based on premises similar to those already described. Patients with poor lung function and/or muscle weakness preoperatively are more likely to require intubation and postoperative ventilation as the lung function deteriorates during the immediate postoperative course. Preparation for the possible need for prolonged ventilation may diminish anxiety and stress for the patient and the family and allow for better planning for facilities and personnel.

The long-term ability to withstand pneumonectomy is believed to be related to the quantity and function of lung tissue removed, and the lung function of the remaining lung. Removal of lung tissue in a severely compromised patient may result in incapacitating dyspnea, failure of gas exchange, and/or severe pulmonary hypertension.

The pulmonary responses to cardiopulmonary bypass are similar to those described above, but often the postoperative changes are minimal when compared to thoracotomy and resection of lung tissue.[67] Postoperative pulmonary complications are related directly to preoperative pulmonary diseases, intraoperative events, duration of cardiopulmonary bypass, and postoperative cardic function. Postoperatively, there may be increases in the (a-A) PaO_2 difference to very high values, increases in respiratory rate, and decreases in tidal volume (V_T) and alveolar ventilation, patchy alveolar collapse, decreases in RV and lung compliance, and increases in airway resistance and work of breathing. The maximum change usually occurs on the first postoperative day with resolution over a 2-week period.[67] As with other types of surgery, preoperative pulmonary function evaluation may indicate the risk and aid in planning for the procedure and the postoperative state.[67]

Several investigators[68,69] have observed severe hypoxemia in normal subjects undergoing thoracotomies for benign esophageal disease. Bainbridge[68] has postulated that the 30% decreases in PaO_2 may be due to postural effects, trauma to lung tissue by collapse, and retraction and possibly fluid administration.

In brief, evidence has accumulated that there is a strong correlation between the risk of postoperative complication and preoperative evaluation of pulmonary function. Although there is impressive evidence for a causal relationship, the statistical data alone are quite convincing[5] and have been accumulated in multiple centers. Because risk recognition is of decisive importance in applying preventive measures and early treatment of pulmonary complications, we may wonder that knowledge of the relationship of risk to preoperative evaluation of pulmonary function is not used more frequently (Table 19-2).

INDICATIONS FOR TEST

There is no general agreement regarding the particular patients to be studied preoperatively nor the specific tests to be performed. Some believe that all patients should be studied, regardless of age and prior to any type of surgery. Others believe the patients should be selected for preoperative lung function studies on the basis of historic and physical examination indicating lung dysfunction. Simple tests of air flow rates have been recommended as the preoperative screen in some laboratories whereas others may prefer extensive studies before and after bronchodilators, including lung volumes, lung mechanics, gas distribution, diffusing capacity, and blood-gas exchange during rest and exercise.

Table 19-3 includes a suggested list of indications for preoperative screening based on current information. Simple screening studies of air flow rates can indicate the risk. More refined studies in some patients, as indicated, can delineate the physiologic abnormalities. Specific spirometry studies that have been utilized to indicate the risk are included in Table 19-4. The asterisks in Table 19-4 indicate that the studies have been demonstrated to be statistically valid indicators.

GUIDELINES FOR ASSESSMENTS OF
INCREASED RISK

The pulmonary function values, any one of which can place the preoperative patient in a poor risk category, are listed in Table 19-5. The data are not available to indicate that abnormal studies of terminal airways function (closing volume, closing capacity, volume of isoflow, $\dot{V}_{50}$, etc.) are more sensitive indicators than the usual spirometric studies of air flow rates. As emphasized by Tisi[19] and others,[13,20,50] there is no single or combination of studies that indicates the risk of a lethal or morbid complication in the individual patient. Thus, a patient with an $FEF_{200-1200} < 200$ liter/min who undergoes laparotomy may have

Table 19-3 Indications for Preoperative Pulmonary Function Screen

1. All thoracic surgery patients.
2. All abdominal surgery patients.
3. History of heavy tobacco use.
4. Known or suspected cardiopulmonary disease.
5. Obesity.
6. Age > 60 yr.

Table 19-4 Preoperative Screening Tests

VC	*$FEF_{25-75\%}$
FVC	*MVV
*$FEV_{1.0}$	FEF_{50}
*$FEV_{1.0\%}$	FEF_{75}
*$FEF_{200-1200}$	Closing volume
	HeO_2 flow-volume

*Statistically valid indicators of risk.

Table 19-5 Pulmonary Function Study Values that Indicate Increased Risk of Postoperative Complications

$FEV_{1.0}$ < 2.0 liter [19]
$FEF_{25-75\%}$ < 40% predicted, < 1.2 liter/sec [48]
$FEF_{200-1200}$ < 200 liter/min [13]
MVV < 50% predicted [15,16,19,74]
Arterial $PaCO_2$ > 45 mm Hg [13,49]

a 90% chance of a postoperative pulmonary complication; and following thoracotomy, 80% chance; the statistical chance falls to 30% following other types of surgery. [13] The importance of these indicators is substantiated by several reports that prophylactic therapy and prompt attention to postoperative pulmonary complications decrease the risk. [19,20,22,45] The pitfalls, artifacts, technical difficulties, and hazards of pulmonary function studies have been discussed in *Pulmonary Function Testing Guidelines and Controversies*. [78] Erroneous information obtained by the improper performance of preoperative evaluation studies implies hazards similar to those that may occur with other types of diagnostic and laboratory testing.

CONTROVERSIES

Postoperative pulmonary complications account for a large number of postoperative mortalities, [45,66] millions of days of hospitalization, great financial expenditure, and anxiety and frustration for patients, their families, and the medical personnel rendering care. However, precise, reliable data are not available and some studies report an incidence of postoperative pulmonary complications that are unbelievably small. The routine or prophylactic use of intensive care units (ICUs) with attendant pulmonary care following certain types of surgery, in part, may be responsible for the low incidence of postoperative pulmonary complications sometimes observed. Many of the studies of preoperative evaluation with subsequent pulmonary complications predate the ready availability of nurses skilled in critical care, physiotherapists trained in chest physiotherapy, and respiratory therapists.

In a recent retrospective study, Cain et al.[70] found no substantial association between preoperative pulmonary function and postoperative complications in a group of 106 patients undergoing cardiovascular surgery. These authors equated length of stay on an ICU with postoperative complications and did not obtain specific data on pulmonary complications. Gracey et al.[22] attempted to improve pulmonary function in patients with preoperative pulmonary disease by a 48–72 hour standardized prophylactic regimen (bronchodilator drugs, chest physiotherapy, and heated aerosol). Although several tests of pulmonary function were improved significantly, they felt the changes were not of functional importance. The preoperative improvement in pulmonary function did not enhance the ability to predict complications in specific patients. Nevertheless, the preoperative preparation did result in a reduction in the frequency of postoperative pulmonary complications when compared to historic controls from the same institution.[71] Severe preoperative reductions of the $FEF_{25-75\%}$ and MVV were associated with prolonged requirements of mechanical ventilation. Schachter[72] has responded to the data of Cain et al. with an emotional defense of preoperative pulmonary function studies, but he presented no data. Snider[73] suggested that Gracey et al.[22] may have been accomplishing improvements of aspects of lung function by their preoperative regimen other than those measured by spirometric techniques, e.g., mucociliary clearance.

The use of noninvasive radionuclide studies combined with spirometry have been shown to be effective predictors of postoperative lung function when pneumonectomy is performed. Boysen[74] has demonstrated that patients with pulmonary disease can survive if their predicted postoperative FEV_1 is between 800 and 1000 ml, although 17% did succumb with pulmonary failure. Ali[75] has indicated that radionuclide and pulmonary function studies may not be reliable in predicting the results of lobectomy. Indeed, the immediate postoperative effect of a lobectomy on lung function may be similar to pneumonectomy. Pecora has stated by letter[76] that clinical impressions and mean pulmonary artery pressure measurements are better prognosticators for the results of pneumonectomy than ventilatory measurements.

Other controversies have been discussed in previous sections. It can be reemphasized that the postoperative pulmonary complications are not directly related to the severity of the preoperative pulmonary function abnormality. Location of surgery is extremely important. Thoracic and upper abdominal surgery are more frequently associated with complications. Age, obesity, and smoking history are important, but lesser factors.

The goal of the preoperative pulmonary evaluation is to alter the outcome with reduction of morbidity and mortality due to pulmonary complications. Although prophylaxis and therapy are beyond the scope of this presentation, proper management of the patient with preoperative ventilatory impairment can result in a decline of postoperative complications to levels similar to those with normal lung function (Fig. 19–4).[20,49,77] The data are not yet available to decide whether these reductions in lung complication rates are due to the administration of specific agents and procedures, additional supervision, improvement in lung function preoperatively, maintenance of lung function postoperatively, or combinations.

REFERENCES

1. Chevers N: An inquiry into certain of the causes of death after injuries and surgical operations in London hospitals. Guys Hosp Rep 1:78–102, 1843.
2. Churchill EG, McNeil D: The reduction in vital capacity following operation. Surg Gynecol Obstet 44:483–488, 1927.
3. Beecher HK: The measured effect of laparotomy on the respiration. J Clin Invest 12:639–650, 1933.
4. Beecher HK: Effect on laparotomy on lung volume: Demonstration of a new type of pulmonary collapse. J Clin Invest 12:651–658, 1933.
5. Ali J, Weisel RD, Layug AB, et al. Consequences of postoperative alterations in respiratory mechanics. Am J Surg 128:376–382, 1974.
6. Anscombe AR, Buxton R: Effect of abdominal operations on total lung capacity and its subdivisions. Br Med J 2:84, 1958.
7. Diament ML, Palmer KNV: Postoperative changes in gas tensions of arterial blood and in ventilatory function. Lancet 2:1980, 1966.
8. Mead J, Collier C: Relation of volume history of lungs to respiratory mechanics in dogs. J Appl Physiol 14:669, 1959.
9. Pasteur W: The Bradshaw lecture on massive collapse of the lung. Lancet 2:1351–1355, 1908.
10. Pasteur W: Active lobar collapse of the lung after abdominal operations: A contribution to the study of postoperative lung complications. Lancet 2:1080–1083, 1910.
11. Elwyn H: Postoperative pneumonia. JAMA 79:2154–2158, 1922.
12. Anscombe AR: Pulmonary Complications of Abdominal Surgery. Chicago, Year Book Publ Inc, 1957, pp. 121.
13. Stein M, Koota GM, Simon M, et al.: Pulmonary evaluation of surgical patients. JAMA 181:765–770, 1962.
14. George J, Hornum I, Mellemgard K: The mechanism of hypoxemia after laparotomy. Thorax 22:382, 1966.
15. Gaensler EA, Cugell DW, Lingren I, et al.: The role of pulmonary insufficiency in

mortality and invalidism following surgery for pulmonary tuberculosis J Thorac Surg 29:163, 1955.

16. Mittman C: Assessment of operative risk in thoracic surgery. Am Rev Respir Dis 84:197, 1961.

17. Miller WF, Wu N, Johnson RL, Jr: Convenient method of evaluating pulmonary ventilatory function with single breath test. Anesthesiology 17:480–493, 1956.

18. Veith FJ, Rocco AG: Evaluation of respiratory function in surgical patients: Importance in preoperative preparation and in the prediction of pulmonary complications. Surgery 45:905–911, 1959.

19. Tisi GM: Preoperative evaluation of pulmonary function. Am Rev Respir Dis 119:293, 1979.

20. Stein M, Cassara EL: Preoperative pulmonary evaluation and therapy for surgery patients. JAMA 211:787, 1970.

21. Peters RM, Brimm JE, Utley JR: Predicting the need for prolonged ventilatory support in adult cardiac patients. J Thorac Cardiovasc Surg 77:175–182, 1979.

22. Gracey DR, Divertie MB, Didier EP: Preoperative pulmonary preparation of patients with chronic obstructive pulmonary disease. Chest 76:2–123, 1979.

23. Laros CD, Swieringa J: Temporary unilateral pulmonary artery occlusion in the preoperative evaluation of patients with bronchial carcinoma: Comparison of pulmonary artery pressure measurements, pulmonary function tests and early postoperative mortality. Med Thorac 24:269–283, 1967.

24. Neuhaus H, Cherniack NS: A bronchospirometric method of estimating the effect of pneumonectomy on the maximum breathing capacity. J Thorac Cardiovasc Surg 55:144–48, 1968.

25. Kristersson S, Lindell SWE, Svanberg L: Prediction of pulmonary function loss due to pneumonectomy using 133^{Xe} radiospirometry. Chest 62:694–698, 1972.

26. Olsen GN, Block J, Tobias JA: Prediction of postpneumonectomy pulmonary function using quantitative macroaggregate lung scanning. Chest 66:13–16, 1974.

27. Hedley-Whyte J, Burgess GE III, Feeley TW et al.: Applied Physiology of Respiratory Care. Boston, Little, Brown, and Co, 1976.

28. Wightman JAK: A prospective survey of the incidence of postoperative pulmonary complications. Br J Surg 55:85–91, 1968.

29. Schlenker JD, Hubay CA: The pathogénesis of postoperative atelectasis. A clinical study. Arch Surg 107:846–850, 1973.

30. Diament ML, Palmer KNV: Spirometry for preoperative assessment of airways resistance. Lancet 1:1251–1253, 1967.

31. Morton HJV: Tobacco smoking and pulmonary complications after operation. Lancet 1:368–370, 1944.

32. Thoren L: Postoperative pulmonary complications. Observations on the prevention by means of physiotherapy. Acta Chir Scand 107:193–205, 1954.

33. Nunn JF: Influence of age and other factors on hypoxaemia in the postoperative period. Lancet 2:466–468, 1965.

34. Fleming WH, Bower JC: Early complications of long-term respiratory support. J Thorac Cardiovasc Surg 64:729–738, 1972.

35. Chalon J, Tayyab MA, Ramanathan S: Cytology of respiratory epithelium as a predictor of respiratory complications after operation. Chest 67:32–35, 1975.

36. Rees AM, Roberts CJ, Bligh AS, et al.: Routine preoperative chest radiography in non-cardiopulmonary surgery. Br Med J 1:1333–1335, 1976.

37. Klidjian AM, Foster KJ, Kammerling RM, et al.: Relation of anthropometric and dynamometric variables to serious postoperative complications. Br Med J 281:899–901, 1980.

38. Gravelyn TR, Weg JG: Respiratory rate as an indicator of acute respiratory dysfunction. JAMA 244:1123-1125, 1980.

39. Leigh JM, Walker J, Janaganathan P: Effect of preoperative anaesthetic visit on anxiety. Br Med J 2:987–989, 1977.

40. Ziffren SE: Management of Aged Surgical Patient. Chicago, Year Book Publ, Inc, 1960, p. 219.

41. Epstein PE: Preoperative evaluation of the patient with pulmonary disease, in Fishman AP (ed): Pulmonary Diseases and Disorders. New York, McGraw-Hill, 1980, p. 1695.

42. Ali MK, Mountain CF, Miller JM, et al.: Regional pulmonary function before and after pneumonectomy using zenon-133. Chest 68:288–296, 1975.

43. Lipscomb DJ, Pride NB: Ventilation and perfusion scans in the preoperative assessment of bronchial carcinoma. Thorax 32:720–725, 1977.

44. McNicol GP: Clinical Thinking and Practice. Diagnosis and Decision in Patient Care. New York, Churchill Livingstone, 1979, p. 80.

45. Bendixen HH: Pulmonary problems in the postoperative patient, in Fishman AP (ed): Pulmonary Diseases and Disorders. New York, McGraw Hill, 1980, pp. 1716-1727.

46. Lockwood P: The principles of predicting risk of post-thoracotomy-function-related complications in bronchogenic carcinoma. Respiration 30:329, 1973.

47. Boushy SF, Billeq DM, North, LB, et al.: Clinical course related to preoperative and postoperative pulmonary function in patients with bronchogenic carcinoma. Chest 59:383, 1971.

48. Lockwood P: An improved risk prediction method in bronchial carcinoma surgery. Respiration 39:166–171, 1980.

49. Milledge JS, Nunn JF: Criteria of fitness for anaesthesia in patients with chronic obstructive lung disease. Br Med J 3:670–673, 1975.

50. Lockwood P, Lloyd MH, Williams GV: The value of a wide range of tests in the assessment of lung function in carcinoma of the bronchus. Br J Dis Chest 74:253, 1980.

51. Shackford SR, Virgili RW, Peters RM: Early extubation vs. prophylactic ventilation in the high risk patient: A comparison of postoperative management in the prevention of respiratory complications. Anesth Analg 60:76–80, 1981.

52. Sloan H, Morris JD, Figley M, et al.: Temporary unilateral occlusion of the pulmonary artery in the preoperative evaluation of thoracic patients. J Thorac Cardiovasc Surg 30:591, 1955.

53. Walkup RH, Vossel LF, Griffin JP, et al.: Prediction of postoperative pulmonary function with the lateral position test. Chest 77:24–27, 1980.

54. Olen GN, Block AJ, Tobias JA: Prediction of postpneumonectomy pulmonary function using quantitative macroaggregate lung scanning. Chest 66:13–16, 1974.

55. Tønnesen KH, Dige-Petersen H, Lund JO, et al.: Lung split function test and pneumonectomy. Scand J Thorac Cardiovasc Surg 12:133–136, 1978.

56. Boysen PG, Block AJ, Moulder PV: Relationship between preoperative pulmonary function tests and complications after thoracotomy. Surg Gynecol Obstet, 152:813–815, 1981.

57. Peters RM, Turner E: Physical Therapy. Indications for the effects in surgical patients. Am Rev Respir Dis 122:2, pp. 147–154, 1980.
58. Skillman JJ: Postoperative respiratory failure, in Fishman AP (ed): Pulmonary Diseases and Disorders. New York, McGraw-Hill, 1980, p. 1682.
59. Rehder, K, Sessler AD, Marsh HM: General anesthesia and the lung. Am Rev Respir Dis 112:541, 1975.
60. Nunn JF: Anesthesia and the lung. Anesthesia 52:107–108, 1980.
61. Potgieter PD: Postoperative pulmonary morbidity. Sa Mediese Tydskrif 18. Maart: 412, 1981.
62. Dueck R, Young I, Clausen J, et al.: Altered distribution of pulmonary ventilation and blood flow following induction of inhalational anesthesia. Anesthesia 52:113–125, 1980.
63. Collins JA: Surgery and chronic obstructive disease of the airways, in Fishman AP (ed): Pulmonary Diseases and Disorders. New York, McGraw-Hill, 1980, p. 1709.
64. Arora NS, Gal TJ: Cough dynamics during progressive expiratory muscle weakness in healthy curarized subjects. J Appl Physiol 51:494–498, 1981.
65. Ali J, Ali Khan T: The comparative effects of muscle transection and median upper abdominal incisions on postoperative pulmonary function. Surg Gynecol Obstet 148:863–866, 1979.
66. Pierce AK, Robertson J: Pulmonary complications of general surgery. Ann Rev Med 28:211–21, 1977.
67. Edmunds LH, Jr, Alexander JA: Effect of cardiopulmonary bypass on the lungs, in Fishman AP (ed): Pulmonary Diseases and Disorders. New York, McGraw-Hill, 1980, p. 1728.
68. Bainbridge ET, Matthews HR: Hypoxaemia after left thoracotomy for benign oesophageal disease. Thorax 35:264–268, 1980.
69. Black J, Kalloor GJ, Leigh CJ: The effect of the surgical approach on respiratory function after oesophageal resection. Br J Surg 64:624–627, 1977.
70. Cain HD, Stevens PM, Adaniya R: Preoperative pulmonary function and complications after cardiovascular surgery. Chest 76:130–135, 1979.
71. Tarhan S, Moffitt EA, Sessler AD, et al.: Risk of anesthesia and surgery in patients with chronic bronchitis and chronic obstructive pulmonary disease. Surgery 74:720–726, 1973.
72. Schachter AJ: Communications to the editor: In defense of preoperative pulmonary function tests. Chest 77:711–712, 1980.
73. Snider GL: Communications to the editor: Preoperative pulmonary preparation of patients with COPD. Chest 77:814–815, 1980.
74. Boysen PG, Harris JO, Block AJ, et al.: Prospective evaluation for pneumonectomy using perfusion scanning. Chest 80:163–166, 1981.
75. Ali MK, Mountain CF, Ewer MW, et al.: Predicting loss of pulmonary function after pulmonary resection for bronchogenic carcinoma. Chest 77:337–342, 1980.
76. Pecora DV: Communication to the Editor: Preoperative evaluation of pulmonary function. Chest 80:249, 1981.
77. Williams CD, Brenowitz JB: "Prohibitive" lung function and major surgical procedures. Am J Surg 132:763, 1976.
78. Clausen JZ (ed). *Pulmonary Function Testing Guidelines and Controversies.* Academic Press. San Diego. 1982.

CHAPTER 20

Pulmonary Function Testing for Occupational Epidemiology and Disability

KAYE H. KILBURN
RAPHAEL WARSHAW

Pulmonary function testing for occupational lung disease was rarely utilized until the latter half of the 1950s. Thus, there is about a quarter century of useful experience upon which to base some conclusions and obtain guidance for the future. An example of early studies that made sensitive and useful observations were those of Schilling, McKerrow, and their colleagues [1,17] of the functional impairments caused by cotton dust in the Lancashire mills. They found, as others have found since, that the forced vital capacity (FVC) maneuver with measurement of the forced expiratory volume in one second (FEV_1) is the most reproducible and least variable pulmonary function test in studies of populations. Spirometry, particularly with waterless spirometers, single-breath diffusing capacity, and even exercise testing using the Master's step test with monitoring by ear oximetry can be performed quickly, in larger numbers of people, and with a high degree of accuracy. Tests requiring body plethysmographs, treadmills, blood sampling, and gas collection are too time consuming, too complex, and require such a high of a degree of cooperation that they are not readily applicable to studying large numbers of subjects under field conditions. Many of them are equally unapplicable to large numbers in the fixed base laboratory. In general, for field use, apparatus should be reasonably rugged and the tests able to be performed without special training or conditioning on the part of the subject.

PULMONARY FUNCTION TESTING
INDICATIONS AND INTERPRETATIONS

THE OBJECTIVES FOR A HUMAN PULMONARY ASSAY SYSTEM

To measure the effect of exposure to occupational or environmental agents upon the human lung, three basic objectives can be distinguished. The first is to determine the worker's level of function compared to predicted normals and thus detect his or her level of impairment. The second is to determine the functional decrements occurring during months or years of exposure for surveillance not only in the individual but of the population. The third application is to assess the overall effectiveness of industrial hygiene measures in a workplace. An example of the last, is to assay a work force collective response to cotton dust over an interval of time, such as 1–5 years, to determine whether a full work life of exposure would be safe.

METHODS

The criteria for choosing methods to be used for this type of large population testing include (1) accuracy; (2) sensitivity; (3) reproducibility versus variability; (4) minimal breakdown, that is, robustness; (5) speed of handling data, which includes on-line collection of data, comparisons, and quality checks, and; (6) a permanent record in a form that can be manipulated for reporting to the individual and assembling population data.

The decision as to what to measure is usually derived from studies of individual workers or from pilot studies. Often, what is essential is to make an initial assessment, determine the procedures to be used, and take these to the field and test them under field conditions. This initial assessment is both useful to orient the staff who will be carrying out the tests and to determine whether they will work satisfactorily under the conditions of mass testing.

MECHANICS OF BREATHING

Spirometry with measurement of flow rates can focus upon large airway effects using FEV_1 or peak expiratory flow rate, or upon small airways disease by measuring forced expiratory flow later in expiration (FEV_{25-75} and FEF_{75-85}). Although the closing volume and closing capacity have been used in the field, their excessive variability has rendered them practically useless. Body plethsmography or measurements of airway resistance using pulsed flow can also be used in the field but are more complex and time consuming and are best utilized for specific studies aimed at smaller groups of selected individuals in which training can be applied and be effective.

Lung Volumes

In addition to standard tests of lung volume—helium dilution and body plethysmography—another test that can be employed in the field to give a prevalence of hyperinflation (emphysema) is measurement of the lung volume using posteroanterior and lateral chest Xrays taken at full inflation (see also Chapter 6, this volume).[5] The films are measured using a sensor pen and a light box for a computer calculation and comparison.

Gas Exchange

The diffusing capacity for CO utilizing the single-breath technique ($DL_{CO}Sb$) and fuel cell analyzers for CO is a portable test that can be done quickly in the field. Fuel cell analyzers for CO are both more robust and more stable than infrared analyzers and fare better in field use. The DL_{CO} procedure also provides a serviceable alveolar volume or total lung capacity (TLC) in subjects without maldistribution of ventilation. In contrast, diffusing capacity using steady-state methods for O_2 or CO are more laborious and eliminate themselves from consideration. Similarly, the measurement of arterial blood or penetration of an artery with a sensor is not practical for large numbers of subjects.

Exercise

The measurement of exercise capacity using the step test or small treadmill, and monitoring with ECG and ear oximeter has been applied successfully in the field in a large number of asbestos-exposed workers with pulmonary impairment.

Thus, the armamentarium that has had the most field testing includes spirometry, single-breath diffusing capacity for CO utilizing a fuel cell analyzer, and exercise using the step test and the new fiberoptic ear oximeter (Hewlett-Packard, Andover, MA). We have used this technique to study over 2000 asbestos-exposed subjects in field studies in several sites in this country. For assessment of impairment for compensation purposes, more extensive exercise studies to define physical working capacity may be helpful.

CONTROVERSIES

The expiratory flow in small airways as evaluated by FEF_{75-85} is more sensitive and more variable than FEV_1. Measuring FEF_{75-85} accurately requires that FVC be continued until the flow ceases, i.e., until the complete VC is registered. Failure to observe this requirement results in a *early termination* artifact, which accounts for much of the disappointment in its use. Also, comparisons of flow rates from time to time in the same individual must be done at the same volume (isovolume). The prediction formulae of Morris are adequate standards although they may be questioned at the seventh and eighth decade.[13]

The closing volume and closing capacity are much more capricious and are difficult to reproduce at a point in time in surveys of people who are naive with regard to pulmonary function testing. However, they may be useful to explore and quantify responses. This same conclusion applies, in my opinion, to helium versus air spirometry or flow-volume loops and to frequency dependent of compliance. These are second-and third-level tests to be used for close mapping of phenomena explored in the field with the recommended measurements.

Comparisons to Determine Differences from Normal

The three measurements of flow rates, lung volumes, and gas exchange by diffusing capacity can be compared to standardized prediction formulae used to compare and assess the results. For example, such cross-sectional studies on a large number of cotton textile workers revealed that workers with several years of exposure had average levels of FVCs and FEF_1 below predicted.[6]

Decrements in functional capacity during the exposure of the workday have been used extensively to examine the response to toluene diisocyanate, cotton dust, red cedar, detergent enzymes,[7] and a host of specific exposures under the rubric of occupational asthma. The measurement of functional residual capacity (FRC) has also been shown by us to be useful in metal fume fever. Where there is widespread exposure to a chemical like formaldehyde, this is an ideal modality but a FEV_1 or FEF_{25-75} measurement is also very sensitive. Similarly, if there is exposure to fungal spores, endotoxin, ozone, or NO_2, the diffusing capacity can be utilized in the same way and may show effects even when the flow rates are unchanged.[18] Finally, the exercise response can be tested before and after work exposure. Although I know of no examples in which this has been applied, it remains a distinct possibility and might be useful for solvent exposures such as methyl ethyl ketone (MEK) or bischlormethylether.

Inhalation Testing for Occupational Asthma

The most specific and diagnostic use of pulmonary function tests is inhalation testing.[15] In a sense, it is the strategy discussed previously called by another name (see also Chapter 5, this volume). The subject provides his or her own baseline. Exposure is either on the job or in the laboratory; retesting may be done at intervals of up to 24 hours.[15] When there are several agents, which may be competing, the procedure frequently helps to dissect the relative contribution of each and helps to find the single responsible agent. Although inhalation testing is not usually applied to groups, it may become a very important tool to detect differences within a group or to specify the pattern of change produced by a given exposure. Thus, one can profile the effects of fungal spores and correlate these findings with the diameter of the spore and thus its probable site of deposition in the airway.

Another example of the value of inhalation testing is in metal fume fever. Zinc, copper, or cadmium oxides are produced where these metals are heated, especially when they are welded. Not only do they have pulmonary effects, but they also have systemic effects such as temperature elevation, white count elevation, and malaise. These features add specificity and improve the ability to characterize the response.

Determining decrements in function across lapsed time in months or years utilizes the individual as his or her own standard for comparison and thus compares the decrement measured with the decrement expected in a population without exposure. Clearly, there are different standards to be applied for age, gender, and smoking history, but these are simple to use. The largest use of such a decrement with time was the Fletcher et al. study of the effect of chronic bronchitis on pulmonary function over 10 years.[4] The recent publication of several series of normals from various sections of the country[3,9,11-13] have produced a much better picture of normality against which to judge working and ambulatory populations than was available 10 years ago. Not only has this made interpretation much easier but it is now possible to recognize degrees of impairment that were not detectable earlier.

The determination of the prevalence of reduction in vital capacity (VC) and forced expiratory flow or other measurements in an occupational group depends upon a suitable comparison population. Working people generally are free of disease and have better function than the population from which they are drawn. Because of this phenomenon, they may lose some function without the loss being noted unless they are compared to well-matched controls. It is in this way that the newer population studies are extremely useful. The employment of each subject as his or her own control for workshift decrement or yearly decrement increases the power of these tests considerably. Thus, not only can one obtain information about individual susceptibility or degree of susceptibility to specific agent exposure, but one can look for decrements occurring without symptoms or without a decrement during acute exposure. Unfortunately, although this theoretical use has been discussed for at least a decade, few studies have been published.

EXAMPLES

COTTON DUST

The definition of workers' pulmonary physiologic response to cotton exemplifies the logical application of the principles covered above. The cross-shift changes in the expiratory flow of groups of workers were nicely assayed with monitoring of FEV_1.[10] There is also a subgroup of workers in which FVC decreases and another group in which FEF_{75-85} falls, suggesting a variation in the type or site of response within the worker group. The decrement of cross-shift changes for the group predicts that an excessive yearly decrement will occur which is not confined to the reactive individuals of the cross-shift comparisons.[1]

Toluene diisocyanate (TDI) exposure also illustrates the temporal connection between the cross-shift decrement in FEV_1 and excessive yearly decreases in exposed workers.[16,21] Such monitoring has provided evidence that the standard adopted for the exposure limit is too high to protect against the excessive decrements per year when compared to unexposed nonsmoking controls. Obviously, in both of these comparisons, cigarette smoking groups must be considered separately. Useful smoking-specific data are gradually becoming available upon which to determine the effect of an occupational exposure by subtraction of the smoking effect.[12]

ASBESTOS EXPOSURE AND ASBESTOSIS

Despite longer observation of the functional and pathologic effects of asbestos exposure, there are almost no data concerning longitudinal changes in radiologic milder grades of the disease. The picture is emerging, however, from large cross-sectional studies in insulators and shipyard workers, which include enough noncigarette smokers to deduce, at least in part, the effects of asbestos as disease evolves. It appears that these asbestos-exposed workers manifest an initial reduction in expiratory air flow in small airways FEF_{75-85}[8]. The next stage is a reduction in FVC (and TLC) as these susceptible peripheral airway units are functionally lost. At this stage, the reduction in FEF_{75-85} disappears. As the lung volume decreases further $DL_{CO}SB$ is reduced, commensurate with the volume loss. Later, as the disease progresses past the moderate radiologic stage (1/1 or 1/2 by ILO U/C criteria), $DL_{CO}SB$ decreases excessively, that is, beyond the degree predicted from the drop in TLC. The helium lung volume measured from 10-second breath holds of the DL_{CO} serves as an excellent estimate of the effective lung volume. After this stage is reached, the FEV_1 decreases. Hence, following exposure to asbestos: first, FEF_{75-85} decreases; second, FVC and TLC decrease and FEF_{75-85} returns toward or to normal; third, $DL_{CO}SB$ decreases, initially proportionately to volume and later excessively and, finally; flow rates as measured by FEV_1, decrease. Data are being assembled in several laboratories from nonsmokers exposed at least 20 years ago to asbestos to complete and verify this sequence of impairment.

IMPAIRMENT AND DISABILITY

The last major use of function tests is to document dysfunction or impairment to help quantify disability. The chief problem is deciding what amount or degree of loss constitutes impairment sufficient to characterize disability. Disability must be related to a particular job or activity. Disability is constituted of several parts of which medical impairment is one. The others include economic dislocation, restricted ability to perform regular work, the likelihood of future medical problems, ability to find work that is reflective of the job market, and the particular definitions, usually legal or paralegal, which are applied to the specific subgroup being evaluated. A major point of importance is that although the medical impairment or medical scientific evaluation of impairment is important and substantial, medical impairment per se, often does not constitute proof of disability without these other factors being considered. The usual steps in completing the exposure impairment equation are to first obtain an occupational history from the onset of employment and place the probable causes in their proper perspective. Second, to assess the impairment, which is usually accomplished by comparison of the individual's performance to that of a population study as described previously. This comparison requires, first, accurate and reproducible assessment of the individual's degree of impairment for air flow, diffusing capacity, and exercise and, then, comparison to the predicted values from a normal control group.

OCCUPATIONAL HISTORY

Occupational history must be taken from the onset of employment, although we now are becoming aware of important exposures within the family, such as to asbestos, which need to be considered and included because bystander exposure in childhood may be productive of disease after a lapsed period of 20 or more years. The best way to take an occupational history is to begin chronologically with any jobs held during school and to take the history year by year until retirement. With many people who have held only one or two jobs this is simple. Others may have had many jobs and exposures. For asbestos, even a month or two may be of sufficient length to be powerfully important. After the chronology is established as a scaffold, then one adds the operations performed, the materials used, their generic, if possible, or trade names, and then the operations concurrently going on in the work area, the building, or the plant in which there may be important bystander exposures. These include, for example, the use of asbestos insulation, welding, painting, sandblasting and metal preparation including grinding. Obviously, it is essential to record the cigarette smoking history and all environmental exposures extending beyond the workplace.

IMPAIRMENT

The assessment of impairment is the next important step. Although pulmonary function tests are emphasized in this discussion of the use of standardized testing, it is clear that for the pulmonary system, the history of dyspnea and its relation to the degree of exertion are essential information. Historic detail must be provided as to what activities performed at what speed cause dyspnea. Finally, recovery time should be noted; it is important to inquire how much rest is required for recovery (the minutes required for recovery can often be used to predict the ability to do standardized exercise and to predict the capability to carry out similar work operations at work). Physiologic testing of impairment has been discussed previously and essentially includes the mechanics of breathing, gas transfer capacity, and exercise ability.

PREDICTED VALUES

The comparison of the data obtained for an individual to his or her peer group is essential in order to interpret the findings. This comparison perhaps should not be made unless composition of the comparison group and the methods used are carefully examined. Finally, it is important to realize that for practically all of these tests there is a wide band of normality rather than simply a mean, and this band is usually almost two SDs above and *below* the mean. Often, the workers, particularly under the age of 40 years, will be above the mean of the comparison population. The racial background of the individual has important influence on the predicted pulmonary functions, for example, blacks have lower VCs and FEV_1 than caucasians, and, in most studies Orientals have even lower values compared to norms for whites,[14,19] Finally, the decrement with time still needs perfection and specificity for age and sex. It is clear that nonsmoking normals have less decrement with time for FVC and FEV_1 than do cigarette smokers as a group, but it is equally true that some cigarette smokers manifest little or no impairment. Exercise testing can be perfected to estimate first the O_2 requirement for a job on a steady-state basis and then to determine the extent to which the worker can meet this requirement.[2,20] Perhaps the most important conclusion is that one should provide clear interpretations of the tests and be unequivocal when possible.

The final step is to summarize the information, both that obtained from history and from measurements, so that a clear expression of impairment may be made. Is the individual impaired for his or her usual job? Is he or she impaired for any job? Or is the impairment for life activities? Finally, an estimate of the degree this impairment is due to occupational exposure should be made. It is an important service to the individual and to society to make a clear and quantitative presentation of the information in language that can be understood by the layperson.

REFERENCES

1. Berry G, McKerrow CB, Molyneaux MKB et al.: A study of acute and chronic changes in ventilatory capacity of workers in Lancashire cotton mills. Br J Ind Med 30:25–36, 1974
2. Brude RA: Exercise testing of patients with coronary heart disease: Principles and normal standards for evaluation. Ann Clin Res 3:323, 1971.
3. Crapo RO, Morris AH: Standardized single breath normal values for carbon monoxide diffusing capacity. Am Rev Respir Dis 123:185–189, 1981.

4. Fletcher CM, Peto R, Tinker C, et al.: The natural history of chronic bronchitis and emphysema. New York, Oxford Press, 1976.

5. Harris TR, Pratt PC: Total lung capacity measured by roentgenograms. Am J Med 50:756-763, 1971.

6. Imbus HR, Suh MW: Byssinosis: A study of 10,133 textile workers. Arch Environ Health 26:183-191, 1973.

7. Kilburn KH (ed): Pulmonary reactions to organic materials. Ann NY Acad Sci 221:1-390, 1974.

8. Kilburn KH, Warshaw RH, Einstein K, et al.: Airway disease in non-smoking asbestos workers. Am Rev Respir Dis, submitted 1984.

9. Knudson RJ, Slatin RC, Lebowitz MD, et al.: The maximum expiratory flow-volume curve: Normal standards, variability and effects of age. Am Rev Respir Dis 113:587-600, 1976.

10. Merchant JA, Lumsden JC, Kilburn KH, et al.: Intervention studies of cotton steaming to reduce biological effects of cotton dust. Br J Ind Med 31:261-274, 1974.

11. Miller A, Thornton J, Warshaw RH, et al.: Single breath diffusing capacity in a representative sample of the population of Michigan, a large industrial state. Amer Rev Resp Dir 127:270-277, 1983.

12. Miller A, Thornton JC, Smith H Jr, et al.: Spirometric "abnormality" in a normal male reference population: Further analysis of the 1971 Oregon survey. Am J Ind Med 1:55-68, 1980.

13. Morris JF, Koski A, Johnson LC: Spirometric standards for healthy nonsmoking adults. Am Rev Respir Dis 103:57-67, 1971.

14. Oscherwitz M, Edlavitch SA, Baker TR, et al.: Differences in pulmonary functions in various racial groups. Am J Epidemiol 96:319-327, 1972.

15. Pepys J: Basic mechanisms in acute and chronic allergic lung disease. Immunol Allergy Pract 3:13-26, 1981.

16. Peters JM, Murphy RLH, Pagnotto L, et al.: Acute respiratory effects in workers exposed to "safe" levels of toluene diisocyanate (TDI). Arch Environ Health 20:364-367, 1970.

17. Schilling RSF, Hughes JPW, Dingwall-Fordyce I, et al.: An epidemiological study of bysinosis among Lancashire cotton workers. Br J Ind Med 12:217-226, 1955.

18. Schlueter DP: Response of the lung to inhaled antigens. Am J Med 57:476-492, 1974.

19. Seltzer CC, Siegelaub AB, Friedman GD, et al.: Differences in pulmonary function related to smoking habits and race. Am Rev Respir Dis 110:598-608, 1974.

20. Wasserman K, Whipp BJ: Exercise physiology in health and disease. Am Rev Respir Dis 112:219-249, 1975.

21. Wegman DH, Musk AW, Main DM, et al.: Accelerated loss of FEV_1 in polyurethane production workers: A four year prospective study. Am J Ind Med 3:209-215, 1982.

Index

Page numbers in *italics* indicate illustrations.
Page numbers followed by *t* indicate tables.

This book may be kept

FOURTEEN DAYS

A fine will be charged for each day the book is kept overtime.

GAYLORD 142			PRINTED IN U.S.A.